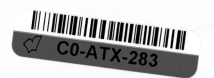

The Athabaskan Languages

Recent Volumes Published

1 Gunter Senft: *Classificatory Particles in Kilivila*
2 Janis B. Nuckolls: *Sounds Like Life: Sound-Symbolic Grammar, Performance, and Cognition in Pastaza Quechua*
3 David B. Kronenfeld: *Plastic Glasses and Church Fathers: Semantic Extension from the Ethnoscience Tradition*
4 Lyle Campbell: *American Indian Language: The Historical Linguistics of Native America*
5 Chase Hensel: *Telling Our Selves: Ethnicity and Discourse in Southwestern Alaska*
6 Rosaleen Howard-Malverde (ed.): *Creating Context in Andean Cultures*
7 Charles L. Briggs (ed.): *Disorderly Discourse: Narrative, Conflict, and Inequality*
8 Anna Wierzbicka: *Understanding Cultures through Their Key Words: English, Russian, Polish, German, and Japanese*
9 Gerrit J. van Enk and Lourens de Vries: *The Korowai of Irian Jaya: Their Language in Its Cultural Context*
10 Peter Bakker: *A Language of Our Own: The Genesis of Michif, the Mixed Cree-French Language of the Canadian Métis*
11 Gunter Senft: *Referring to Space: Studies in Austronesian and Papuan Languages*
12 David McKnight: *People, Countries, and the Rainbow Serpent: Systems of Classification among the Lardil of Mornington Island*
13 Penelope Gardner-Chloros, Robert B. Le Page, Andrée Tabouret-Keller, and Gabrielle Varro (eds.): *Vernacular Literacy Revisited*
14 Steven Roger Fischer: *Rongorongo, the Easter Island Script: History, Tradition, Text*
15 Richard Feinberg: *Oral Traditions of Anuta: A Polynesian Outlier in the Solomon Islands*
16 Bambi B. Schieffelin, Kathryn A. Woolard, and Paul V. Kroskrity (eds.): *Language Ideologies: Practice and Theory*
17 Susan U. Philips: *Ideology in the Language of Judges: How Judges Practice Law, Politics, and Courtroom Control*
18 Spike Gildea: *On Reconstructing Grammar: Comparative Cariban Morphosyntax*
19 Laine A. Berman: *Speaking through the Silence: Narratives, Social Conventions, and Power in Java*
20 Cecil H. Brown: *Lexical Acculturation in Native American Languages*
21 James M. Wilce: *Eloquence in Trouble: The Poetics and Politics of Complaint in Rural Bangladesh*
22 Peter Seitel: *The Powers of Genre: Interpreting Haya Oral Literature*
23 Elizabeth Keating: *Power Sharing: Language, Rank, Gender, and Social Space in Pohnpei, Micronesia*
24 Theodore B. Fernald and Paul R. Platero (eds.): *The Athabaskan Language: Perspectives on a Native American Language Family*

The Athabaskan Languages

Perspectives on a Native American Language Family

Edited by
Theodore B. Fernald
Paul R. Platero

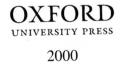

OXFORD
UNIVERSITY PRESS

2000

OXFORD

UNIVERSITY PRESS

Oxford   New York

Athens   Auckland   Bangkok   Bogotá   Buenos Aires   Calcutta
Cape Town   Chennai   Dar es Salaam   Delhi   Florence   Hong Kong   Istanbul
Karachi   Kuala Lumpur   Madrid   Melbourne   Mexico City   Mumbai
Nairobi   Paris   São Paulo   Singapore   Taipei   Tokyo   Toronto   Warsaw

and associated companies in
Berlin   Ibadan

Library of Congress Cataloging-in-Publication Data
The Athabaskan languages : perspectives on a Native American language family/
edited by Theodore B. Fernald and Paul R. Platero.
p.   cm. — (Oxford studies in anthropological linguistics : 24)
Papers presented at or closely related to the Athabaskan Conference
on Syntax & Semantics, held Apr. 25–28, 1996, Swarthmore College.
Includes bibliographical reference.
ISBN 0-19-511947-9
1. Athapascan languages—Congressed.   2. Navajo language—Congresses.
I. Fernald, Theodore B.   II. Platero, Paul R.   III. Athabaskan Conference on
Syntax & Semantics (1996 : Swarthmore College)   IV. Series.
PM841.A93   1999
497'.2—dc21   98-36532

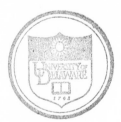
1 3 5 7 9 8 6 4 2

Printed in the United States of America
on acid-free paper

To the memory of Gladys Reichard,
Swarthmore College class of 1919.

ACKNOWLEDGMENTS

We gratefully acknowledge the support of the Wenner-Gren Foundation for Anthropological Research, which provided major funding for this conference, and of Swarthmore College, which provided space, office support, and housing for the conference participants. We also appreciate the support of the Eugene M. Lang Foundation for making it possible for Paul Platero to come to Swarthmore as the Visiting Professor for Social Change in the spring of 1996 and for funding Herb Benally's participation in the conference. We are also grateful to the William J. Cooper Foundation for funding Ken Hale's participation.

Special thanks go to Swarthmore College President, Alfred Bloom; to the Provost, Jennie Keith; to Donna Jo Napoli, Naomi Nagy, and Dagmar Jung; and to the many Swarthmore students who assisted in running the conference.

We particularly wish to thank Chris Couples, Susan Blair Das, Jennifer Freeman, Eric Raimy, and Tom Stenson for substantial assistance in preparing the camera-ready copy of this volume. Finally we thank the two anonymous Oxford reviewers.

CONTENTS

CONTRIBUTORS

Melissa Axelrod is an assistant professor in the department of linguistics at the University of New Mexico.

Leonard M. Faltz is an associate professor in the department of computer science at Arizona State University.

Theodore B. Fernald is an assistant professor in the linguistics program at Swarthmore College and a member of the board of directors of the Navajo Language Academy, Inc.

Ken Hale is a professor emeritus in the department of linguistics and philosophy at Massachusetts Institute of Technology and a member of the board of directors of the Navajo Language Academy, Inc.

Eloise Jelinek is an associate professor emerita in the department of linguistics at the University of Arizona.

Dagmar Jung is a lecturer at the University of Cologne.

Jeff Leer is an assistant professor at the Alaska Native Language Center, University of Alaska, Fairbanks.

Joyce McDonough is an assistant professor in the department of linguistics at the University of Rochester.

William Morgan is retired in Fort Defiance, (Arizona) Navajo Nation.

Paul Platero is the tribal administrator in Canyoncito, New Mexico.

Keren Rice is a professor in the department of linguistics at the University of Toronto.

Carlota S. Smith is a professor in the department of linguistics at the University of Texas at Austin and a member of the board of directors of the Navajo Language Academy, Inc.

Chad Thompson is an associate professor at the Indiana University–Purdue University, Ft. Wayne.

MaryAnn Willie is an assistant professor of linguistics and American Indian studies at the University of Arizona.

Robert W. Young is a professor emeritus in the department of linguistics at the University of New Mexico.

The Athabaskan Languages

INTRODUCTION

Theodore B. Fernald and Paul R. Platero

The Athabaskan language family stretches from Alaska through northwestern Canada and also appears in the American Southwest and in isolated regions of Washington, Oregon, and California. Navajo is currently the most widely used with somewhere between 90,000 and 150,000 speakers. The reason for the high margin of error in the estimated number of speakers is easily imagined by people who are familiar with what happens with endangered languages. In the case of Navajo, it is difficult to decide whom to count as a Navajo speaker: many people spoke it fluently when they were children but no longer do. They may understand some Navajo when they hear it, but they may no longer attempt to speak the language themselves. The other Athabaskan languages are numerically far worse off than Navajo and are very unlikely to survive the coming century.

The chapters in this volume range from technical analyses of the grammars of these languages to issues involved in trying to preserve Navajo. They were all presented at, or are closely related to, the Athabaskan Conference on Syntax and Semantics held at Swarthmore College (Pennsylvania) from April 25 to 28, 1996. Most of the essays in this collection are technical works of scholarship, making a contribution to the ongoing effort to understand human language in general and the Athabaskan languages in particular. These articles represent the current state of the art, and it would be very difficult for people with no background in linguistics to make sense of them. The volume contains two nontechnical essays that might appeal to a wider audience. The first is this introduction, which will describe in some detail what the conference at Swarthmore was all about. It will conclude with a brief overview of the other chapters in this volume. The second nontechnical essay is a summary of a discussion of the interaction of sacred and secular aspects of Navajo culture and its effects on efforts to use the Navajo language in public education. This discussion took place at the Swarthmore conference. The nontechnical essays are presented in this volume alongside the theoretical chapters for two main reasons. One is that including them provides a reflection of the conference at which they were presented. The other is that linguists need to do everything we can to help preserve the languages we work with.

The Swarthmore conference was unusual in that it brought together people and issues involved with intellectual, practical, political, and cultural work on Athabaskan. These issues are interrelated, but it is rare for theoretical linguists to get so deeply involved in them. (It is not rare for the linguists who are Navajos themselves to get so involved; one must confront fears of language shift every day.) This was a conference which combined work in theoretical linguistics with a series of discussions about ways to assist the speakers of Navajo with some of the problems surrounding the efforts to sustain it as a modern language. In addition to the linguists who work on Athabaskan syntax and semantics, we invited several educational professionals who are involved in teaching Navajo language and literacy to other Navajos. Our original goal was to have a discussion of a thesis of Paul Platero's, that efforts to preserve the Navajo language and culture would benefit from a separation of religious and secular cultural matters in educational settings. (A summary of this discussion is included in this volume.) Since we were inviting linguists and native speakers of Navajo to a conference, and since in the past it has been difficult for linguists to get consistent judgments on quantification data in the field, it was natural for us to have a discussion of data of this sort. As plans for the conference became more specific, it became clear that there was a need for a discussion of the gulf between academic theorists and language educators, so we added a discussion of these issues. The difference between theorists and educators does not quite coincide with the Navajo-Anglo distinction. Five Navajos who have doctoral degrees have produced linguistic work on Navajo. Four of them were present at the conference, and their presence changed the dynamics of the discussion. One of the high points of the conference came when the theoretical issues of Navajo linguistics were discussed in Navajo. This was a lengthy and sustained discussion of certain quantificational and scope taking particles and nuances of interpretation of sentences containing them. This may have been the first time ever that such a discussion took place in Navajo. It was a significant moment for those of us who seek to preserve the strength of Navajo language and culture; scientific investigation was being conducted about Navajo in Navajo.

This conference was unusual in a number of ways. To the Navajo educators, the strangest thing was its location in Pennsylvania, far from traditional Athabaskan territory. This is odd since many Athabaskans have a close personal connection to the land they inhabit. The conference was also unusual in that the participants consisted of theoretical linguists and language educators, and the topics under consideration covered two fairly distinct domains of inquiry.

The conference was held in Pennsylvania for a number of circumstantial reasons. Swarthmore College is where both of us were working at the time. Paul was invited here as the Eugene M. Lang Visiting Professor for Social Change to coteach a course on the structure of Navajo with Ted. In conversations between the two of us and also with Ken Hale and Clay Slate, the idea emerged of taking advantage of the opportunity in other ways. We decided to have a broader discussion of certain issues affecting the strength of the Navajo language. We realized that Pennsylvania was an odd location for a meeting about the Navajo language and culture, but we did not want to miss the opportunity with which we were presented. In fact, there is a historical connection between Swarthmore College and the Navajo Nation: Gladys Reichard, the anthropologist and linguist who produced numerous works on Navajo grammar and culture, completed her undergraduate education at Swarthmore in 1919. Swarthmore is a college that is proud of its heritage. Holding the Athabaskan Conference on Syntax and Semantics at Swarthmore continues Reichard's legacy.

There were several reasons for creating a conference which focuses on both theoretical linguistics and issues of the interaction of education with language and culture. In the particular case of the groups involved in this conference, there had already been a fair amount of interaction going in both directions. Linguists have been involved in putting to pedagogical use the insights of their analyses, and professional educators have attended linguistics conferences in the past, to add insights from practice and to further their understanding of grammatical theory. In general, linguists and language educators have some very important common goals. For both groups, it is of tantamount importance that the speech community with which they work should survive. In the past, linguists have benefited the speakers of the languages on which they work by analyzing how the language works and sometimes by writing descriptive grammars. The product of linguistic analysis may be beneficial to members of the speech community if it can be used in pedagogical settings, in teaching grammatical analysis, for example. Although this is valuable work, in many cases it is not enough to help preserve the strength or even the existence of the speech community. Linguists need to be more deeply involved, both in an effort to maintain linguistic diversity and as a matter of fair exchange for the valuable data we obtain. Linguists customarily provide monetary compensation for the time and expertise of native speakers who are the source of their data. But money gets spent and disappears, often without providing a significant benefit to the community where the language is spoken. The discussion sessions at this conference represented an effort to offer something more useful to the Navajo culture by providing a forum for educational and cultural issues and by getting linguists more deeply involved in these concerns. The discussion of quantificational sentences, in addition to being useful linguistic research, was an effort to get Navajo language educators more deeply involved in work on theoretical linguistics, in hopes of stimulating their interest in the scientific study of the Navajo language.

The article reporting the discussion session of the conference considers the thesis that public schools in the Navajo Nation would benefit from a separation of secular and religious elements in Navajo culture. This separation would allow public schools to provide instruction of and inquiry into the secular domains, which would include the grammar of Navajo. This would make it possible for a portion of the culture to be discussed and investigated in schools without violating the doctrine of the separation of church and state. This would also make it possible for students who do not hold traditional Navajo religious beliefs to study secular aspects of Navajo culture. The proposal to make a distinction between the secular and the religious may be opposed in a different direction by those Navajos who believe that it would be impossible or improper to separate religion from other aspects of culture. The thesis is controversial, but it deserved to be discussed. We are not doing anything so presumptuous as to recommend policy, but we hope that our discussion will be of some benefit to the Navajo

Nation by clarifying certain issues. It is likely that other groups of American Indians are faced with similar difficulties in their schools. We hope that our discussion will be of use to them as well. Finally, we hope that linguists will be inspired to become more involved in finding ways to be of service to communities that are the source of the data we need. This conference has done this in two ways: by providing a forum for a discussion of language education issues and by involving language educators in the work of linguistic theory.

Both groups of participants in this conference view the endangerment of a language and a culture with great sadness. Languages are natural systems for encoding information in a way that makes sense to people. There are many different ways in which a human language can be configured, but these do not encompass every logical possibility. This apparently is due to the architecture of human brains. To figure out all that language can teach us about human cognition, we need to be able to study as many languages as possible. When a language dies, researchers lose a piece of the puzzle. The Athabaskan languages differ from the heavily studied Indo-European languages in a great variety of ways. This makes them especially valuable to linguists and cognitive scientists.

There is an intimate interaction between a culture and the language it uses. When a language is lost, the culture loses many of its art forms and possibly some of its concepts. The decline of a culture and a language involves many complex issues that we cannot cover adequately here. Although we are indulging here in generalizations, we hope the point is clear and uncontroversial. When a culture is lost, humanity loses a unique perspective of the universe and how people fit into it. The worldview of a culture is the result of a collective effort to follow assumptions about the universe to their logical conclusions. As our species faces technological, social, ethical, and political issues it has never faced before, we need every consistent set of assumptions about the universe that we can get. An example of this is the effort being made by Herb Benally and others at Navajo Community College to develop an educational curriculum that is consistent with Navajo philosophy. It was noted that the Anglo-American system of education has not been generally successful at providing Navajo young people with a basis for leading wonderful and exciting lives. We think the same can be said, in general, for Anglo-American young people. At a time when so many Americans are concerned with the state of education in our country, the perspective offered by another culture may make a valuable contribution.

These comments provide a view of the motivation behind this conference. The goals are consistent with those of a good number of educators and linguists. The Athabaskan Conference on Syntax and Semantics certainly did not address all the issues raised here, but the conference was designed to contribute in a modest way to their resolution.

The collection of chapters that this volume comprises may strike some as unusual, since it includes a discussion of certain sociological issues alongside theoretical work in linguistics. The volume reflects the unusual character of the conference. This was more than a traditional linguistics conference in which the speakers of the languages under scrutiny participate at best as observers. In organizing this conference, we tried to find a way to be of service to the community of native speakers who are our sources of data. They are from a culture that has been exploited in the past by European-American culture, and their culture and language are struggling for survival. It behooves linguists to make contributions where we can. We would like to argue that what is unusual about the conference and this volume ought not to be so unusual. Linguists have a responsibility to any endangered speech community. Where there is a theoretical conference that focuses on the language of any such community, there ought to be sessions addressing ways to be of better service to the goal of preserving that community and its language.

Linguists are convinced of the value of linguistic diversity, but many other people are not. Linguists are, then, the most likely outsiders to care whether a speech community survives. This alone is reason for involvement, but there is a further matter. Aside from disease and war, the main challenges to the survival of a language come from economic pressures on the native speakers. Consider Navajo as a relevant case in point. Although there are a number of ways to make a living in Navajo country today, in nearly every case a worker will be more successful if he or she knows English, and there are fairly few jobs in which not knowing Navajo is a serious impediment. Tourism has been significant in the Navajo economy, but economic development in that direction adds pressure to stop using Navajo.

The Navajo language itself is one resource that is highly valued outside the Navajo community which could add pressure to retain the language. Unfortunately or not, the main market for this resource consists of linguists who depend on the existence of the speech community for data. Unfortunately, linguists do not command adequate financial resources to offset the economic pressures that push a speech community to abandon its traditional language. Although it is customary for field linguists to compensate their consultants, these arrangements never have a significant economic impact on the community: as far as we know, no one has made a career as a consultant for a field linguist. We are sure that many linguists would love the state of academic finance to allow such eventualities to obtain, but we cannot get off the hook so easily. We are obligated to do everything we can to contribute to the survival of an endangered speech community.

The theoretical essays in this volume focus mostly on issues of syntax and semantics. There is a major linguistic controversy surrounding the Athabaskan family, among certain others. The question is whether nominal expressions should be analyzed as arguments, as is traditionally assumed, or whether they are better treated as adjuncts coindexed with pronominal arguments that are incorporated into the verb. Chapter 11, by MaryAnn Willie and Eloise Jelinek, adds an important argument to this debate in support of the claim that nominals are adjoined. Chapter 2, by Leonard Faltz, extends these assumptions to account for various idiosyncrasies of Navajo semantics. Supporting the other side of the debate is Chapter 4, by Ken Hale and Paul Platero, considering facts about negative polarity items in Navajo. Ted Fernald, in chapter 3, article does not take sides in this debate but investigates some issues in genericity and the contrast between individual- and stage-level predicates. A better understanding of quantification in Navajo may eventually be relevant to the syntactic controversy.

Chapter 10, by Chad Thompson. and Chapter 5, by Dagmar Jung, deal with questions of word order in Koyukon and Jicarilla Apache, respectively. Keren Rice, in Chapter 8, considers issues of argument structure and subject in three

Athabaskan languages. She concludes that the position in which a subject appears depends on semantic properties of the subject rather than on any subcategorization mechanism. Melissa Axelrod, in Chapter 1, lays out nominal and verbal aspectual classification in Koyukon and draws parallels between them. Chapter 9, by Carlota Smith, concerns the interpretations of Navajo verb bases.

In Chapter 7, Joyce McDonough, argues that the position class does not exist as a morphological type. Her work is on Navajo, which in the past has been taken to be a canonical example of position class morphology. In Chapter 6, Jeff Leer takes a historical linguistics perspective leading to the reconstruction of negative/irrealis morphemes in Proto-Athabaskan-Eyak-Tlingit. There are numerous comments throughout on the syntactic and aspectual effects of these morphemes.

In addition to these articles, which were presented as papers at the conference, this volume includes an additional a chapter that figured prominently in several of the conference discussions. Chapter 12, "The Function and Signification of Certain Navaho Particles" was written in the 1940s by Robert Young and William Morgan. The paper was published by the Education Division of the United States Indian Service, with an intended audience of Anglo educators of Navajo children. The original introduction was designed to explain to English teachers why their Navajo students seemed to sound monotonous when they spoke English. It explained that Navajo is a tone language and that emphasis and association to focus are accomplished by adding particles to sentential constituents rather than giving them intonational stress, as is done in English. The remainder of the article is a catalogue of Navajo particles with copious example sentences reflecting various nuances of meaning. This catalogue has been highly sought after by linguists who work on Navajo natural language semantics, but copies of it have been very hard to locate. This volume includes the original article in its entirety along with a new introduction by Robert Young. It is being included in this volume as a service to scholars and because it figured prominently in the discussion sessions of the conference.

1

THE SEMANTICS OF CLASSIFICATION IN KOYUKON ATHABASKAN

Melissa Axelrod

The aspectual system of Koyukon[1] is perhaps the most elaborate of the Athabaskan languages. It has a complex network of four modes, 15 aspects, four superaspects, four postaspectual derivations, and some 300 aspect-dependent derivational prefix strings, allowing thousands of distinct and very precise characterizations regarding the time frame and type of verbal notion expressed.

Koyukon also has an extensive system of classifying both nouns and verbs. Its noun classification system consists of six gender classes (including a zero class), which categorize nouns according to size, shape, consistency, and material. The language also has a set of the classificatory verbs, which are a well-known feature of Athabaskan languages. These verbs specify the shape, material, consistency, size, location, arrangement, and number of their nominal arguments.

I will suggest here that the aspectual system of the language classifies verbal actions in a manner that is parallel to the way that gender and classificatory verbs classify nouns. I'll begin with a brief summary of Koyukon noun classification, and then go on to demonstrate how aspect works to classify verbs into categories or types of action. The second part of the chapter will explore parallels between the semantic features used to class verbs and those used in noun classification. The final section of the chapter will point out similarities in the discourse-pragmatic uses of both classificatory systems, both noun classification and aspect, in discourse.

1.1 Noun Classification

Beginning with Koyukon noun classification, I will briefly describe here both the classificatory verb system and the gender system. Koyukon verbs in general show a wide range of classificatory functions. Some verbs are specialized according to whether the subject of the action is singular (or dual) or plural. Others are specialized for singular vs. plural objects. Still other actions are referred to by different stems depending on the physical characteristics of the subject or object involved. These stems are the classificatory verb stems.

In most noun classification systems, the extralinguistic factors that speakers consider important in distinguishing categories are material, shape, consistency, size, location, arrangement, and quanta (Allan 1977). These are the categories delineated by the Koyukon classificatory verbs. The following list[2] shows the 11 intransitive verb themes[3] that classify objects in position.[4]

Koyukon Classificatory Verbs

G+ø+'o	'compact object is in position, is sitting there'
G+ø+ton	'flat, rigid, or sticklike object is there'
G+ø+lo	'plural objects are there'
ø+kko	'object in an open, shallow container is there'
G+ł+ton	'bag or enclosed object is there'
G+ł+kooł	'flat, flexible, or clothlike object is there'
G+ł+koot	'food, edible object is there'
de+ł+t'on	'burning object is there'
G+de+dzok	'disorderly, scattered plural objects are there'
G+de+tlaakk	'mushy, wet, messy object is there'
de+de+nokk	'granular or powdery substance is there'

The first of these themes, *G+ø+'o*, is used to describe such diverse items as beads, buckets, hills, typewriters, hats, and houses—it is the largest category of objects referred to by classificatory verbs. What these so-called compact objects have in common is that each has a height, length, and width that are roughly comparable, no protruding or extending parts, and extremities which are close to the center of gravity. This is, however, the least specified category and seems to contain all those objects whose characteristics are not clearly specified by one of the other classificatory verbs.

The second theme in the preceding list, *G+ø+ton,* describes the second-largest category of objects. In addition to flat, rigid objects such as sheet iron, trays, or snowshoes and elongated objects such as sticks or spoons, this theme also describes sleds and canoes (and by extension all other vehicles, e.g., cars, snow machines, ships) and shallow containers such as dishes, cups, or roasting pans.

The classificatory verbs are combined with the gender system of the language to allow very explicit reference to particular sorts of objects. There are six gender classes, marked by the verb prefixes shown:

Koyukon Gender Prefixes

1. ne-   *faces, berries, beads, thimbles, string, rope*
2. de-   *wood, plants, furniture, mittens, boots, rigid containers*
3. dene- round, heavy objects: *animal heads, cabbages, apples, rocks;*
          long, cylindrical objects: *pipes, bridges, pencils, guns*
4. hʉ-   the areal prefix, used also to classify *areas, events, abstract ideas*
5. hede- *weather*
6. zero   *people, animals*

Many verbs, including the majority of the classificatory verbs, are obligatorily marked for gender. The interaction of gender and classificatory verb stem can be seen in the items classified by the first two themes listed above. With *de-* gender, derivatives with the stem - *'on* refer to bottles, jars, and cans, as in example (1):

(1)   *boogee daal'onh*
       boogee de + le + ø + *'onh*
       flour   G   + M/A + CL + classif.: compact objects
       'A canister of flour is there.'

Derivatives with *de-* gender and the stem *-ton* refer to boxes, as in example (2):

(2)   *boogee daaltonh*
       'A box of flour is there.'

The stem *-kkon* is used to describe the contents of all such containers, but its focus is not on the container itself.

The examples that follow give an idea of the range of meaning of the classificatory verbs:

Semantics of Classificatory Verbs

boogee le'onh	'A lump of flour is there.'
boogee daal'onh	'A canister of flour is there.'
boogee daaltonh	'A box of flour is there.'
boogee etltonh	'A bag of flour is there.'
boogee lekkonh	'A bowl of flour is there.'
boogee ledlo	'Lumps of flour are there.'
boogee etlkoot	'Flour is there (stored as a provision).'
boogee ełetlaakk	'Dough is there.'
boogee daałenokk	'Loose flour is there.'

1.2 Aspectual Verb Classification

The combination of classificatory verbs and gender acts to categorize the nominal portion of the Koyukon lexicon. As nouns are classified and described via the gender and classificatory verb system, verbal notions in Koyukon are grouped and described via aspect (see Axelrod 1993 for a fuller description of verb classification in Koyukon). In addition to the four modes of Koyukon (imperfective, perfective, future, and optative), there are 15 aspects (or aktionsarts) which can be classed into three general groups. The first group is made up of those aspects which are used in referring to an entity's state, condition, position, or existence. State aspects include the neuter and the transitional. The second and third groups are made up of aspects used in the expression of activities or events. The second group, motion aspects, refer specifically to the path or manner of an activity through time or space: momentaneous, perambulative, continuative, persistive, and reversative. The third group, the activity aspects, contains those aspects which refer to the durativity, cyclicity, or punctuality of an activity; these aspects are the durative, consecutive, repetitive, directive-repetitive, semelfactive, bisective, conclusive, and onomatopoetic.

As in other Athabaskan languages, mode and aspect in Koyukon are marked morphologically by prefixation and also by suffixation and/or vowel lengthening and/or ablaut of the verb stem. The mode and aspect system can be diagrammed, as in figure 1.1, to illustrate this intersection of mode and aspect. Notice that mode in this figure forms a horizontal axis and aspect a vertical axis.

A verb will have four possible stems for each aspect that it allows: an imperfective stem, a perfective stem, a future stem, and an optative stem. The stem set for the verb 'chop' thus has four momentaneous stems: *tlaał* (imperfective), *tlaatl* (perfective), *tlełtl* (future), and *tlaał* (optative). It also has four durative stems: *tlaał, tlaatl, tlaał,* and *tlaał*. This verb allows eight different aspects and thus has 32 stems (i.e., eight times four) in all, though many of these stems are homophonous (and disambiguated by prefix morphology).

It has been suggested that noun classifiers group nouns according to their inherent properties (Lee 1988:228; Paprotte 1988:457), while aspect groups verbs by perceived characteristics. In fact, while the speaker does choose how to classify an activity, the choices are often quite limited or constrained by the external character of the activity or event in question. A speaker of English, for example, can't choose to categorize the verb 'know' as an event or as a process with discrete intervals; it must be categorized as a state because of inherent properties of the concept the verb expresses. Similarly, 'cough' can't be expressed with the aspectual marking associated with states because the inherent semantics of the verb naturally require it to be considered a punctual activity. These constraints on choice are perhaps more overt in Koyukon than in other languages because there is such an elaborate system of morphologically marked aspect and aktionsart.

Each verb in Koyukon allows only a particular set of the 15 possible aspects. The verb 'chop', for example, allows semelfactive ('do it once') derivatives in addition to durative and momentaneous (motion) ones. The verb 'eat' permits durative and momentaneous derivatives, but not semelfactives, while the verb 'go by foot' allows momentaneous derivatives but neither semelfactives nor duratives. Koyukon aspect is thus tied to the inherent properties of verbal concepts in much the same way that noun classification is tied to the inherent pro-

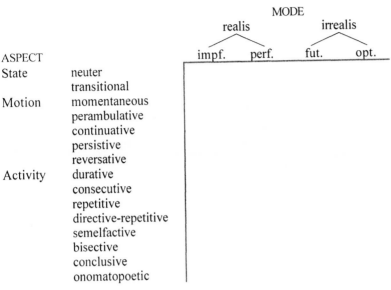

FIGURE 1.1. *The Koyukon Modes and Aspects*

perties of nominal concepts. We can, however, view a concept from different perspectives in both kinds of systems. In Koyukon the difference between 'bite' and 'chew', for example, is indicated by different aspectual derivatives of the same verb root. Similarly, the difference between a lump of flour and a bowl of flour is indicated by gender prefix and classificatory verb.

In Koyukon we can clearly distinguish categories of verbs defined by semantic constraints on aspectual choice, and these are the categories we call aspectual verb theme categories. Verb themes are the bases from which all verbs in the language are derived. Each theme consists of a verb root plus a classifier prefix and perhaps other thematic, or lexical, prefixes. A verb form derives from the addition of derivational and inflectional material to the basic theme. These verb themes are grouped into larger categories on the basis of shared formal and semantic characteristics. Formally, each of the seven major categories is characterized by a particular aspect—that is, the primary (or least marked) derivative of each is of a particular aspect or mode and aspect combination (e.g., the primary aspectual derivative of 'eat' is durative, and the primary aspectual derivative of 'go by foot' is momentaneous). Because each verb theme category is associated with a particular aspect or group of aspects, each can also be characterized as having a particular semantic core. Table 1.1 shows the primary (or diagnostic) aspect and the semantic range associated with each of the categories. Verb theme categories are a means of describing or symbolizing the morphological and semantic similarities shared by a group of verb themes.

In the kind of aspectual classification we see in Koyukon, six important features used to distinguish categories can be identified:

movement	Is motion an integral part of the verbal expression?
direction	Does it have a particular direction, bearing, or course?
countability	Can the activity/event be considered a discrete or bounded unit, or does it have persistence and duration without bounds?
telicity	Is it an activity that leads to a particular goal?
orientation	Is location, arrangement, or alignment a defining factor?
essence	Can it be predicated as inherent to the entity, or is it a temporary or contingent characteristic?

Figure 1.2 illustrates how these distinguishing features are associated with each of the verb theme categories. (Features are shown in lowercase type and theme categories in capital letters.)

As figure 1.2 is intended to illustrate, the feature "movement" distinguishes the motion theme category and the three activity categories (successive, conversive, and operative), all of which are [+movement], from the state theme categories (extension, descriptive, and stative), all of which are [−movement]. The motion theme category is distinguished from the active categories by the feature [±direction]: verbs of the motion theme category (e.g., 'go by foot', 'swim') generally specify the direction, bearing, or course of the movement, while this specification is not a primary semantic feature of verbs of the other activity categories. The other activity categories are distinguished from one another by the features of countability and telicity. Verbs of the successive category (e.g., 'chop', 'kick') specify actions that are punctual—countable and discrete units. Verbs of the conversive theme category (e.g., 'make a single object') are telic, goal-directed. Verbs of the operative theme category (e.g., 'eat', 'see') refer to durative ongoing activities which are neither countable nor telic.

The state verb theme categories, on the right of figure 1.2, do not specify movement. Verbs of the extension category (such as 'ridge extends', 'land slopes') generally refer to the orientation of an object, i.e., location, arrangement, and/or alignment, while verbs of the descriptive and stative categories do

TABLE 1.1. *Diagnostic Aspect and Semantic Characteristics of Verb Theme Categories*

Category	Primary Aspect	Semantic Range	Example
STATE			
Stative	le- neuter	location contingent quality	'sit'
Descriptive	ø neuter	inherent quality	'good'
Extension	ne- neuter	position extending over space	'ridge extends'
ACTIVE			
Motion	momentaneous	movement over space or time	'go by foot'
Activity			
Operative	durative	process	'eat'
Conversive	conclusive	goal	'make one object'
Successive	semelfactive	punctuality	'chop'

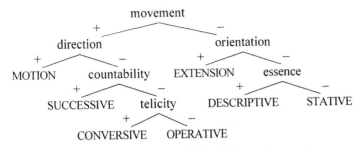

FIGURE 1.2 *Semantic Features and Verb Theme Categories*

not. The descriptive category is comprised of verbs which refer to essential or inherent characteristics of an object (e.g., 'good', 'big') while stative verbs are used to refer to noninherent qualities (such as 'sit', 'be in a particular position').

1.3 Semantic Parallels between Verb and Noun Classification in Koyukon

Many of these semantic features shown in figure 1.2 can be seen as parallel to those illustrated for the classification of nouns via gender and classificatory verbs listed previously. In the next sections, I will sketch how these six features inform both noun classification and aspectual verb classification.

1.3.1 Movement, Direction, and Orientation

The aspectual features of movement, direction, or orientation are comparable to the features of shape and arrangement most commonly associated with noun classification. Orientation or arrangement is the defining feature of extension verbs. An example of an extension verb is shown in (3), which describes the position and alignment of an item:

(3)   *neek'et* (extension neuter)
       'It is stretched out.'

Orientation or arrangement is an important feature throughout the noun classification system. Compare, for example, *boogee eɬetlaakk* and *daaɬenokk,* 'the flour is there as dough' vs. 'as loose flour.' Compare, too, the spatial orientation implied by the shape characteristics specified by the gender prefixes. The shape of an object, whether long, flat, round, is an essential classifying feature for both the gender prefixes and the classificatory verbs. Similarly, the shape of an activity is what is marked in the aspectual system, both by orientation, in extension verbs such as example (3), and also by direction in motion verbs. For example, the momentaneous describes a linear path of motion, motion up to a particular point in time and/or space, as in example (4):

(4)   *neebaanh* (momentaneous)
       'S/he arrived swimming.'

The continuative, another motion aspect illustrated in (5), expresses a round trip motion, tracing an elliptical path to goal and then returning to its source.

(5)   *eeyet nelbaanh* (continuative)
       'S/he swam there and back, made a round trip to there swimming.'

The perambulative, on the other hand, expresses a wandering movement, a path with a more free-form shape. A perambulative derivative is shown in example (6):

(6)   *kk'o'eedebaayh* (perambulative)
       'S/he is swimming around going here and there.'

Both motion and extension verbs focus on shape, as do many of the gender prefixes and noun classifying verbs. In the aspectual expression of shape, the motion aspects indicate the shape, or direction, of movement while the state mode and aspect combinations can indicate shape or orientation of a more static verbal concept.

1.3.2   Countability and Telicity

Countability is a feature that has long been recognized as applying to both verbal and nominal components of the lexicon. Bolinger (1975:147), for instance, says,

> *Mass* and *count* do more than cut the noun class in half—they do the same with verbs, in a very special way. Any verb can be either mass or count according to its form. In *too much talking*, the verb is mass. In *He talked for a moment* it is count, in the sense that there can be many such moments of talking. Grammarians refer to this distinction in verbs as aspect. If a noun or verb refers to one instance of something (*a flash, he jumped*), the instances are countable; if not, the sense is mass (*light, jumping*).

Countability is a defining feature of Koyukon successive verbs, where the distinction between punctual and ongoing activity is primary. Compare the punctual semelfactive example in (7) with the consecutive example in (8):

(7)   *yeeltleł* (semelfactive)
       'S/he chopped it once, gave it a chop.'

(8)   *yegheetletl* (consecutive)
      'S/he chopped it repeatedly, gave it a series of chops.'

Activities expressed within the successive verb theme category are viewed as discrete countable units, as in (7) and (8), or they are viewed as ongoing rather than countable, as in the durative example in (9):

(9)   *yegheetlaatl* (durative)
      'S/he was chopping it (for a while).'

Both the semelfactive derivative in (7) and the consecutive derivative in (8) refer to the activity of chopping from the viewpoint of punctuality—we're conceptualizing separate instances of activity, single chops. The successive category encompasses as well the possibility of seeing the activity as nondiscrete, as in the durative example in (9). The activities expressed via the successive category are those that can be conceptualized from either viewpoint (as opposed to verbs of the operative category, which can only be viewed as nondiscrete and durative). The semelfactive and consecutive aspects allow the specification of countability.

Countability is also specified for nouns via the classificatory verbs, as in the singular *boogee le'onh* 'a lump of flour is there' and the plural *boogee ledlo* 'lumps of flour are there.' Just as activities can be described as countable (with the semelfactive and consecutive aspects) or as a noncount whole (with the durative aspect), nominal objects can be characterized as countable ('a single lump' vs. 'several lumps') or as noncount masses with the classificatory verbs. This mass characteristic is expressed by *boogee daałenokk* 'loose flour is spread around' and by the derivatives with *-tlaakk* 'mushy, wet object' and *-dzok* 'disorderly, scattered objects.' The gender prefixes **hu** 'areal' and *hede* 'weather' likewise refer to mass or abstract notions, while the first three gender prefixes listed in section 1.1 refer to countable entities.

Telicity is a defining feature of verbs of the conversive theme category, which describe activities leading to a goal, such as 'cutting out a shape' or 'making a sled', as shown in examples (10) and (11).

(10) *yeghedaaltlaatl* (conclusive)
      'S/he hewed it into a shape.'

(11) **hu**tl *etltseenh* (conclusive)
      'S/he made a sled.'

These verbs provide a view of the activities of 'chopping' and 'constructing' from the perspective of their outcome, purpose, or goal. The notion of purpose and goal can also be specified for nouns using classificatory verbs. Compare *boogee daałenokk* 'loose flour is spread around', an expression which focuses on the mass characteristic of the flour, with *boogee lekkonh* 'a bowl of flour is there' and *boogee etlkoot* 'flour is there stored as a provision' which focus more directly on the purpose or intended use of the flour.

1.3.3   Essence

The last feature indicated in figure 1.2, essence, is the feature that distinguishes descriptive verbs like 'good', from stative verbs which refer to derived or temporary characteristics like 'be lying down.' This feature is an important feature in noun categorization in Koyukon as well. Notice that *'o* 'compact object', *ø+ton* 'rigid flat or stick-like object', and *kooł* ' flat, flexible object' all specify the essential shape of the object they refer to—these verbs are required in referring to objects of a particular shape in a nonmetaphorical manner. These verbs have counterparts in other verbs in the lexicon; for example, the motion themes *G+ø+gheł* 'rigid flat or sticklike object moves independently, falls' and *G+ø+nekk* 'flat, flexible object moves independently, falls' refer specifically to objects of the same characteristics as do *ø+ton* and *kooł.*

The other classificatory verbs do not emphasize the essential shape of an object. Four of the classificatory verbs clearly refer to achieved or derived characteristics of the objects they are used to describe: *kko* and *ł+ton* refer to contained objects, *koot* refers to the object's use as a foodstuff, and *t'on* refers to an object which is burning. The remaining four classificatory verbs are more ambiguous as to whether they refer to essential or derived physical characteristics: *lo* 'plural objects' draws attention to the plurality of the object referred to, while *dzok* 'disorderly, scattered objects', *tlaakk* 'mushy, wet object', and *nokk* 'granular or powdery substance' emphasize mass nature or amorphous condition of the object to which they are used to refer.

1.4   Discourse Functions of Classification

The previous section argued that the semantic features by which Koyukon nouns are classified spatially have parallels with those by which verbs are classified both temporally and spatially. We shall see in the following discussion that the uses of both noun class and aspectual verb classification in discourse also have similarities; both provide strategies for maintaining referential and structural cohesion.

1.4.1   Discourse and Noun Classification

It has been said (e.g., Denny 1986:303; Aikhenvald 1993) that noun classifiers serve an anaphoric function in referring to items introduced via nominal reference earlier in a discourse. Noun classifiers also have an additional but related role: they establish expectations about what verb predicate the speaker is likely to use and about what other predicates are likely to be relevant in subsequent discourse. "A noun classifier," writes Denny, "expresses the speaker's claims as to the sort of thing he is going to talk about. This sort communicates expectations about the predicates which he might assert for that thing—this is the classificatory role" (pp. 306–7). Hence, noun classifiers serve both a cognitive and a discourse function.

Mithun (1986:395) agrees that "the modification of these predications in terms of the classes of entities they involve permits speakers to deal with large quantities of information in efficient ways." Like other anaphoric strategies, classifiers allow speaker and hearer to reliably track the referents in a conversation or narrative, and they provide cohesion between the structural parts of a discourse. Example (12) is from the personal historical narrative of Chief Henry, *Chief Henry Yugh Noholnigee*, "The Stories Chief Henry Told." Here we see an example where the classificatory verb for handling plural objects (*-lo*) is used with a *de-* gender prefix to refer back to the boxes of shells mentioned three lines earlier and thus maintain referential continuity:

(12)　*Ts'uh bugh yooghskkaat ts'uh*
　　　'And so I bought it from him and'

　　　k'edotlaa' yaasek neteekk'ee yaan',
　　　'just two boxes of shells.'

　　　"Go es huyaan' kk'udaa bedotlaa' be'est'aanee," yelnee.
　　　'"These are the only ones I have to go with it [a gun]," he said.'

　　　Ts'uh eeydee
　　　'So there'

　　　yeyel setl'odegheelo.
　　　'he gave me those [the shells] along with it [the gun].'

Example (13), from the folktale "She's Dragging Her Bag," told by Catherine Attla, again shows the use of the classificatory verb for handling plural objects (*-lo*) with a *de-* gender prefix, referring anaphorically to a stick of skewered fat left for a child.

(13)　*Dehoon k'ekk'uh beghunk'edaal'oy yetolts'ooz laaghe,*
　　　'And he left skewered fat for him to suck on,'

　　　yetolt'uga laaghe soo' yugh needaaneelo.
　　　'he left that there for him to lick.'

These examples show, as Mithun suggests, that noun classification allows efficient tracking of referents within a stretch of speech. Another way of making the flow of information more efficient is by providing a context. Gender and classificatory verb stem derivatives are used both to refer anaphorically to referents introduced earlier and also to introduce a new referent or context without its being named explicitly. Bransford and Johnson (1973), among others, have demonstrated the utility of visual contextual information in improving comprehension, providing retrieval cues, and thus improving recall. Koyukon noun classification, with its focus on shape, number, purpose, and condition, can provide an important visual frame or context for speakers' utterances. They allow the hearer to integrate new information with prior perceptual knowledge about the world. For example, in (14), Chief Henry uses the classificatory verb for handling plural objects to refer to gutting an animal. We have a visual image of plural objects being taken out of the animal's body; with no explicit mention of guts, we have a clear understanding of the activity.

(14)   *Ts'ʉh, "Ggenaa',*
        'And so, "My friend,'

        eey daaggoo ghenee tlaa nohʉdeenɫkk'oyh dehoon
        'build a fire for that ptarmigan and meanwhile'

        dodegge
        '(I'll go) up there'

        dedaayee tlee' eenaaghst'uɫ konh ts'aak'etaaghslaaɫ," seɫnee.
        'and I'll cut off the bull's head and gut it," he said to me.'

Classificatory verbs, then, are a means of providing explicit contextual cues and in this way serve an important function in concept formation and comprehension. Gender is also used to provide contextual information. These prefixes are often used to further specify the shape of a item previously introduced in the discourse. Example (15) is from Chief Henry, and shows the use of the *de-* gender prefix, used to refer to rigid containers, to specify that the milk he had was in a can:

(15)   *Doo',*
        'Well,'

        doogh Eagle milk yaan' daaghs'oɫ ts'ʉh
        'carrying just a can of Eagle milk'

        nonotaalseyo.
        'I started back across the river.'

Example (16), also from Chief Henry's narrative, shows the use of the classificatory verb for compact objects to specify that the snow he had was compact or hard-packed:

(16)   *Eeydee yee*
        'And over that'

        tseetl dol'onh
        'he put some hard-packed snow.'

1.4.2 Discourse and Verb Classification

The functions of verbal aspectual distinctions in discourse and cognitive processes are actually quite similar to those outlined for noun classification. As is the case with noun classification, aspect too serves to provide a visual context or frame for the speaker's utterance. Examples (4)–(6), repeated here as (17) –(19), demonstrate this use of aspect in specifying the path and thus providing a spatial frame for the movement:

(17)   *neebaanh* (momentaneous)
      'S/he arrived swimming.'

(18)   *eeyet nelbaanh* (continuative)
      'S/he swam there and back, making a round trip.'

(19)   *kk'o'eedebaayh* (perambulative)
      'S/he is swimming around going here and there).'

This extra visual information about shape, number, purpose, and condition of states and events that aspect provides can make ideas less abstract and thus easier to comprehend and establishes expectations about what may come up in later discourse.

Aspectual classification then can assist in integrating the new information about participants and events that the hearer is absorbing with what she/he already knows about what events look like. According to Reed (1988:146), classification can "determine what we emphasize in a text and can provide a framework for recalling ideas." In this sense, verb classification also has an anaphoric function. This function is achieved in large part through the use of repetition. It is the repetition of particular aspects with different verb roots and the repetition of particular roots in different aspectual derivatives that provide the means for maintaining referential continuity and textual cohesion in Koyukon discourse.

In their analysis of cohesion in English, Halliday and Hasan identify repetition as an important factor. According to Maynard (1982), "Halliday and Hasan list three types of cohesion, namely, (1) relatedness of form, (2) relatedness of reference, and (3) semantic connection." Cohesion occurs, they say, "when the interpretation of some element in the discourse is dependent on that of another" (1976:4; cited in Maynard 1982:20).

Tannen (1987) also argues that repetition is an essential strategy in cohesion and in meaning-making. Repetition is a strategy used in both literary and conversational discourse to involve the audience in the speaker/writer's theme and to effect their participation in creating or negotiating meaning (1987:575).

Each time a word or phrase is repeated, its meaning is altered. The audience reinterprets the meaning of the word or phrase in light of the accretion, juxtaposition, or expansion; thus it participates in making meaning of the utterance. (1987:576)

This participation of the audience in meaning-making facilitates the cognitive effect of comprehension by creating coherence (the link between structure and meaning) in the discourse.

Tannen claims four purposes for repetition, which are very similar to some of the purported uses of pronominal or classifier anaphora:

1. *Production.* The automaticity of repetition allows a speaker more efficient and more fluent production of language.
2. *Comprehension.* Repetition allows semantically/lexically less dense discourse with less new information.
3. *Connection.* Tannen, like Halliday and Hasan 1976, refers to the "referential and tying function" (1987:583) of repetition, its ability to link utterances and show relationships between concepts or referents. She also points to the evaluative use of repetition, allowing the speaker to point to what is important by focusing attention simultaneously on both the similarities and differences between instances of a repeated utterance.
4. *Interaction.* Repetition is a strategy for conversational management, e.g., for linking speakers' and hearers' ideas and for ratifying contributions. It acts to tie participants to the discourse and to each other.

This use of repetition as a cohesive device has been studied in a variety of languages and dialects (see Tannen 1987 for a summary of these studies). It is also well documented in English (e.g., Halliday and Hasan 1976, and discussed in Rosen and Behrens 1994, and Lunsford and Connors 1995). In Athabaskan, McCreedy's (1989) study of cohesion in Navajo discourse examined such devices as pronominal reference and lexical repetition, synonymy, and collocation in three genres of Navajo texts. Gómez de García and Axelrod (1998) examined the use of repetition and its implications for curriculum building in the Mescalero, Chiricahua, and Plains Apache languages.

As is noted in Gómez de García and Axelrod (1998), the structure of Athabaskan languages may make repetition strategies especially available to speakers: "The structure of the verb lends itself to repetition and, because verb roots can be repeated with different prefixal derivations and prefixal derivations can be repeated with different verb roots, Apachean allows this repetition without excess redundancy. It is a strategy that provides cohesion within a text and also allows for increased learnability" (1998:123).

Repetition in Apache texts was found to account for between 30 and 40% of the verbs used. The use of repetition in Koyukon may be even more frequent. In a sample of conversation between Bessie Henry and Catherine Attla of Huslia (used here for examples (26) and (29)), there are a total of 59 verbs. Of these, 23 represent new instances and 33 are repetitions of one or another of those 23 previously introduced verb roots. Excluding the verb 'to say', of which there are twelve occurrences, there are 58 verbs; 22 of those, or 37%, are instances of repetition. In the popular Koyukon folktale *Tobaan Etseh,* as told by Catherine Attla (discussed in Axelrod 1993), there are a total of 108 verbs (excluding instances of 'say' in its reportative or evidential uses); fully 65, or 60%, of these contain repeated verb roots.[5]

Variation in aspectual marking is an important strategy for providing cohesion in Athabaskan languages. An examination of Koyukon folk stories, personal narrative, and conversation shows a frequent pattern of the repetition of a particular verb with alternating aspectual derivations. A second common pattern is the repetition of a particular aspectual derivation with different verb roots. Like anaphora, these patterns of repetition serve to tie referents to the prior discourse and provide cohesive ties.

The following examples (20) and (21) from *Tobaan Etseh*, "She's Crying on the Beach," told by Catherine Attla, illustrate the first of these patterns. In (20) the action of slapping the tail (by the porcupine woman) is expressed first in the semelfactive and then, some 10 lines later, in the consecutive:

(20) *Huyeł bekaayeedleghuł*
    'Then she slapped (semel. perf.) him with her tail . . .'

    yekaaghelghułtl ts'uh
    'because she'd hit (cons. perf.) him again and again with her tail.'

Notice that this kind of verb repetition provides cohesion and referential continuity over the intervening stanzas. Example (20) also illustrates the use of the feature of countability to provide explicit visual images of an activity from different perspectives. A second illustration is given in example (21), which shows the verb 'eat' expressed first in a momentaneous derivative and then, in the next line, in a durative derivative:

(21) *Degheel go ledo degheel edaak'uhdeedon'.*
    'I guess around there where she was living, she had eaten (mom. perf.) everything there was to eat.'

    Et'eeyło dekenh kkotsel yeen' ehonh.
    'Apparently she ate (dur. impf.) only tree bark.'

Often, rather than an entirely different aspect, a verb root is repeated with a different aspectual prefix string within the same aspect, as shown in examples (22) and (23), from a folk tale called *Kaazene*, 'The Lynx'. Example (22) is from a version of the story told by Chief Henry of Koyukuk, and example (23) is from the telling by Catherine Attla of Huslia. Notice that in both examples, the motion verbs (for 'go by canoe, paddle' in (22) and for 'go by foot' in (23)) are repeated with varying aspectual derivations.

(22) *Ts'e kkudaa hulookk'ut*
    'And now it was spring'

    gheel en notedekkaayh, go denaa.
    'when he customarily goes (by paddling a canoe) (customary) hunting, this man.'

    Ts'e nodekkaayh.
    'And then he usually comes (by paddling a canoe) (mom. perf.) home.'

(23) *Dehoon nonoo' haadeeyo.*
'And she took off (sing. 'go by foot') (mom. perf.) upriver.'

Ts'e yoogh ghehoł.
'So she was walking (sing. 'go by foot') (progressive) along.'

Example (24), from a folktale called "Great Raven Who Shapes the World," also told by Catherine Attla, shows the same pattern.

(24) *Ts'uh kk'udaa yeyeł notaałeyo.*
'And now he started home (iterative incept. perf.) with it.'

Ts'uh go hedaadletl'ee de no'eedeyo.
'And he came back (iterative perf.) to where they were staying.'

Ts'uh go yuh eet neeno'eedeyo

'And he got back (iterative mom. perf., with *nee#ne-* 'up to a point') there.'

This pattern can also be found in personal narrative. In the example in (25) from Chief Henry, the verb for 'dual go by foot' is used first in the momentaneous perfective, and then repeated in the progressive:

(25) *Ts'uh koon an nosaałet'ots go seggenaa' J.O. yeł.*
'So my friend J.O. and I went ('dual go on foot') (perfective) out hunting.'

Ts'uh yoogh dzaank'ets'o'ustl
'And we had walked (dual 'go on foot') (progressive) all day.'

The pattern shows up also in conversation. Examples (26) and (27) are taken from a conversation between Bessie Henry and Catherine Attla of Huslia:

(26) B: *Ts'e gheel go kk'udaa k'enhoonaaldlaa'.*
'So it was then that they started trapping (reversative conative inceptive).'

       C: *Oho'.*
'Yes.'

       B: *K'ehooneelaa'.*
'They were trapping (reversative conative perfective).'

(27) B: *Dehoon heɬde kk'udaa noneelnoos . . .*
'By this time his face had swollen up (transitional impf.) . . .'

    C: *. . . go dekk'un kk'aa. Tl'ogho Grandma gheelaa' kkaa dehedegheenee' tsen'.*
'. . . for want of tobacco. That's just what Grandma and them used to say.'

        Yooghedon heɬde genee laaghe heyehʉtaadle'aan go daakk'un kk'aa heɬde noheneeghelnus hedegheenee'?
'How did they get so addicted that long ago to that tobacco that they said their faces would swell up (customary perf.) for want of it?'

Notice in this last example, the two women are collaborating in constructing a coherent narrative with this kind of verb repetition with aspectual variation. B. uses a verb in the transitional imperfective, and C. repeats it but expresses it in a customary derivative.

These latter examples (22)–(27) which use different aspectual prefixes rather than an entirely different aspect, permit referential and structural coherence by varying the expression of the spatial and temporal shape of the activity. The aspectual system, like the noun classification system, allows shape, number, purpose, and condition to be used for very explicit reference.

Another pattern of aspect used as a cohesive device is the repetition of a particular aspectual derivation with different verb roots. Like the preceding pattern, this pattern too was found in all the genres of text examined. The example in (28) is from the version of *Kaazene* told by Catherine Attla:

(28) *Yaalo'ooghenaaltset.*
'His hands shrank around it.'

    Belo'ooghenaadledzoyh.
'His hands just shriveled up.'

Example (29) is from the conversation in Huslia and shows both patterns, both repetition of a particular verb that means 'to shake', with different aspectual derivations, and the repetition of a particular aspectual derivation, the inceptive (marked with a *te-* prefix and a *le-* perfective prefix), with two different verb stems, 'shake' and 'fart':

(29) *"Hʉn detaaɬeneenh detaaɬeneenh,*
'"Pretty soon he started to shake and shake (incept.),'

    dedeneenh dehoon detaadletl'et," yeɬnee.
'he was shaking (durative) and then he began farting (inceptive)," he said.'

1.5   Conclusions

Aspectual verb classification, then, is like noun classification in its semantic structure and in its discourse function of providing strategies for text cohesion. The two components of the noun classification system and the aspectual system have, of course, different diachronic sources and different synchronic uses and ranges. The similarities between them, though, suggest that the salient semantic features of a language will surface in more than one area of the grammar. This look at the semantics of classification in Koyukon provides another illustration of the functionalist principle that elements of grammatical structure (such as noun classifiers and verbal aspect) both shape and depend on discourse pragmatic and semantic requirements of communicative interaction.

Notes

1. Koyukon is an Athabaskan language spoken in Central Alaska. It is a moribund language with about 650 speakers, who are all over the age of 30. The data presented here come mostly from Eliza Jones of Koyukuk, who is a linguist and native speaker of the language.
2. Abbreviations are as follows:

CL	classifier	G	gender
M/A	mode and aspect	perf.	perfective mode
impf.	imperfective mode	incept.	inceptive
+	conjunct morpheme boundary	#	disjunct morpheme boundary
mom.	momentaneous aspect	dur.	durative aspect
cons.	consecutive aspect	semel.	semelfactive aspect

3. Verb themes are the lexical bases from which inflected verbal forms are derived. The themes in Figure 1 have the root at the far right. Preceding the root is a classifier prefix and, preceding that, usually a G indicating that gender marking is required by the theme.
4. The discussion here is drawn from Thompson, Axelrod, and Jones 1983.
5. Lexical repetition in English prose is generally much lower. The first three paragraphs of Jane Austen's *Emma*, for example, contain 22 verbs and only three (13%) of them are repetitions (of the verb 'to be'). Repetition is much more frequent, however, as a cohesive strategy in English oral narrative. In the first two paragraphs of Book 1 of Studs Terkel's *Working* (Pierce Walker, Farmer), for example, there are 31 verbs; of these, 10 (or 32%) are repetitions.

References

Allan, K. 1977. Classifiers. *Language* 53(2):284–310.
Aikhenvald, A. 1993. Classifiers. *Language* 53(2):284–310.
Axelrod, M. 1993. *The Semantics of Time*. Lincoln: University of Nebraska Press.
Bolinger, D. 1975. *Aspects of Language* (2nd ed.). New York: Harcourt Brace.
Bransford, J. D., and M. K. Johnson. 1973. Considerations of Some Problems of Comprehension. In W. G. Chase (ed.), *Visual Information Processing*. New York: Academic Press.

Denny, J. P. 1986. The Semantic Role of Noun Classifiers. In C. Craig (ed.), *Noun Classes and Categorization*. Amsterdam: Benjamins.

Gómez de García, J., and M. Axelrod. 1998. Rhetorical Strategies and Language Learning in Apache. *Proceedings of the 1997 Mid-America Linguistics Conference*.

Lee, M. 1988. Language, Perception and the World. In J. A. Hawkins (ed.), *Explaining Language Universals*. Oxford: Blackwell.

Lunsford, A., and R. Connors. 1995. *The St. Martin's Handbook*. New York: St. Martin's Press.

Maynard, S. K. 1982. Analysis of Cohesion: A Study of the Japanese Narrative. *Journal of Literary Semantics* 11(1):20.

McCreedy, L. 1989. Cohesion and Discourse Structure in Three Genres of Navajo Discourse. In E.-D. Cook and K. Rice (eds.), *Athapaskan Linguistics: Current Perspectives on a Language Family*, pp. 439–486. Berlin: Mouton de Gruyter.

Mithun, M. 1986. The Convergence of Noun Classification Systems. In C. Craig (ed.), *Noun Classes and Categorization*. Amsterdam: Benjamins.

Paprotte, W. 1988. A Discourse Perspective on Tense and Aspect in Standard Modern Greek and English. In B. Rudzka-Ostyn (ed.), *Topics in Cognitive Linguistics*. Amsterdam: Benjamins.

Reed, S. K. 1988. *Cognition*. Pacific Grove, Calif: Brooks/Cole.

Rosen, L. J., and L. Behrens. 1994. *The Allyn and Bacon Handbook*. Boston: Allyn and Bacon.

Tannen, D. 1987. Repetition in Conversation: Towards a Poetics of Talk. *Language* 63(3):574–605.

Thompson, C., M. Axelrod, and E. Jones. 1983. *Han Zaadlitlee*. Nenana: Yukon-Koyukuk School District.

2

A SEMANTIC BASIS FOR
NAVAJO SYNTACTIC TYPOLOGY

Leonard M. Faltz

This chapter is intended as an exploration of the approach found in Faltz (1995) as applied to a number of typological features of the Navajo language. The intent is to show that a significant collection of such features, including features discussed in Faltz (1995) and Speas (1995), as well as some additional ones, form a coherent collection that can be understood by examining the way semantic interpretation is related to syntactic structure.

Faltz (1995) showed that a number of typological features followed from the assumption that a language satisfies the pronominal argument criterion, namely:

(1)   A language is said to be a *pronominal argument language* if only pronouns are permitted to occupy argument positions.

The reasoning was roughly that if the condition in (1) holds, then, making the reasonable assumptions that semantic interpretation depends on syntactic structure and that only argument-position NPs can be semantically functional on the (denotations of the) predicate-denoters they are combined with, we derive the fact that a nonpronominal NP cannot be interpreted as a generalized quantifier. From this, various conclusions can be drawn, two significant ones being the nonexistence of determiner quantification (i.e., all quantifiers must float) and the nonexistence of English-style relative clauses (by which term I mean predicate-denoting phrases derived from sentences with one argument understood as bound by a lambda). In fact, both of these conclusions stem from the impossibility of a predicate-denoting common-noun-phrase category in languages satisfying (1).

Now, another way of interpreting facts like this is to notice that what is impossible is a syntactic category, namely the category of common-noun-phrase, which denotes a predicate none of whose arguments is specified—we can call such a denotation a *fully unsaturated predicate*. But saying it this way reminds us that in Navajo there are no verbs which constitute syntactic units on the surface (i.e., which are independent words) that denote fully unsaturated predicates, for the simple reason that Navajo verbs always have pronominal arguments attached to them. Now, this does not quite follow from assuming that Navajo satisfies (1): we can certainly conceive of a language in which (1) holds but where the pronominal arguments of a verb are separate syntactic elements not attached to the verb. This suggests that it might be productive to consider the following somewhat different generalization as a typological fact about Navajo:

(2)   Syntactically visible constituents never denote fully unsaturated predicates.

By *syntactically visible constituents* I mean words and phrases; what I intend to exclude are bound forms that cannot constitute words by themselves.

For convenience, let's rephrase (2) slightly. By a *pure predicate phrase* (or PPP) I'll mean a syntactically visible constituent (that's the "phrase") which denotes a fully unsaturated predicate (a "pure predicate"). We can then rewrite (2) as:

(2')   *Non-PPP parameter:* Navajo does not contain PPPs.

Let's take a look at this parameter a bit.[1]

To some extent the categorization of Navajo as a non-PPP language is problematical: there are a number of cases in Navajo where the issue of whether we are dealing with one word or more than one is unclear. As an example, consider the following three Navajo phrases:

(3)   *báá'díílgeed*
        'I uncovered it by digging.'

(4)   *yaa yiní'á*
        'He/she gave it to him/her.'

(5)   *dah dííyá*
        'I set out' (that is, 'I started to go').

In (3)–(5) the phrases are presented as conventionally written. However, we might ask why the phrase in (3) was written as one word rather than as two. One could write, for example:

(6)   *báá adíítgeed*

Of course, we can see just by comparing (6) with (3) that a phonological process has applied in one of these expressions, either deleting an *a* vowel in (3) or else inserting it in (6) depending on the analysis. This process, which appears to be sensitive to the presence (or absence) of a word boundary, suggests that, since the expression is usually heard without this vowel, we are dealing with a single word.

But arguments like this could be adduced for (4) and (5) as well. For example, in common speech, (4) is usually pronounced:

(7)   *yeiní'á*

The change from *a(a)i* to *ei* is not something that we would expect to be possible with an intervening word boundary. (Alternatively: if such a process is possible with an intervening word boundary, then perhaps the process illustrated in (3) and (6) is, too). Similarly, the expression

(8)   *dah jidííyá*
       'One set out.'

which is the form that corresponds to (5) when the fourth-person subject is used instead of the first-person singular subject, is usually pronounced

(9)   *dashdííyá*

again exhibiting a phonological process that might suggest either the absence of a word boundary in (5) or else the presence of a word boundary in (3).

However, cases like these are not going to be problematic for us, for it is clear that none of the elements—*báá, adíítgeed,* or *báá'díítgeed* (whichever is ultimately right)—denotes a fully unsaturated predicate (the *b-* of *baa* is an overt marker of a pronominal argument, and similar pronouns can be found in the other forms). The same can be said for the forms *yaa, yiní'á, dííyá,* and *jidííyá.* Elements like *dah* are less clear; I'll come back to them later.

What is the real content of the assumption in (2) or (2'); that is, what is the content of the non-PPP parameter? For one thing, (2) only makes sense against the background of the classical analyses of natural language semantics that treat the semantic content of verbs (and other similar words) as predicates whose arguments correspond only to the participant roles of the events, actions, or states that are named by the verbs but not including those events, actions, and states themselves. This is not necessarily a problem; for example, (2) can be reformulated to allow for an event-logic semantics. But let's stick to the formulation in (2) for our discussion; if, say, an event logic is preferred, the formulation in (2) would have to be adjusted accordingly.[2]

We noted earlier that the non-PPP parameter does not quite follow from the pronominal-argument parameter (in (1)). What about the reverse: is any non-PPP language necessarily a pronominal-argument language? To try to clarify this, at least for Navajo, let's note that at some level the portion of a Navajo verb that represents the class of action, event, or situation that is being predicated must be interpreted as a fully unsaturated predicate. By assumption (2), this portion of a Navajo verb, which we can call the *verb base*, cannot be a word or phrase; rather, it must be a bound element. Any word or phrase containing this element must contain other bound elements whose referents are the major participants in the event or situation named by the verb base. That is, in order to have an actual verb in Navajo, pronominal elements have to be attached to the verb base.

We saw before that this is not exactly what is meant by "pronominal argumentness", which classically requires that nonpronominal referring expressions be adjuncts in a coreference relation with the pronouns that are the true (and obligatory) arguments of the verb. The notion of pronominal argumentness makes no reference to bound forms or words: it leaves open the possibility of a pronominal-argument language where the pronouns are independent words. In Navajo, of course, this is definitely not the case. But does that automatically mean that Navajo is a pronominal-argument language?

Here is an argument that at least suggests that any language that satisfies (2) satisfies (1). A verb without arguments is necessarily a fully unsaturated predicate denoter; therefore, by (2), arguments to a verb must be affixed to it. We can exclude the idea of a language where all argument NPs are verb affixes, since NPs form an infinite class.[3] We are left with the idea of a finite class of possible argument NPs; but this is just what a class of pronouns is. Thus, we are forced into the pronominal argument scheme: only members of this special finite class of NPs, namely the pronouns, can be arguments at all.

Let's return to the question of what typological consequences follow from the non-PPP parameter. Recall that in the approaches that were popularized by Montague and further developed in the theories of generalized quantifiers, boolean semantics, and other similar developments, verbs, common nouns, and common noun phrases are the kinds of syntactic units that denote fully unsaturated predicates. We have already seen that Navajo (surface) verbs are not fully unsaturated predicate denoters. What about common nouns and common noun phrases? By (2), a Navajo common noun cannot denote a fully unsaturated predicate, a conclusion that also follows from (1), as shown in Faltz (1995), where we also showed that a Navajo NP cannot denote a generalized quantifier and in fact cannot consist of a quantifier combined with a common noun or common noun phrase. So we immediately have the following questions: What *does* a Navajo NP denote? What *does* a Navajo common noun denote? What *does* a Navajo NP consist of?

To answer these questions, let's start by remembering that in any language an unadorned proper noun constitutes an NP. Since the denotation of a proper noun can always be understood as being (a representation of) the entity who/which carries that proper noun as a name,[4] we see immediately that the semantic combination of a proper-noun-type NP with a verb is necessarily a case of coreference-binding.[5] For example, starting with the verb:

(10)   *naané*
       'He/she is playing.'[6]

whose denotation could be diagrammed

(11)   play(e_1)

where e_1 is the denotation of the pronoun element represented by the subject prefix hidden in (10), the interpretation of the sentence

(12)   *John naané*
       'John is playing.'

can be gotten by binding the denotation of *John*, say, john, with e_1:

(13)   play(e_1) & john=e_1

I'll sometimes speak of this arrangement metaphorically by saying that the semantic connection between *John* and *naané* in (12) is via the "pronominal bus."[7]

Having gotten this far, we can now ask about other NPs. It appears that all languages have common nouns as a class of word, and Navajo is no exception. How can a common noun be used as the head of an NP if only a minimal amount of required additional material is combined with it? In a language with fully unspecified predicate-denoters, such as English, the common noun will denote a fully unspecified predicate, and something will be combined with it to create a generalized quantifier. In Navajo, the non-PPP parameter forces us into the position that a common noun all by itself cannot, as it is used in a real utterance, denote a fully unspecified predicate. But at some level a common noun *has to* denote such a predicate: what else could the word *ashkii* denote, for example, than the fully unspecified predicate $(\lambda x)(boy(x))$?

We can answer this by combining two principles. The first one is this: while not exactly forced on us, let's make the reasonable guess that, as used in a real utterance, a common noun is similar to a verb in that it must have a pronominal element in it. From this idea only, we conclude that the word *ashkii* as used in an utterance must have the following denotation:

(14)   boy(e_2)

that is, something which is equivalent to "he is a boy."

Our second principle is simply that the semantic function of an NP is to refer, not to predicate. Applying this to (14), we conclude that if the word *ashkii* can be an NP at all, its denotation must be:

(15) (ιe_2)boy(e_2)

that is, something which is equivalent to "the one who is a boy." Note that our reasoning has led us to a remarkable prediction:

(16)   If a common noun can be used all by itself as an NP in Navajo, then it must be understood as having undergone definite closure; that is, it must be understood as though it is being used to refer to a contextually defined member of the class of entities that satisfy the predicate which the common noun, as a lexical but not syntactic unit, denotes.

In (16), the idea is that as a lexical item we are indeed allowing common nouns to denote fully unspecified predicates, but that as soon as a common noun becomes part of a syntactic structure, it must have had a pronominal element affixed to it.[8]

It might be objected that this pronominal element is never visible. In the case of third person (which is the most common case for a noun used as the head of an NP), an invisible pronoun is no problem: third-person markings are often zero for Navajo verbs, so why not for common nouns? However, Navajo nouns have no non-third-person pronominal affixes, either. For example, a sentence like "I am a boy" does not involve affixing any visible first-person singular affix to the noun *ashkii*; rather, a copular verb is used, much as in English (where *nishłį́* contains an overt 1sg affixed pronoun.[9]):

(17)   *ashkii nishłį́*
　　　boy　　1SG=be
　　　'I am a boy.'

But this is not necessarily as damaging as it might seem at first. Let's examine what happens with a similar situation when, instead of an ordinary common noun like *ashkii*, we use a word created according to the very common Navajo arrangement known colloquially as a "descriptive noun". This is a nominalized, verb-based construction that acts as a noun. Navajo speakers often make these up as nonce expressions, but quite a few of them have become lexicalized, particularly to serve as nouns that name entities that are not part of traditional Navajo life and for which new terms were needed. An example of such a "noun" is:

(18)   *bá'ólta'í*
　　　'teacher'

whose structure can be unpacked into a meaning somewhat as follows: "an entity such that reading activity is performed for that entity"; note that the teacher is the entity for whom the reading is done.[10] Since (18) is constructed using standard verb morphology, the entity for whom the reading is done is marked in (18) in the usual way, which, for an argument that corresponds to the object of the adposition that means "for", is explicit; in fact, it's the initial consonant *b*. Now, note how "I am a teacher" is expressed:

(19)   *bá'ólta'í nishłį́*
       teacher   1SG=be
       'I am a teacher.'

The affixed pronoun in the descriptive noun which refers to the referent of the noun itself remains third person, even though the actual referent is the speaker.[11] This might be viewed as evidence that the word for teacher has become lexicalized, and hence frozen, but further examination shows that the situation is not so simple. First of all, the general verb pluralizing prefix *da* can be inserted into the word for "teacher" in order to create a noun meaning "teachers":

(20)   *báda'ólta'í*
       'teachers'

Second, if we think about the unpacked meaning of the word in (18), we'll realize that to express a meaning involving a possessive, such as "my teacher", the possessive 1sg entity corresponds to the one who does the reading. This suggests the possibility that inserting a 1sg subject prefix into (18) would be the way to express this idea. In fact, subject prefixes *can* be inserted into (18) in order to express such possessives:

(21)   *bá'íínίshta'í*
       'my teacher'

(22)   *yá'ółta'í*
       'his/her teacher'

Example (22) also shows the regular shift from *b* to *y* that occurs (for direct forms) when a subject and a nonsubject are both third person. (The barred *ł* in (22), as compared with the plain *l* in (18), is due to the fact that in (22) we have a "real" third-person subject, namely the referent of "his/her", as opposed to the unspecified third-person subject in (18).)

With examples like these, a better explanation for the third-person marking in (19) is to posit that Navajo common nouns are necessarily third person. This also explains why normal common nouns never show any visible pronominal affixes.[12] Thus, if we assume that the occurrence of a common noun in a syntactic utterance necessarily involves an invisible third-person pronoun affix, then

(2) remains true for this case, and we can still say that Navajo is a non-PPP language.

Let's proceed with our survey of the consequences of (2) for Navajo. First of all, if a common noun phrase syntactic type does not exist, and in particular, if common nouns by themselves can be referring expressions, it would appear that there cannot be a determiner phrase type with which common nouns can combine. Is this true?

This is almost true. The possible counterexample is provided by a closed class of demonstratives which can occur directly in front of common nouns, apparently in syntactic construction with them:

(23) *díí   ashkii*
      this   boy
      'this boy'

(24) *naghái   łíí'*
      that   horse
      'that horse'

I do not believe that it is possible to separate the demonstrative from the noun by material extraneous to the referring material headed by the noun, so syntactically we are probably really dealing with a phrase.[13] I have no real explanation for this, although the fact that a bare common noun undergoes default definite closure suggests that a demonstrative can combine with a common noun because a demonstrative can be interpreted as a kind of modifier of the definiteness operator.

Apart from this case, though, it is true that determiners do not form phrases with the head nouns they are semantically understood as applying to. The classical case of such determiners are the quantifiers. The relative freedom of positioning of Navajo quantifiers is well known. Here are a few examples:

(25) *John   awéé'   díkwíí shíí   yiłhozh.*
      John   baby   a few $3 \rightarrow 3$=tickle=I[14]
      'John is tickling a few babies.'

(26) *John díkwíí shíí awéé' yiłhozh.* (same)

Here we see that a quantifier can precede or follow the common noun that it is understood to apply to. The following examples illustrate some additional facts:

(27) *Awéé'   t'áálá'í nítínígo   deiłhozh.*
      baby   3=each $1SG \rightarrow 3$=PL=tickle=P
      'I tickled each baby.'

(28) *T'áálá'í nítínígo awéé' deiłhozh.* (same)

(29) *Awéé   adą́ą́dą́ą́'   t'áátá'í nítíntgo   deíthozh.*
       baby   yesterday   each   1SG→3=PL=tickle=P
       'I tickled each baby yesterday.'

(30) *T'áátá'í nítíntgo adą́ą́dą́ą́' awéé' deíthozh.*   (same)

Sentences (27)–(30) illustrate three additional facts about Navajo quantifiers, facts which further suggest that a quantifier is not in construction with its common noun.

First of all, a quantifier may be separated from its common noun by material extraneous to the reference of that noun. This is seen in (29) and (30), where the word *adą́ą́dą́ą́'* 'yesterday' intervenes between the quantifier and the noun.

Second, many Navajo quantifier expressions contain overt pronominal elements, just like verbs. The form for 'each' in (27)–(30) is marked for third person, for example. That form should be compared with the form for 'each' in:

(31) *T'áátá'í niitíntgo   nihidaané'é   bee   nideii'né.*
       1PL=each   1PL=toy   3=INST   1PL=PL=play=I
       'We are each playing with our toys.'

The presence of an explicit pronominal element in a quantifier is an indication that the semantic combination of a quantifier with other phrases, including the noun over which it is quantifying, is of the same sort as the semantic combination of a verb and an explicit referring expression, namely, by means of the pronominal bus. This is another striking piece of evidence that the quantifier does not form a phrase with its noun.

And third, it is possible to use the plural prefix *da* (indicated by PL in the gloss) in a verb if one of its arguments is quantified by 'each'. This is in strong contrast to English where an NP with the determiner *each* or *every* is necessarily singular.

Let's look at this last issue a bit. To do so, it will be helpful to know a little about the Navajo plural verb prefix *da*. An exact rule governing its usage is not, I believe, completely known, but the following seems to be approximately correct.

First, a given verb either contains the plural prefix *da* or it does not. It is not possible for a verb to contain more than one occurrence of *da*. Moreover, if a verb does contain *da*, this prefix can appear only in one position in the verb, no matter what argument it refers to.

As hinted in the last sentence above, the plurality marked by the *da* prefix can be understood to apply to one of potentially several different arguments of a verb. The following rules seem to be more or less true.

(32) If the subject of a verb is a set of three or more entities, if this plurality is not shown by the use of a special verb stem,[15] and if the set of entities is not being viewed in some special way as a single entity itself, then *da* is required.

(33) Apart from the circumstances listed in (32), if any argument of a verb is a
      set of three or more entities, and if the verb is to be understood as apply-
      ing distributively over the members of that set, then *da* may be put into
      the verb, to call attention to the distributivity.

The optionality spoken of in (33) remains to be fully explored: it may be the
case that *da* is more strongly felt to be required in some circumstances than in
others due to additional relevant conditions that would have to be determined.

    (Incidentally, in examining the examples, note that a regular phonological
process changes *da* to *de* when an *i* vowel immediately follows.)

    Examples (27)–(30) are all examples of rule (33) at work: the *da* prefix in the
verbs in those examples appears to call attention to the distributivity of the verb
over the members of the set named by the direct object, which in those sentences is a set of babies.

    The optionality mentioned in (33) can be illustrated as follows:

(34) a.   *John   t'ááłá'í nítínígo   awéé'* *yiyííłhozh.*
           John   each   baby   3→3=tickle=P
           'John tickled each baby.'

      b.   *John   t'ááłá'í nítínígo   awéé'* *deiyííłhozh.*
                                                3→3=PL=tickle=P

           (same)

Comments by a Navajo speaker suggest to me that, in the case of plural objects
such as (34), *da* is marking event plurality; but this can just be viewed as the
result of (or the meaning of) distributivity over the plural object. We cannot
regard *da* as an event pluralizer (from which the argument plurality results by
means of inference) because, as far as I can tell, *da* cannot be used *unless* there is
at least one plural argument.

    Getting back to the plurality marking of arguments with the quantifier 'each',
note that with our non-PPP assumption (2) we would expect that the English
arrangement, where an NP in the scope of *each* is everywhere treated as a singular, should be impossible. The reason is that since the (syntactically visible)
verb has to include a pronominal registration of the argument referred to by the
noun being quantified over (since the verb cannot denote a fully unsaturated
predicate), this registration can only be interpreted as referring to the set over
which the quantification is occurring. And, of course, with *each*, this is a plurality. Note that this means that we are claiming that even in cases like (34a),
where the verb doesn't have *da* in it, the object "looks" plural to the verb; otherwise put, any connection between the verb and a quantified argument is still
via the pronominal bus. And, again, this goes along with the nonconstituency
of the quantifier together with its noun.[16]

    Apart from demonstratives and quantifiers, another possible determiner is a
possessive. In English, full possessive NP's can be (syntactic) determiners, a
situation which is perhaps somewhat marked typologically. Semantically,
possessors are better viewed as modifiers of the head noun; and they are treated
as such syntactically in many languages. Many languages provide a genitive

case-marking arrangement for NPs that are to denote possessors,[17] which means that such NPs are interpreted as predicates (e.g., *John's* means $(\lambda x)R(x, john)$, where R is an abstract relation that sometimes reduces to ownership) which are combined (via *and*) with the predicates denoted by the common noun phrase with which the genitive is in construction. Now, we cannot regard this denotation as a fully unsaturated predicate, since the predicate R is saturated in one argument by *john*; in other words, (2) does not directly rule out genitive structures (but see the discussion of (48) below). However, in a language that satisfies (2), the denotation of a genitive structure would have nothing to combine with, since it would require (in general) a fully unsaturated predicate as its conjunct. The situation is exactly parallel to the situation with quantifiers: (2) does not directly rule out the possibility of expressions that denote generalized quantifiers, but if there were such an expression, it would have nothing to combine with.

Thus, such an arrangement is predicted to be impossible in Navajo, and this is true. Navajo uses another common arrangement instead, in which any possession is registered pronominally by an affix (a prefix in Navajo) on the noun. A full referential expression that is intended to refer to a possessor is then coreferent with the pronominal possessive prefix. Here are some examples:

(35) a.   *ł{í'*
          horse
          'horse'

   b.   *shi-ł{í'*
        1SG-horse
        'my horse'

   c.   *bi-ł{í'*
        3-horse
        'his/her horse'

   d.   *John bi-ł{í'*
        John 3-horse
        'John's horse'

This means that the semantic connection between *John* and *bilį́į'* in (35d) is via the pronominal bus, just as in the case of the semantic connection between a referring expression and a verb or between a quantifier and a referring expression. Given this, and given the facts illustrated for quantifiers in (27)–(30), we might ask about the relative ordering possibilities of possessor referring expressions with the possessed noun. In the case of possessors, it appears that a possessor is not permitted to follow a possessed noun; however, it is perhaps permitted to be separated from its possessed noun by extraneous material. The following sentences illustrate this:

(36)   *Baa' bi-yáázh   Kinłání-di   naalnish.*
        Bah 3-son   Flagstaff-LOC   3=work=I
        'Bah's son works in Flagstaff.'

(37) *Baa' Kinłání-di*   *bi-yáázh*   *naalnish.*
    Bah Flagstaff-LOC   3-son   3=work=I
    (same)

(38) **Bi-yáázh*   *Kinłání-di*   *Baa'*   *naalnish.*
    3-son   Flagstaff-LOC   Bah   3=work=I

The unacceptability of orderings such as (38) is not surprising if we recall that Navajo is a verb-final language. If *Baa'* in (36)–(38) is viewed as an argument referrer for *biyáázh*, then the requirement that *Baa'* precede *biyáázh* can be subsumed into a general word-order pattern for the language according to which argument referrers have to precede the words that contain pronominal registrations of those arguments. The possibility of a quantifier preceding its noun does not invalidate this, since the noun is not a referring expression that further specifies an argument of the quantifier. However, we should note that it is more usual for quantifiers to follow their nouns than to precede them; that is, the (apparently acceptable—see (28) and (30)) order in which a quantifier precedes its noun is somewhat marked.[18]

Of course, the common-noun-phrase-modifying phrases par excellence are the relative clauses. Classically, a relative clause denotes the lambdaized version of an arbitrary sentence; its canonical use is to denote a predicate which will be conjoined with the predicate denoted by the head noun of an NP to create a complex predicate denoted by the common-noun-phrase consisting of that noun together with the relative clause. Since by (2) a common noun in actual use cannot denote a fully unsaturated predicate, a classical relative clause would not be able to find a phrase whose denotation it could combine with. We therefore predict that such a relative clause arrangement should be impossible in Navajo, and in fact we do not find it. Instead, we find a nominalization construction which allows relative-clause-like semantic combinations to be expressed, but without actually involving syntactically visible phrases that refer to lambdaizations of sentences. Traditionally, these constructions have been analyzed as internally headed relative clauses, although it is not at all clear that this is the right analysis. Let's look at some examples. A simple one is:

(39) *Ashkii*   *hastiin*   *yiztałée*   *at'ééd*   *yizts'os.*
     boy   man   3→3=kick=P=NOM   girl   3→3=kiss=P
     'The boy that kicked the man kissed the girl.'
     'The man that the boy kicked kissed the girl.'

If we think of the first three words of (39) as an internally headed relative clause, then the two readings of (39) fall out naturally. There are two choices for the internal head, *ashkii* and *hastiin*. If *ashkii* is the internal head, then the first three words correspond to 'the boy that kicked the man', whereas if *hastiin* is the internal head, then the first three words correspond to 'the man that the boy kicked'. In both cases it is the boy who is doing the kicking and the man who is getting kicked; this follows directly from standard rules of Navajo thematic role interpretation, based on the order of the two nouns and the fact that the verb displays the direct object form (*y*) rather than the inverse object form (*b*).

But there are potentially other ways in which the structure of (39) might be analyzed. For example, suppose we bracket the words in (39) in the following relatively flat manner:

(40) [*ashkii*] [*hastiin*] [*yiztałę́ę́*] [*at'ééd*] *yizts'ǫs.*

The word *yizts'ǫs* registers two arguments, so we can expect two syntactically visible referring expressions. Since *at'ééd* is the last bracketed expression preceding the verb, and since the verb *yizts'ǫs* has the direct form of the object prefix, *at'ééd* is understood to be coreferent with the object of *yizts'ǫs*. The question now is, How are the first three bracketed expressions interpreted and related to the rest of the sentence?

The first thing to note is that the expression *yiztałę́ę́*, coming as it does as the next farther expression from the verb *yizts'ǫs*, will be understood as coreferent with its subject. But what does *yiztałę́ę́* mean? One possibility is: 'the one that kicked him/her.' This interpretation of this word gives us so far: 'The one that kicked him/her kissed the girl.' To get the remaining two expressions into the semantics, all we have to do is apply the standard rules of coreference and ordering and note that *hastiin* must be coreferent with the object of *yiztał*, since it immediately precedes it and *yiztał* has the direct object pronoun prefix; *ashkii* ends up coreferent with the subject of *yiztał*. This gives us the first reading of (39).

But the second, and probably less likely, reading of (39) can also be gotten from the bracketing in (40). All we need to do is interpret the expression *yiztałę́ę́* as 'the one that s/he kicked.' Attaching *hastiin* and *ashkii* as before, this will give us the second reading of (39).[19]

Note what we have done. We have retained (somewhat) the idea of an internally headed relative clause, but according to the discussion above, the internally headed relative clause in (39) is just the word *yiztałę́ę́*, not the first three words. Clearly, this is a substantial confirmation of the reality of the pronominal argument character of Navajo: surely, only a "real" argument can be the head of an internally headed relative clause, so the "real" internal head of such a clause would have to be the pronominal registration on the verb, not the noun.

This line of thinking helps clarify other data. Since there is a moderate amount of expression-order freedom that is permitted in Navajo, we can get sentences like the following:

(41) *Ashkii   at'ééd   yizts'ǫs   hastiin   yiztałę́ę́.*
       boy   girl   3→3=kiss=P   man   3→3=kick=P=NOM
      'The boy that kicked the man kissed the girl.'
      'The boy kissed the girl that kicked the man.'

Starting with the interpretation 'the one that kicked him/her' for *yiztałę́ę́*, the last two words of (41) can be interpreted as 'the one that kicked the man.' To bind the subject pronoun in this expression, we necessarily have to disregard the next previous word, namely the verb *yizts'ǫs*, since this word is not a referring expression (it is a verb without a nominalizing suffix). The next word before that is *at'ééd*; coreference with this word gives us the second interpretation listed for (41) above. As long as we're skipping over words, though, we can skip over *at'ééd* as well, which leads to the binding with *ashkii* and the first interpretation.

Note that the interpretation in which the girl is involved in the relative clause is impossible in (39) because the positioning of the words makes it impossible to consider *at'ééd* as an afterthought expression. In (41), of course, *hastiin yiztałę́ę* is an afterthought expression. The fact that *at'ééd* has occurred somewhere to the left of this expression is what makes it possible for the girl to be involved in the relative clause in (41).

If we examine our analysis above of (39) and (40), we'll see that potentially there might be two other readings for (41). What if we interpret *yiztałę́ę* in (41) to mean 'the one that s/he kicked'? The afterthought phrase *hastiin yiztałę́ę* would then be interpreted as 'the man that s/he kicked,' since *hastiin* would still be coreferent with the object of *yiztał*. Now, we could conceivably bind the remaining pronoun (the subject of *yiztał*) with either *ashkii* or *at'ééd*, but any coherent reading that would result would require major assumptions of word-order freedom. For example, suppose we bind the pronoun to *at'ééd*. The reading would be 'The boy kissed the man that the girl kicked.' But this would mean that a noun immediately in front of a transitive verb would not only not be bound to the object pronoun of that verb but also would be construed together with an afterthought phrase, even though it wasn't itself in an afterthought position. Apparently, this sort of structural bending is too much: the reading is (apparently) ruled out. Similar considerations apply if we bind the subject of *yiztał* (with *yiztałę́ę* interpreted as 'the one that s/he kicked') to *ashkii*, a binding that would result in the reading 'The man that the boy kicked kissed the girl' if it were possible, which it appears not to be.

The argument in the preceding paragraph turned on the impossibility of interpreting a noun as bound to part of an afterthought expression if that noun is itself not in afterthought position and if that interpretation would conflict with a standard binding for that noun. This level of conflict is not present in the case of sentences like the following:

(42) *Hastiin yiztałę́ę*   *ashkii*   *at'ééd*   *yizts'ǫs.*
      man   3→3=kick=p=nom   boy   girl   3→3=kiss=p
      'The boy that kicked the man kissed the girl.'

Our discussion predicts at least some possibility for the indicated reading. Platero (1974) indicates that at least for some speakers (42) is a possible sentence, with the reading shown in there. I have, however, heard other Navajo speakers claim that (42) is impossible; for those speakers, the conflict between the postposed position of *ashkii* vis-à-vis *yiztał* (suggesting, perhaps, an afterthought arrangement) and the nonafterthought functioning of *ashkii* vis-à-vis *yizts'ǫs* is presumably what rules (42) out.

We have earlier mentioned the fact that at least sometimes referring expressions can be separated from the pronominal registrations that they are coreferent with by extraneous material; examples of this are shown in (29), (30), and (37). At least for some speakers, some striking possibilities of this sort can involve relative clause arrangements as well; note that this possibility is further support for the idea that the internally headed relative clause actually consists only of the verb with its nominalizing suffix. Here are two examples relevant to this notion:

(43) *Łééchąą'í   t'áá ałtso   ashkii   deishxashígíí*   *nidahał'in.*
       dog   3=all   boy   3→3=PL=bite=P=NOM   3=PL=bark=I
       'All the dogs that bit the boy are barking.'

(44) *John Bill t'áá ałtso   chidí   yaa   nayiisnii'ę́ę*   *t'éiyá*
       John Bill 3=all   car   3=from   3→3=buy=P=NOM   only
             nizhónígo   nidaajeeh
             well   3=PL=run.PL=I
       'All the cars that John bought from Bill (and only those) run well.'

For example, if we analyze (44) using an older-fashioned notion of internally headed relative clause, then we have a problem. The relative clause (that is, the referring expression which is coreferent with the subject of *nidaajeeh*) would be [*John Bill t'áá ałtso chidí yaa nayiisnii'ę́ę*], so that *t'áá ałtso* would be positioned inside the relative clause even though its interpretation is at the main clause level: we'd have to ignore *t'áá ałtso* while interpreting the relative clause and then come back to *t'áá ałtso* when interpreting the main clause. But if the relative clause is only *nayiisnii'ę́ę* (or probably: *yaa nayiisnii'ę́ę*, but that's another issue), this is not a problem. While *John Bill t'áá ałtso chidí* are processed, their referents can be set up on the pronominal bus (which is independent of any phrase structure), and then the proper combinations can be made when each of the pronominal registrations come along.

I should point out that while the speaker who provided me with (44) did so on a number of separate occasions and insisted that this was a good sentence, other speakers have claimed that (44) is hard to understand. Perhaps this should be compared with (42), which also elicits different reactions from different speakers. But this is just what we'd expect when dealing with a system where semantic combination is effected by means of binding on the pronominal bus, as opposed to by means of some process tied to syntactic phrase structure. In the simplest cases, speakers agree; but when the sentences become complex, different speakers generalize the binding system differently. It is interesting to note, in this connection, that speakers who have difficulty with complex sentences usually say that such sentences are hard to understand, rather than rejecting them as ungrammatical.

Note, though, that I am not suggesting that syntactic phrase structure is necessarily irrelevant to such interpretations. What I am suggesting is that the cross-speaker variation that we find with these relative clause interpretations is likely to be understood better if we approach these interpretations procedurally. Such interpretations might be sensitive to configurational characteristics, but the preceding discussions suggest the possibility that they aren't driven by them.

As a penultimate example of a prediction deriving from (2), let's examine the matter of the kinds of relations specified in languages like English by adpositions. Strictly speaking, the denotation of an adposition *is* the relation; that is, it's a (usually) two-place fully unsaturated predicate. By (2), Navajo cannot have any adpositions as syntactically visible expressions; in particular, there cannot be independent Navajo words which correspond to adpositions. In fact, there are (at least) four ways in which the relations normally denoted by adpositions are expressed in Navajo. In none of these constructions is the adpositional relation by itself denoted by a syntactically visible word or phrase.

The Navajo arrangement which perhaps comes closest to an adposition (specifically, to a postposition) is a bound form to which a pronominal prefix must be attached to register the entity which would correspond to the object of the postposition. Such a word is comparable to a verb whose arguments have been registered pronominally or to a possessed noun whose possessor has been so registered. Any further specification of the object is provided by a referring expression understood to be coreferent with the pronominal prefix. A simple example is:

(45) *Jooł   bee   naashné.*
      ball   3=INST   1SG=play=I
      'I'm playing with the ball.'

In context, one can say:

(46) *Bee   naashné.*
      3=INST   1SG=play=I
      'I'm playing with it.'

In the literature words like *bee* are commonly referred to as postpositions. But we have seen that it is possible for a referring expression to be separated from its pronominal registration by extraneous material. The same can happen with these postpositions:

(47) *Báda'ólta'í   áłchíní   bilagáanak'ehjí   yich'į'   yádaałti'.*
      PL=teacher   children   in-English   3=to   3=PL=speak=I
      'The teachers speak to the children in English.'

which means that the term "postposition" is slightly misleading for such words, since this term tends to suggest that these words are in syntactic construction with the referring expressions that constitute their objects. (Of course, this is true for Navajo if the pronominal prefixes are what we identify as the objects of these postpositions.)

Before moving on to the other three adposition-like constructions in Navajo, let's briefly take a side trip that will explain something about the postpositions we've just been talking about.

Throughout our discussion, what we've been assuming is that independent words, such as verbs or common nouns, cannot denote fully unspecified predicates. But something stronger is undoubtedly true for Navajo. For example, looking at verbs for a moment, we can say that not only can there not exist an independent Navajo word that denotes, say, $(\lambda x)(\lambda y)(see(y, x))$, but there also cannot even be an independent Navajo word that denotes $(\lambda x)(see(e_1, x))$. For example, there is no Navajo verb that is the semantic equivalent of the Spanish verb *vió*, whose denotation includes reference to a contextually specified third-person entity as subject but no reference to an object. This suggests amending (2) to something like:

(48)   Syntactically visible constituents never denote predicates that are not fully saturated.

The formulation in (48) opens up at least two cans of worms. One of these is the issue of what to do with the actual event or situation denoted by the verb; but this can be deferred until such time as this exploration is recast using event logic. The other is the fuzzy boundary that encircles the potential arguments of a verb. For example, is the instrument referred to in (45) and (46) an argument of the verb "play"? This is not the place to resolve this matter, but to the extent that it is, (48) would lead us to expect that in Navajo we would find this instrument registered on the verb, in some sense. In fact, there are (at least) six pieces of evidence that the postpositions which carry pronominal registrations of arguments such as instruments are either prefixes to the verb or at least in close combination with the verb, namely: (i) the strong tendency for postpositions like *bee* in (45) and (46) or *yich'į'* in (47) to appear immediately before the verb; (ii) the rhythm of sentences like (45) and (47) in speech, which shows the postposition to be strongly associated with the verb; (iii) the phonological processes which we saw in our discussion of (3)–(9); (iv) the fact that the pronominal registration on such postpositions displays the normal *yi/bi* alternation found with nonsubject arguments of verbs; (v) the possible positions of the negative marker *doo* (which must precede the verb and may optionally precede other elements, but which typically cannot be interposed between postposition and verb in the cases we are considering); and (vi) the fact that such postpositions sometimes enter into idiomatic combinations with the verbs they are combined with. These six traits can be explained directly as consequences of (48), if we take (48), or something like it, as a reasonable extension of (2), which is true for Navajo. (Note, incidentally, that (48) provides further justification for the impossibility of a genitive construction in Navajo, since the denotation of a genitive construction is a partially but not fully saturated predicate.)

Let us return to the remaining three Navajo constructions that correspond to adpositions. We have first the suffixed locative/temporal relators such as the *-di* seen already in (36) and (37) suffixed to *Kinłání*, 'Flagstaff'. Another example is:

(49)   *Kintah-góó   déyá.*
         town-DIR   1SG=go
         'I'm going to town.'

which shows *-góó*, meaning (here) 'motion to', suffixed to *kintah*, 'town'.[20] These suffixes attach only to nouns and postpositions (which are perhaps nouns at some level of analysis). Some of them at least can never be combined with a some level of analysis). Some of them at least can never be combined with a pronominal affix. That they are not independent words appears to be uncontroversial.

Another Navajo construction that corresponds (somewhat) to the sort of thing sometimes expressed by adpositions is furnished by certain disjunct verb prefixes, such as *ch'í-* 'out' or *'a* 'off', as in:

(50)   *ch'íníyá.*
      out=1SG=go=P
      'I went out.'

Since these are clearly affixes, they cannot be counterexamples to (2) (or (48)) no matter how we analyze their semantics.

Finally, there are those pesky particles such as *yah, dah, yoo'* that contribute path information to motion verbs, as in:

(51)   *yoo' ííyá.*
      away   off=3=go=P
      'He/she went away.' *or* 'He/she disappeared.'

The formal nature of the semantics of these particles is not clear to me; it would appear that they denote functions that apply to motion events. Possibly they do denote predicates of such events; but in the case of these words, we noticed near the beginning that they also tend to drift close to the verb (see especially (5), (8), and (9)). In fact, these words share with postpositions the six properties mentioned earlier as evidence that those postpositions are prefixes or quasi prefixes to verbs, except for the *yi/bi* alternation fact, which doesn't apply here, since these words do not carry any pronominal registration at all. Thus, these words ought to be regarded possibly as prefixes as well, which would mean that they are not distinguishable as a class from the third class of adposition-like structures.

As a last example of the significance of (2) for Navajo syntax, let's briefly look at the matter of attributive adjectives.

In languages like English, it is reasonable to analyze attributive adjectives as part of the common noun phrase projected from the head noun. Semantically, an attributive adjective might be viewed either as a predicate or a function; for those adjectives whose semantics is nonintersecting (i.e., for the majority of them), a predicate denotation in the simplest sense is impossible (although it could be defined as parametrized by the denotation of the head noun). In any case, though, (2) predicts that an attributive adjective-noun combination, with normal common-noun-phrase denotation, cannot exist in Navajo; for one thing, we saw earlier that a noun occurring as an independent word has to be understood as having a third-person registration that links the noun to the pronominal bus. How does Navajo grammar get around this in order to express the notion of adjectival attribution? There appear to be two methods.

First, there exist a limited number of noun suffixes whose semantics can be

understood as functional on the semantics of the noun to which they are suffixed. Often, these really create new lexical items; for example:

(52)   a.   *chidítsoh*
            'truck'

       b.   *chidí*
            'car'

       c.   *-tsoh*
            'big'

(53)   a.   *shashyáázh*
            'bear cub'

       b.   *shash*
            'bear'

       c.   *-yáázh*
            'small'

A syntactically visible common-noun-phrase constituent is avoided by having
the adjectival element be an affix to the noun. Words like *chidítsoh* and
shashyáázh are treated just like any other common noun; predicate-denoting
parts of these nouns do not occur as independent words.
   The second method of avoiding a visible common-noun-phrase constituent is
simply to use the nominalization arrangement that Navajo grammar uses normally to express the meaning corresponding to relative clauses; for example:

(54)   *ashkii   nineezígíí*
        boy   3=tall=NOM
        'the tall boy'

The semantic arrangement that underlies (54) is no different from the semantic
arrangement that underlies any other such construction in Navajo—see the earlier
section on relative clauses for discussion. However, in the case of adjectival
elements, we find in Navajo a substantial use of the alternate nominalizers *-í* and
-ii. These can be used with "ordinary" verbs as well (i.e., verbs that do not
express particularly adjectival notions) but not generally in relative-clause-like
contexts.[21] With adjectival words, we find constructions such as:

(55)   *ashkii   yázhí*
        boy   (3?)=little=NOM
        'the little boy'

Some such constructions involve lexicalizations, too. To the extent that they
can be productively formed as syntactic constructions, they represent an arrangement different from the usual relative clause construction. In any case,

these combinations deserve further study; but we can at least say here that the presence of the nominalizing suffix on words like *yázhí* is what renders such words possible (as independent words) given the assumption in (2).

All in all, the assumption (2), or perhaps its generalization in (48) (or a more adequate generalization), can be seen as a unifying principle leading to an interesting assortment of grammatical characteristics found in Navajo. It would be very instructive to examine how the Athabaskan languages in general vary with respect to these characteristics. A hierarchy of predictability might emerge, for example, or further light might be shed on the general notion of pronominal argumentness.

Notes

My thanks to the following persons for data, ideas, criticisms, and encouragement: Emmon Bach, Elroy Bahe, Bernice Casaus, Ted Fernald, Ken Hale, Eloise Jelinek, Alexis Manaster-Ramer, and Peggy Speas.

1. Thinking ahead, a stronger parameter is likely valid for Navajo: not only are fully unsaturated predicates not allowed as denotations of syntactically visible constituents, but, as we'll see later, partially unsaturated predicates appear not to be so allowed, either. Some complications arise in those cases, which I will discuss later.

2. In a classical logic, a sentence like (i) could be represented as (ii):

(i)   A boy played.

(ii) $(\exists x)(boy(x)$ & $play(x))$

whereas in an event logic we might have something like:

(iii) $(\exists x)(\exists y)(boy(x)$ & $play(y)$ & $agent(y, x))$.

In (iii), the predicate 'play' still has only one argument, but this argument represents the event, not the player. A transitive event would, in event logic, also have only one argument (representing the event), even though it would have two role-bearing participants. If event-logic representations such as (iii) were used, then the notion of saturation would have to be redefined so that it applies to the participants of an action or event.

Note that this concept of event logic is a bit different from the semantic unpacking of event types as described, for example, in Smith (this volume), since a representation like (iii) chunks the entire event into one unit. Intuitively, the elements that constitute the building blocks of event semantics in analyses such as those in Smith (this volume) are part of a domain different from the domain of those elements that can saturate a predicate (in the sense of (2) and (2')), so that we are justified in proceeding with our discussion the way we have done. But a precise definition of these domains is hard to come by.

3. Noun incorporation is something else; in particular, there can be lots of noun incorporation in a language where verbs do denote predicates.

4. I am ignoring the issue of type-raising, since it doesn't affect the discussion here.

5. See Willie and Jelinek (this volume) for a discussion of the notion that this binding is a case of discourse anaphora.

6. Verb-only sentences require a sufficiently articulated context to be acceptable in actual usage. This does not affect the discussion.

7. The "pronominal bus" is a metaphor in the making. Roughly, the image is that of a bus wire in an electrical device which allows communication between randomly located circuits. In the case of a structure such as (13), the symbol e_1 can be identified with the wire. We then imagine that "play(e_1)" means that the argument of "play" is connected to the e_1 wire. Similarly, "john=e_1" means that "john" is connected to the same wire. Thus, the argument of "play" is identified as being the same as "john". It is not assumed a priori that bus connections suffice to determine semantics uniquely—see Note 16.

8. Definite closure can, apparently, be usurped by other processes in certain contexts.

9. In the discussion at the conference, it was suggested that some speakers may have forms in which nouns like *ashkii* contain overt non-third-person pronominal markers that denote subjects. I believe this issue must be looked at more carefully before making any statements about it.

10. The morphology of *bá'ólta'í* can be diagrammed roughly as follows:

(iv)   *b*   *á*   '   *ó*   *l*   *ta'*   *í*
       3   for   UNSPEC   3-SUBJ   CL   read   NOM

In this diagram, a number of morphological complexities have been finessed in order not to confuse things unnecessarily. Note that "3" means third-person pronominal element; "UNSPEC" refers to a pronominal element that denotes an unspecified argument, usually the object when the verb is transitive; "CL" denotes the classifier; the element denoted "NOM" has been traditionally called a nominalizer, but it has also been analyzed as a moved pronominal element, in this case coreferent with the initial *b* (see Hale and Platero, this volume). The initial *b* must be understood as the object of the adpositional element that means "for".

11. If we were to try to express the meaning of (19) by using a first-person pronominal element instead of the third-person one in the word for "teacher", we'd get the word "*shá'ólta'í*". Some native speakers at the conference suggested that such a word does not exist.

12. Affixed pronouns are indeed attached to ordinary common nouns for the purpose of indicating possessives. This is a different process which is not relevant to the discussion at this point. We will return to this phenomenon later on.

13. It is possible to find expressions such as:

(v)   *díí*   *k'ad*   *ak'eed-ígíí*
      this   now   autumn-NOM

Note that *k'ad* does apply semantically to the noun which follows it. The full range of possible expressions like this remains to be studied.

14. In this and succeeding glosses, the symbol = connects morpheme meanings that correspond to identifiable categories in the actual word but that are not shown as separate morphemes in the actual word due to morphophonemic complexity. I means imperfective mode, and (later on) P means perfective mode. By itself, PL names the so-called distributive plural prefix, whose basic form is *da* (more on this later). x →y means the verb form is transitive, with an x subject and a y object. Also, LOC means locative, INST means instrumental, and DIR means directional, and, as I said, NOM means nominalizer.

15. For example, verbs that denote certain versions of "go"-events have three sets of stems, corresponding to singular, dual, and plural agents. Such verbs normally do not use *da* with plural stems. However, as claimed by (33), *da* can indeed be used with such stems to indicate true distributivity.

16. A semantic "pronominal bus" representation of (34a) might be:

(vi)   john(e_1) & each(e_2) & baby(e_2) & tickle(e_1, e_2)

At least two issues concerning (vi) have been finessed: (a) Which pronominal elements get wired to which bus? and (b) How do we determine from (vi) that 'baby' denotes the set over which 'each' ranges (rather than 'tickle')? Issue (a) is (at least for sentences like this one) not particularly problematical, nor is it relevant to our discussion. On the other hand, issue (b) is important; minimally, a formal semantic-interpretation theory applicable to objects such as (vi) would be called for. What is important for the discussion at hand is that e_2, as "seen" by 'tickle' in (vi), is also wired both to 'baby' and to 'each', which means that 'tickle' sees a plurality. Incidentally, this fits well with the hypothesis of Willie and Jelinek (this volume) that the binding of the second argument of 'tickle' to e_2 can be viewed as a case of discourse anaphora.

Facts similar to (34) can be seen with verbs where different verb stems are used according to whether one of its arguments is singular or plural (or, for some verb stems, dual). For example, the transitive notion of leading an animal is represented by distinct verb stems according to whether one animal is being led or a plurality of animals is being led. As we would expect, the plural stem is used if the object is quantified by 'each':

(vii)   *łį́į́'   t'ááłá'í nítínígo   łį́į́' bighangóó   nílóóz.
        horse each   corral   1SG→3=lead.SG=P

(viii) łį́į́'   t'ááłá'í nítínígo   łį́į́' bighangóó   ní'eezh.
                                                        1SG→3=lead.PL=P

'I led each horse to the corral.'

The verbs in (vii) and (viii) see a plural object, so the plural stem verb is required. (Thanks to Ken Hale for suggesting this point.)

17. The "genitive arrangement" can as easily be an adpositional phrase as an overtly case-marked NP. In either case we get a phrase of the sort we want to claim is impossible in languages such as Navajo.

18. The facts involving possessives would also follow (more or less) from (1) if we assume that a possessive is an argument of the possessed head noun. With this assumption, (1) tells us that only pronouns can be possessives, which means that when a nonpronominal NP is a possessor, there would have to be a coreferent pronominal possessor in the picture. This rules out the genitive arrangements in favor of the arrangement by means of which a nonpronominal possessive NP is an ordinary NP in an adjunct position. That possessive pronouns have to be attached to their possessed heads could then be viewed as following from (2) if we recall that the semantics of a possessed head necessarily involves the relation called R in the text. If a pronominal possessor were *not* attached, the unmarked head could be claimed to denote the fully unsaturated predicate $(\lambda x)(\lambda y)(R(x, y)$ & $P(y))$, where P is the predicate which is "really" the denotation of the head noun.

19. The discussion here allows all the readings in Willie (1989), but it (apparently) allows more—possibly Willie doesn't get the second reading of (39), for example. The more complicated the syntax gets, the more variation can be found from one speaker to the next.

20. This noun is itself formed from such a suffix, namely -*tah*, whose meaning is something like 'among', attached to the noun *kin,* 'building; store'.

21 When attached to verbs, the nominalizers -*í* and -*ii* form lexicalizations. They are also found in certain particular syntactic patterns—see for example Hale and Platero (this volume).

References

Bach, Emmon, Eloise Jelinek, Angelika Kratzer, and Barbara Partee (eds.). 1995. *Quantification in Natural Languages.* Dordrecht: Kluwer.

Barwise, Jon, and Robin Cooper. 1981. Generalized Quantifiers and Natural Language. *Linguistics and Philosophy* 4:159–219.

Cook, Eung-Do, and Keren D. Rice (eds.). 1989. *Athapaskan Linguistics.* Berlin: Mouton de Gruyter.

Faltz, Leonard M. 1995. Towards a Typology of Natural Logic. In Bach et al. (eds.). 1995.

Jelinek, Eloise. 1984. Empty Categories, Case, and Configurationality. *Natural Language and Linguistic Theory* 2:39–76.

Jelinek, Eloise.1987. Headless Relatives and Pronominal Arguments: A Typological Perspective. In Kroeber and Moore (eds.). 1987.

Jelinek, Eloise. 1995. Quantification in Straits Salish. In Bach et al. (eds.). 1995.

Keenan, Edward L., and Leonard M. Faltz. 1985. *Boolean Semantics for Natural Language.* Dordrecht: Reidel.

Kroeber, Paul D., and Robert E. Moore (eds.). 1987. Native American Languages and Grammatical Typology. Papers from a Chicago Linguistic Society parasession. Indiana Linguistics Club.

Lehmann, Christian. 1984. *Der Relativsatz.* Tübingen: Günter Narr.

Montague, Richard. 1974. *Formal Philosophy.* New Haven, Conn.: Yale University Press.

Platero, Paul. 1974. The Navajo Relative Clause. *International Journal of American Linguistics* 40:202–246.

Speas, Margaret. 1990. *Phrase Structure in Natural Language.* Dordrecht: Kluwer.

Speas, Margaret. 1995. Remarks on Clause Structure in Athapaskan. Paper presented at the Workshop on Athapaskan Morphosyntax, University of New Mexico, Albuquerque.

Willie, Mary Ann. 1989. Why There Is Nothing Missing in Navajo Relative Clauses. In Cook and Rice (eds.). 1989.

Young, Robert W., and William Morgan. 1987. *The Navajo Language: A Grammar and Colloquial Dictionary.* Revised edition. Albuquerque: University of New Mexico Press.

3

GENERALIZATIONS IN NAVAJO

Theodore B. Fernald

This essay investigates the interaction of generic quantification with the interpretations of nominals and predicates in Navajo and in English. For the first time, evidence is presented of a distinction between individual- and stage-level predicates in Navajo. Kratzer's (1988) Prohibition against Vacuous Quantification and de Hoop and de Swart's (1989) Plurality Condition on adverbs of quantification are two leading explanations of the well-formedness of generics. Data considered here require contextual information to be added to the restrictions of quantifiers and they require the Plurality Condition to be extended to the nuclear scope in addition to the restriction of a quantifier.

This chapter is laid out as follows. Section 3.1 introduces the basic facts of Navajo syntax and provides background on the nominal interpretations with respect to (in)definiteness. Two kinds of uses of -*go* clausal adjuncts are then discussed. These adjuncts can be interpreted as reporting that two eventualities with overlapping run times occurred or they can be interpreted as generalizations. Background about the interaction between genericity and the individual-/stage-level predicate distinction is presented in section 3.2 along with the analyses of Kratzer (1988) and de Hoop and de Swart (1989). Section 3.3 demonstrates the interaction between genericity and predicate status in Navajo, including data that are challenging for both previous analyses. Two new analyses are proposed and evaluated in section 3.4. Section 3.5 presents another type of Navajo generic sentence involving adverbial quantification. The data in this section require an independent modification of the Plurality Condition. Section 3.6 is the conclusion.

3.1   Background

3.1.1   Basic Navajo Syntax

It is widely known that Navajo sentences need not contain any overt nominal expressions. Examples (1) and (2) show that a single verb can be a whole sentence.

(1)   *Neiniłché.*   'S/he/It is chasing him/her/it.'

(2)   *Bits'áníką.*   'I took him/her/it away from him/her/it.'

When sentences contain overt nominals, the word order tends to be SOV (but see discussion of the inverse voice construction Willie and Jelinek, this volume).[1]

(3)   *Náshdóí   bįįh   neiniłché.*
      wildcat   deer   3-3-chase
      'The wildcat is chasing the deer.'

(4)   *Naa'ołí   yishbézhéé   kǫ'   bits'áíką.* (Young and Morgan 1987)
      beans   3-1-cook-REL   fire   3-3-1-take-away-from
      'I took [the beans I was cooking] away from the fire.'

An additional feature of Navajo is that verbs show "agreement" with every NP "argument" in a sentence, as shown in (3) and (4). Quotation marks are used here because the analysis of the basic phrase structure of Navajo is currently a matter of some controversy. Work following from Jelinek (1989) and Willie (1989) assumes that overt nominals are adjuncts rather than being in argument positions. The arguments of the verb are taken to be pronouns that have incorporated into the verb. In other work (e.g., Perkins 1978; Platero 1978, 1982; Speas 1990), these morphemes are taken to be agreement markers and overt nominals are taken to be arguments. This chapter does not take a position on this issue (see Speas and Yazzie 1996 for a paper on Navajo quantification that does) but nevertheless aims to contribute to its resolution; the analysis of the interpretations of nominal expressions in quantificational sentences is likely to be of relevance as this debate develops.

3.1.2 Definiteness and Indefiniteness in Navajo

It is widely recognized that indefinite and definite nominals show a contrast of interpretation or grammaticality under the scope of a quantifier (see e.g., Krifka et. al. 1995, de Hoop and de Swart 1989, Kratzer 1988). Work following Lewis (1975), Kamp (1981), and Heim (1982) accounts for these differences by assuming that indefinites have variable reference and that definite nominals do not. Because of these differences, it is necessary to review what has been established in previous work on nominal interpretation in Navajo. It has frequently been observed that, with a few exceptions, bare nouns (those appearing without any determiner or focusing particle) are unmarked for number and can be construed as definite or indefinite depending on syntactic context. Thus, the nominals in (5–7) are may be interpreted as definite or indefinite, although the definite readings tend to be preferred.

(5) *Dzaanééz   łį́į́'   yiztał.*
     mule   horse   3-3-Pf-kick
     'The/a mule kicked the/a horse.'

(6) *Dzaanééz   łį́į́'   deiztał.*
     mule   horse   pl-3-3-Pf-kick
     'The/some mules kicked the/some/a horse(s).'

(7) *Łį́į́'   dadijáád.*
     horse   pl-3-fast
     '(The) Horses are fast.'

The verbs in (6) and (7) contain a plural marker indicating that the subject is plural and, in (6), that the object may have a plural interpretation.

A nominal in Navajo can be overtly marked as either definite or indefinite (Willie 1991). *Léi'* marks *'ashkii* as indefinite in (8), while the demonstrative *díí*, for example, forces *'ashkii* to be definite in (9).

(8) *'Ashkii léi'   'at'ééd   yizts'ǫs.*
     boy   indef   girl   3-3-kissed
     'A boy kissed the/a girl.'

(9) *Díí   'ashkii   'at'ééd   yizts'ǫs.*
     this   boy   girl   3-3-kissed
     'This boy kissed the/a girl.'

Another way for an argument to have an indefinite interpretation is if the verb bears a morpheme for an unspecified argument (Willie 1991, Jelinek and Willie

1993). In such cases, overt nominals are ungrammatical, and the unspecified argument must be interpreted as indefinite:

(10)   a.   *'Ajiyá.*   'a- absolutive
            3indef-4-eat
            'He's eating something.' (YM 1987:67)

cf.

      b.   **Dah díníilghaazh 'ajiyá.*
            fried-bread   3indef-4-eat.
            'He's eating fried bread.'

(11)   a.   *Yah*   *'ashi'dooltį.*   '(a)d- agentive passive
            inside   1-3indef-carried
            'I was carried inside by someone.' (YM 1987:78)

cf.

      b.   **Jáan*   *yah*   *'ashi'dooltį.*
            J.   inside 1-3indef-carried
            'John carried me inside.'

Finally, Willie (1991) points out that the external argument of verbs bearing *bi*-third person morpheme must be construed as definite, unless the verb is plural:

(12)   *'Ashkii 'at'ééd léi'   bizts'ǫs.*
      boy   girl   indef 3-3-kissed
      'The boy was kissed by a girl.' (=Willie's (46))

(13)   ** 'Ashkii léi'   'at'ééd bizts'ǫs.*
      boy   indef girl   3-3-kissed
      'A boy was kissed by the girl.' (=Willie's (47))

(14)   *'Ashiiké 'at'ééké   dabiiłtsá.*
      boys   girls   pl-3-3-saw
      'The boys were seen by the girls./Some boys were seen by some girls.'
      (=Willie's (65a))

Willie (1991) goes on to show that the subject of a *bi*-verb cannot serve as the restriction of a generic operator. Note that (15) contains a *bi*-verb in the adjunct clause and that it cannot be interpreted as a generalization. Example (16), which contains a *yi*-verb is grammatical as a generalization.

(15) *Łééchąą'í mą'ii   biiłtsą́ągo,   bikéé'   nídiilwod.*
dog   coyote   3.3.sees=when 3.follow 3.runs
'When the dog$_i$ was seen by the coyote$_j$, it$_i$ was chased by it$_j$.'
(=Willie's (53))

(16) *Łééchąą'í mą'ii   yiyiiłtséehgo,   yikéé   nídiilwo'.*
dog   coyote   3.3.sees=when 3.follow 3.runs
'When a dog$_i$ sees a coyote$_j$, it$_i$ chases it$_j$.' (=Willie's (52))

3.1.3 Clausal Complements and Modifiers

Various clitics can be attached to the verb at the end of a clause in Navajo to
allow the clause to be used as a modifier or as an argument (or coindexed with
an argument, following Jelinek and Willie). Schauber (1975) discusses *-go* at
length, arguing that it is a subordinator that has no semantic content of its own.
(17) gives an example of *-go* attached to a clause denoting the event seen in a
perceptual report.[2]

(17) *Bill Baa' neiniłchéego yiiłtsą́.*   An "argument"
B.   B.   3-3-chase   3-1-saw
'I saw Bill chasing Baa'.'

The next example shows that *-go* can also be used to derive an adverbial from
the predicate *nizhóní*:

(18) *Mary nizhónígo French bizaad yee   yáłti'.* An adverbial
M.   well-GO French language 3-P speaks
'Mary speaks French pretty well.'

Clauses bearing the clitic *-go* can also be used as non-arguments. In the sentences below, the *-go* clause is adjoined to the main clause at the sentential
level:

(19) *Mary bilį́į́   holǫ́ǫgo bił   hózhǫ́.*
M.   3-horse exist-GO 3-P   I-happy.
'Mary has a horse and is happy.' ('Because Mary has a horse, she is
happy.')

(20) *Sarah*   *'azee'ííłíní bitsi'*   *nilį́įgo ayóo   dilwo'.*
      S.   doctor   3-daughter   3-be   very   3-run
      (*yitsi'* for *bitsi'* in some dialects)
      'Sarah is a doctor's daughter and she runs fast.'
      ('Because Sarah is a doctor's daughter she runs fast.')

The examples in (19) and (20) strongly suggest a causal connection between the
eventualities denoted by the two clauses. The suggestion of causation, however,
is only implicated (the implicature can be defeated); the interpretation mechanism in the grammar should require only that the denotations of the two clauses
be logically conjoined. Stump (1985:60ff., 325ff.) discusses certain English
absolutes in which, he argues, the logical relationship between the adjunct and
the main clause is underdetermined by the semantics and left to be resolved by
pragmatic considerations. The same considerations seem to be involved with
these examples from Navajo. Since the weakest plausible relationship is logical
conjunction, that is what I am assuming for the semantics of (19) and (20). The
association between the two clauses is in fact a bit stronger than simple conjunction since, as Eloise Jelinek pointed out to me, the *-go* clause is presupposed in
those sentences. It will turn out that this reading, which I will call the conjunction reading, is always in principle a possibility with *-go* adjuncts but that other
readings are sometimes available or preferred for pragmatic reasons.

      The causality suggested by (19) and (20) can be overtly entailed by adding
biniinaa between the two clauses:

(21) *'Adą́ą́dą́ą́'*   *'ayóo   deesdoigo   biniinaa   shibéégashii   'ałtso*
      yesterday   very   hot-go   because   my-cattle   all
                   taah   yikai.
                   into-water   got-into
      'It was so hot yesterday that my cattle all got into the water.' (YM
      1987:795)

(22) *Shich'oozhlaa'* *yiłnáadgo*   *biniinaa   chidí naat'a'í   biyidę́ę́'*
      my-elbow   3-1-licked-go   becauase   airplane   out-from
                       ch'íníłłizh.
                       1-fell
      'Because I licked my elbow I fell out of the plane.' (Hale 1972:6)

These sentences have the same structure of a *-go* clause adjoined to a main
clause that we have been discussing.

      Adjuncts bearing the *-go* subordinator can also be interpreted as eventualities
that overlap in time, with the eventuality denoted by the main clause. An example of this, in which the verbs are in perfective aspect, is shown in (23).

(23)   *Tsé*   *sétałgo*   *chą́ą́h*   *dégo'.*
      rock   on-1-Pf-stub-*go*   on.the.face   1-Pf-fell.flat
      'I stubbed my toe on a rock and fell flat on my face.' (YM 1987: 801)

In cases like this, the sentence entails that both eventualities of the speaker stubbing his or her toe and falling flat on his or her face occurred.

When the verbs appear in the imperfective, a generalization is often possible:

(24)   <u>*Mary*</u>   <u>*yidlohgo*</u>   *hoodiits'a'go*   *yidloh*   *(łeh).*
      M.   3-I-laugh-GO   loudly   3-I-laugh   (usually)
      'When Mary laughs, she (usually) laughs loudly.'

(25)   <u>*Náshdóí*</u>   <u>*ła'*</u>   <u>*bįįh*</u>   <u>*neiłkaahgo*</u>   *ayóo*   *dilwo'*   *(łeh).*
      wildcat   indef   deer   3-3-I-chase   very   run   (usually)
      'When a wildcat tracks deer, it [the wildcat] (usually) runs fast.'

(26)   <u>*Éí*</u>   <u>*dzaanééz*</u>   <u>*łį́į́'*</u>   <u>*neintałgo*</u>   *bił*   *hozhǫǫ*   *(łeh).*
      that   mule   horse   3-3-I-kick-GO   3-P   happy   (usually)
      'When that mule is kicking a horse, it is (usually) happy.'

These have a conditional reading that does not entail that the eventualities denoted by either clause hold in the universe of discourse. Thus, for example, (24) does not mean that Mary is laughing at the time the sentence is spoken, only that, generally speaking, when Mary laughs, she laughs loudly. The ambiguity between the conjunction and conditional readings is very similar to what Hale (1976) found for several Australian languages that have an adjoined clause type that is ambiguous between relative and temporal readings.

3.1.4   Basic Assumptions

In the analysis of (24–26), I will assume the analysis of indefinite descriptions that has emerged from Lewis (1975), Kamp (1981), and Heim (1982). The basic assumptions are that indefinite nominals are interpreted as restricted variables that have no quantificational force on their own. Adverbs of quantification are taken to be unselective quantifiers, binding any free variable in their domain. Quantifiers create tripartite structures as shown in (27).

(27)   G   [restriction]   [nuclear scope]
           adjunct   main clause

The interpretations of (24–26) can be derived by positing the optional existence of a null generic adverb[3] (following among others Stump 1985, Kratzer 1988,

Diesing 1992, Krifka et al. 1995) and by mapping the adjoined *-go* clause to the restriction of the operator and the main clause to its nuclear scope.[4]

3.2 Genericity and Individual- and Stage-Level Predicates

The distinction between individual-level predicates and stage-level predicates (ILPs and SLPs) has been seen to have grammatical reflexes in a wide variety of languages, but evidence for the distinction has not previously been sought in Navajo. A rough characterization of the distinction is that SLPs are characteristics of individuals that are crucially located in space and time (e.g. *kick the chair*) while ILPs denote properties that have nothing to do with time and space (e.g. *know French, be human*). In English, this distinction is evident in contrasts in grammaticality and interpretation. A contrast in grammaticality appears in the existential construction (Milsark 1974):

(28) a.   There are chairs available. (SLP)
            cf. *There are chairs wooden (ILP)

     b.   There were people sick. (SLP)
            cf. *There were people tall. (ILP)

It has been know since Carlson (1977) that there is an interaction between generic sentences and the distinction between ILPs and SLPs. The following paradigm, illustrating this interaction, is from Kratzer (1988):

(29) a.   *When Mary knows French, she knows it well.
            *G [knows (Mary, French)] [knows well (Mary, French)]

     b.   When a Moroccan knows French, she knows it well.
            G_x[Moroccan(x) & knows (x, French)] [knows well (x, French)]

     c.   When Mary knows a foreign language, she knows it well.
            G_x[foreign language(x) & knows (Mary, x)] [knows well (Mary, x)]

     d.   When Mary speaks French, she speaks it well.
            G_l[speaks (Mary, French, l)] [speaks well (Mary, French, l)]

     e.   *When Mary speaks French, she knows it well.
            *G_l[speaks (Mary, French, l)] [knows well (Mary, French)]

Kratzer analyzes (29a) is a case of vacuous quantification, and posits the following prohibition to account for it:

(30) *Prohibition against Vacuous Quantification*
For every quantifier Q, there must be a variable x such that Q binds an occurrence of x in both its restrictive clause and its nuclear scope.

A canonical example of vacuous quantification is shown in (31b) and is contrasted with the fully acceptable example in (31a).

(31) a.   Every man is such that he is tall.
      b.   #Every man is such that John is tall.

Parallel examples in Navajo are shown next:[5]

(32) a.   *Í'neezígíí*   *diné t'áá nízínígo*   *yee   hadít'é.*
           indef-tall-COMP man each-individually 3-P   has-characteristics-of
           'Being tall is a characteristic every man has.'

      b.   *#Jáan nineezígíí*   *diné t'áá nízínígo*   *yee   hadít'é.*
           John   3-tall-COMP man each-individually 3-P   has-characteristics-of
           #'John being tall is a characteristic every man has.'

In Kratzer's analysis, the reason (29a) is odd is that the generic quantifier has no variable to bind in either its restriction or its nuclear scope. When the indefinite nominal *a Moroccan* is introduced in place of *Mary*, as in (29b), the sentence becomes felicitous. The tradition of Lewis (1975), Kamp (1981), and Heim (1982) of treating indefinites as restricted variables allows (30) to make the correct prediction for (29b). (29c) is acceptable for the same reason: *a foreign language* introduces the variable that is bound by the generic operator.

Given this account of (29a–c), it is at first a bit surprising that (29d) is acceptable: there are no indefinite nominals in the sentence and yet it has the interpretation of a generalization. The crucial difference between (29a) and (29d) is that (a) contains an ILP and (d) contains a SLP. This difference leads Kratzer to propose that the relevant difference between ILPs and SLPs is that the latter introduce a spatiotemporal (or "Davidsonian") variable into the logical representation and the former do not. (29d), then, is a generalization about spatiotemporal locations at which Mary speaks French. (29a) cannot be a generalization about spatiotemporal locations at which Mary knows French because *know French* is not located in space and time and does not introduce a spatiotemporal variable. (29e) is noteworthy for its oddness. Even though the adjunct contains a SLP, the main clause does not introduce any variable, so the quantification is vacuous.

De Hoop and de Swart (1989) pointed out that certain SLPs sound just as odd in *when*-adjuncts as (29a):

(33) a. *When a Moroccan kills Fido, she kills him quickly.
      b. *When Anne makes the film "Dangerous Liaisons," she makes it well.

What is odd about these sentences is that the predicate in the adjunct clause, in its ordinary usage, denotes an eventuality that can take place only once. The difficulty these 'once-only' examples pose for Kratzer's analysis is that the SLPs introduce variables into the logical representation, so the prohibition against vacuous quantification is not violated. De Hoop and de Swart propose that the problem with ILPs and with once-only SLPs is that they do not form an adequate restriction for a generalization; forcing them into the restriction results in a trivial generalization about only one eventuality. For reasons having to do with their analysis of tense and aspect, de Hoop and de Swart reject Kratzer's proposal that ILPs do not have a spatiotemporal argument; their solution allows all predicates to have such arguments. The crucial assumption for the interaction of the ILP/SLP distinction with genericity is the idea that each ILP and each once-only SLP is presupposed to be associated with only one spatiotemporal location, while other SLPs are potentially associated with many. This proposal is implemented as follows:

(34) *Uniqueness presupposition on the Davidsonian argument* (de Swart 1991:59) The set of spatiotemporal locations that is associated with an individual-level or a 'once-only' predicate is a singleton set for all models and each assignment of individuals to the arguments of the predicate.

(35) *Plurality condition on quantification* (de Swart 1991:118) A Q-adverb does not quantify over a set of situations if it is known that this set has cardinality less than two. A set of situations is known to be a singleton set if:

      1) the predicate contained in the sentence satisfies the uniqueness presupposition on the Davidsonian argument, and
      2) there is no (in)definite NP in the sentence which allows indirect binding by means of quantification over assignments.

These conditions require the restrictions of quantificational adverbs to have cardinality of greater than or equal to two. The null generic operator posited for the data in (29) is subject to these conditions, as are other adverbs of frequency.

3.3 Navajo Generalizations with ILPs and SLPs

We now turn to consider Navajo data that parallel the English examples in (29). The examples in (36) indicate that Navajo shows a contrast between ILPs and SLPs in the interpretation of *-go* adjuncts.[6]

(36) a. #*Mary* *diné* *bizaad* *bił bééhózingo* *hastóí* *bił*
  M. Navajo language 3-P 3-3-know-GO men 3-P
  danilį́ *łeh*.
  pl-3-respect usually
  #'When Mary knows Navajo, men respect her.'[7] (ILP)

  b. *Mary* *diné k'ehjí* *yáłti'go* *hastóí* *bił*
  M. Navajo 3-speak-GO men 3-P
  danilį́ *łeh*.
  pl-3-respect usually
  'When Mary speaks Navajo, men respect her.' (SLP)

Example (36a) in Navajo seems just as odd as (29a) does in English. As with English, adding an indefinite nominal to an ILP makes the generalization reading possible:

(37) a. *Sáanii* *diné* *bizaad* *bił* *béédahózingo* *hastóí* *bił*
  women Navajo language P-3 3pl-know-GO men 3-P
  danilį́ *łeh*. (ILP)
  pl-3-respect usually
  'When a woman knows Navajo, men usually respect her.'

  b. *Mary* *ał'ąą ana'i* *bizaad* *bił* *bééhózingo* *hastóí* *bił*
  M. foreign language P-3 3-know-GO men 3-P
  danilį́ *łeh*. (ILP)
  pl-3-respect usually
  'When Mary knows a foreign language, men usually respect her.'

Below is another pair of examples with an ILP in the adjunct.

(38) a. *Sarah* *'azee'ííł'íní yitsi'* *nilį́igo* *.ayóo* *ółta'* *łeh*.
  S. doctor 3-daughter 3-be very 3-study usually
  Sarah, being a doctor's daughter, studies a lot.'
  #'When Sarah is a doctor's daughter, she studies a lot. (ILP)

b. *At'ééké ła'   'azee'ííł'íní yitsi'   nilį́įgo ayóo   ółta'*
    girls   indef   doctor   3-daughter 3-be   very   3- study
    łeh.
    usually
    'When a girl is a doctor's daughter, she studies a lot.'   (ILP)

Consultants indicate that (38a) is acceptable on the first gloss given. The second interpretation, like the English gloss, suggests that sometimes Sarah is a doctor's daughter and sometimes she is not. Example (38b), on the other hand, is an acceptable generalization about girls who are doctors' daughters.

There is a fair amount of speaker variation in judgments among the examples in (36–37) with respect to the interpretation of *łeh*. Everyone's judgments are consistent with what I have argued about the basic logic of generics, but how that interpretation is expressed syntactically varies. For some speakers, generalizations are usually possible without *łeh*, although this is not always the case. For them, *łeh* is interpreted as 'usually'. This dialect appears to have a null generic quantifier, since a generalization is possible even when *łeh* is not present. For other speakers, if *łeh* is not in the sentence, the examples in (36–37) cannot be interpreted as generalizations. This dialect has no null generic quantifier (or it is ineffective in this syntactic context.) *Łeh* has the interpretation of the generic quantifier in this dialect. We will examine the effects of *łeh* in section 3.5.

The data in (36–37), both the Navajo examples and their English counterparts, appear to indicate that Kratzer's prohibition against vacuous quantification is too strong. In (36b) and (37b), the main clause appears to contain an ILP. The standard English diagnostics for *respect* indicate that it heads an ILP:

(39) a.   Firefighters respect Mary. (no existential reading)
      b.   *I saw Robin respect Mary. (cf. I saw Robin reach a decision.)

For more on these, see Carlson (1977), Fernald (1994, 2000), Kratzer (1988), or de Swart (1991). Unless we take *respect* to be the head of a SLP, there will be no variable in the nuclear scope that also appears in the restriction. The following would be the representation for (36b):

(40)   G [speak (Mary, Navajo, l)] [G_x [men(x)] [respect (x, Mary)]]

The generalization in the main clause ('Men respect Mary') is well-formed: the generic operator G in the main clause (the second one in the formula above) binds the variable x. The problem arises with the first generic operator in the formula since it has no variable to bind. Thus, our assumptions would seem to make the incorrect prediction that (36b) should be ill formed.

3.4 Contextualized Restrictions and Coercion

There are two kinds of solutions to the problem seen in section 3.3. One, as already suggested, treats *respect* as a stage-level predicate in (36b). It would analyze the problematic examples as cases in which the main clause ILP has been coerced into an SLP, resulting in an inchoative interpretation. The other solution admits contextual information into the restrictions of quantifiers. It thus departs from classical theories in which there is a pristine mapping from syntactic trees to logical representations. However, such a departure is required for many ordinary quantificational sentences. Such an account would need to allow the missing variable to be accommodated under just the right circumstances. We will consider the coercion solution first.

3.4.1 Coercion

When recalcitrant data are discussed in scholarly writing on the ILP/SLP distinction, one frequently finds a speculation that a predicate of one variety is "being used" as a predicate of another variety. Perhaps the ILP in (36b) is being used as a stage-level predicate. We might think such a thing because *respect* is the sort of thing that ordinarily builds over time. There may be something a bit odd about making it depend on particular eventualities of Mary speaking Navajo. Perhaps the oddness results from using respect in a slightly unusual way, from coercing it to be a SLP.

All ILPs are stative. Moens and Steedman (1988) pointed out that stative predicates can be "coerced" into having a change of state reading in certain syntactic environments.[8] A change of state predicate, of course, is not stative itself since it is telic. Since it is not stative, it cannot be an ILP. But then the predicate must be stage-level. And Kratzer (1988) analyzes SLPs as having a spatiotemporal argument. Returning now to the analysis of (36b), if *respect* is a coerced SLP, then we no longer have a problem with vacuous quantification: both *speak* and *respect* will have spatiotemporal arguments that can be bound by the generic quantifier.[9] It seems plausible that (36b) has a change of state (inchoative) interpretation, which may be paraphrased as, 'When Mary speaks Navajo, men in the area come to respect her'. Since *come to respect* is stage-level, it should introduce a spatiotemporal variable into the nuclear scope. The following formula is the result of this assumption along with existential closure of the nuclear scope:

(41) G_l [speak (Mary, Navajo, l)] [$\exists x$ [men(x) & come-to-respect (x, Mary, l)]]

Chierchia (1992) noted that donkey sentences (of which *-go* generics are an example) can, in principle, have two interpretations, although many individual sentences strongly favor one interpretation over the other. Thus, (42) has what

Chierchia calls an $\exists$-reading, shown in (b), and the more obvious $\forall$-reading shown in (c):

(42) a. When a farmer has a donkey he beats it.
      b. G_x [farmer(x) & $\exists$y(donkey(y) & has(x, y))]
             [$\exists$y(donkey(y) & has(x, y) & beat(x, y))]]
      c. G_x [farmer(x) & $\exists$y(donkey(y) & has(x, y))]
             [$\forall$y[donkey(y) & has(x, y) & beat(x, y))]]

Example (41) is the $\exists$-reading of (36a), and in fact this is a fairly unlikely reading for the sentence. The more likely $\forall$-reading would entail that it is a general property of locations at which Mary speaks Navajo that all men at those locations come to respect her there. This interpretation is shown below:

(43) G_l [speak (Mary, Navajo, l)]
          [$\forall$x [men(x) & at(x, l)][come-to-respect (x, Mary, l)]]

Notice what was needed to produce this formula. In addition to coercion, we had to add the contextual information *at(x,l)* to the restriction of the embedded quantifier. We will see that this is exactly the contextual information required by our other proposal.

    Let us now hone our intuitions about (36b) to see whether (43) is a valid interpretation of it. It would appear that (36b) conversationally implicates (44), but that (44) is not a truth-condition of the sentence.

(44) Men do not always respect Mary.

Note that it is not contradictory to say:

(45) When Mary speaks Navajo, men respect her, and in fact, they always respect her.

This shows that, on at least one reading, (36b) does not entail (44). We can show that (44) may be conversationally implicated by (36b) in the right sort of context: if the speaker knew that it is always true that men respect Mary then the speaker could have said so. But since we take (36b) to be a weaker claim than *Men respect Mary*, the speaker must not have adequate evidence for the latter. So by the Maxim of Quantity, we infer that it is not always true that John respects Mary.

    The fact that (36b) does not entail (44) has fatal consequences for appealing to coercion as an explanation for (36b). At least one reading of (36b) does not entail that men ever fail to respect Mary, but (41) does (as long as Mary speaks

Navajo around men at some time) since it entails a change of state to respect for Mary from lack of respect for her. On the other hand, if a context supports the conversational implicature that men do not always respect Mary, it might well support an inference of (41), and this is why (41) might initially seem to be a plausible interpretation for (36b).

Notwithstanding this line of reasoning, Moens and Steedman had solid reasons for positing the existence of inchoative coercion. If we were really convinced that the coerced reading had to be a possible interpretation, we would be forced by (45) to believe that (36b) is ambiguous:[10] (45) shows that there is at least one reading of (36b) that does not entail (44). Thus we conclude that, even with the possibility of coercion, (36b) still poses a challenge for our theory since it must have an uncoerced reading. In the next section we will develop such a reading.

First, however, it should be pointed out that Fernald (1994, 1999, 2000) predicts an additional coerced reading for this sentence. In this earlier work, I claimed that sentences such as *Robin is usually intelligent* exhibit what I called "Evidential Coercion." Like inchoative coercion, evidential coercion can happen when an ILP is used in a spot that is more compatible with a SLP. If a hearer is obliged to produce an interpretation for such a sentence, somehow a spatiotemporal variable must be added to the predicate. Below is a formal account of this:

> **Evidential Coercion:** Let α be an ILP with interpretation α'. α can be used as a SLP with the following interpretation:
> $$\lambda l_i \, \lambda x \, \exists Q \, [Q(x,l_i) \, \& \, G_{y,l}[Q(y,l)] \, [\alpha'(y)]]$$

A proposition using an ILP α that has been coerced by the above rule will entail that the subject has some stage-level characteristic Q at location l, and that, in general, if Q holds of someone, that person has the individual-level property α. Evidential Coercion is predicted, in principle, to be a successful coercion anytime an ILP needs to satisfy the Plurality Condition without the help of an indefinite nominal. Certainly there are particular predicates that are more difficult to coerce than others. Nevertheless, we expect that a pair of evidential coercion readings (a $\forall$-reading and a $\exists$-reading) should be available for (34b). This reading follows:

(46) a. G_l [speak (Mary, Navajo, l)]
   $[\exists x \, [men(x) \, \& \, \exists Q,l \, [Q(x,l) \, \& \, G_y \, [\exists l \, Q(y,l)]$
            $[respect \, (y, Mary)]]]]$

 b. G_l [speak (Mary, Navajo, l)]
   $[\forall x \, [men(x)] \, [\exists Q,l \, [Q(x,l) \, \& \, G_y \, [\exists l \, Q(y,l)]$
            $[respect \, (y, Mary)]]]]$

By these formulas, (36b) is taken to express the generalization that when Mary speaks Navajo at a location, men display some characteristic at that location that generally would be taken to mean that they respect her. In other words, the men display some outward sign of respect for her.

The same considerations that applied to the readings obtained by Inchoative Coercion apply to the readings in (46):

(47)   When Mary speaks Navajo, men respect her, but they do not show it.

The fact that (47) is not a contradiction shows at least that there is another reading for (36b). Now we will see how that reading can be predicted.

3.4.2   Contextualized Restrictions

It is widely known that the restrictions of quantifiers need to allow contextual information to be added if they are to reflect the intended interpretations of quantificational sentences.[11] Let us consider some examples:

(48)   a.   Men respect Mary.
        b.   Robin always eats steak.

The first example is a generalization ranging over men. However, this would never be taken to be a generalization over all men that have ever existed, including those that have never even heard of Mary. We would not want to predict that a sentence like (a) is always false and therefore unusable. The best we could do would be to hope for a Gricean explanation for why it is possible to utter (a) informatively. But a Gricean analysis would predict that using (a) would always involve flouting the Maxim of Quality. Surely this is not the correct way to go. Rather, we must allow context to contribute to the restriction of the quantification so that only those men that are contextually relevant count as cases for quantification.

The example in (b) is a universal quantification. What is understood to be its restriction? It may in fact have an unrestricted reading, which would entail that for all spatiotemporal locations in the universe it is the case that Robin eats steak. However, again the most plausible use of the sentence is one that is taken to be a quantification over contextually relevant spatiotemporal locations. These would normally not include locations at which Robin is sleeping, and they would certainly not include locations at which Robin does not exist.

Example (36b) is ordinarily taken not to mean that all men in the universe respect Mary when she speaks Navajo, but only that the men who are present when she speaks Navajo respect her. The restriction of the embedded quantification has the contextual information $at(x,l)$ added to it:

(49) a. G_l [speak (Mary, Navajo, l)]
        [$\forall$x [man (x) & at (x, l)] [respect (x, Mary)]]

      b. G_l [speak (Mary, Navajo, l)]
        [$\exists$x [man (x) & at (x, l)] [respect (x, Mary)]][12]

Notice that *respect*, lacking a spatiotemporal variable, is not a stage-level predicate in this analysis. Since the variable *l* appears in both the restriction and the nuclear scope in (49), the formula is well formed, and the interpretation is consistent with our intuitions about the meaning of the sentence.

The contextualization strategy used to produce the formulas in (49) has a different effect from what happened with (48a). The latter was well formed prior to contextualization, but the formulas in (49) were not, as we have seen. (48b) is more like the cases in (49) since little if any of the information that ends up in the restriction is represented in the syntax of the sentence.

Clearly a great deal of work needs to be done to see exactly when and where contextual information can be added. Here, I will only add the observation that it is not always the case that contextual information in an embedded restriction can save a generalization the way it seems to in (36b):

(50) #When Mary speaks Navajo, men are tall.

This problem is independent of the issue of contextualization, however. Note that example (a) below is just as odd as (50):

(51) a. #When Mary speaks Navajo to Apaches, they are tall.
      b. When Mary speaks Navajo to Apaches, they understand her.

I can only speculate about an explanation for this. Somehow, it is less easy to see how the height of people could be relevant to Mary speaking Navajo than it is to see how people understanding or respecting her could be relevant to those events. This suggests that the ways in which relevance is involved in contextualizing the restriction can be fairly complex.

In this section we have seen that two kinds of coercions result in possible interpretations for sentences like (36b) but that a pair of noncoerced readings are required as well. To produce these readings it was necessary to contextualize the restriction of the adverbial quantifier.

3.5 The Quantificational Adverb *łeh* 'usually'

Kratzer (1988) pointed out that English ILPs sound odd with frequency adverbials such as *sometimes* and *usually*. This is demonstrated by the English counterparts to the Navajo sentences below, which sound equally odd:

(52) #Jáan nineez łeh
     J.   3-tall   usually
     #'John is usually tall.'   (ILP)

(53) #Mary diné bizaad bił bééhózin łeh.
     M.   Navajo language 3-P 3-know   usually
     #'Mary usually knows Navajo.' (ILP)

As we would expect, changing one of the arguments to be construed as an indefinite makes these acceptable:

(54) Ha'a'aahdéé' hastóí danineez łeh.
     east   men   pl-3-tall usually
     'Eastern men are usually tall.'   (ILP)

In contrast, SLPs sound perfectly natural with frequency adverbials:

(55) Mary diné k'ehjí yee yáłti' łeh.
     M.   Navajo   3-P   3-speak usually
     'Mary usually speaks Navajo.'   (SLP)

(56) Éí   łį́į́'   dzaanééz neintał   łeh.
     That   horse mule   3-3-I-kick usually
     'That horse usually kicks mules.'   (SLP)

In these examples, *łeh* is interpreted as 'usually'.

Kratzer's analysis of this is that frequency adverbials must bind some variable, and therefore they are able to quantify over only those clauses which contain indefinite nominals or SLPs. For de Hoop and de Swart, we would think that the Plurality Condition in (35) should have a role in the analysis of (52–56). Note, however, that (35) is a condition on the *restrictions* of quantifiers, not on their nuclear scopes. Examples (52–56) are interesting cases since all the material in these sentences is mapped to the nuclear scope; the restrictions arise entirely from context. Thus, (55) means that usually, in contextually relevant situations, Mary speaks Navajo. Examples (52–56) show that the nuclear scopes of adverbial quantifiers are just as susceptible to the ILP/SLP distinction as the restrictions are. The question that arises is whether the oddness of (52) and (53) can be predicted by the kinds of contexts in which they could be uttered. If so, the Plurality Condition can cover these cases as currently stated. The alternative is to extend the Plurality Condition to cover the nuclear scope as well as the restriction:

(57)   *Plurality Condition on Quantification* (modified)
The restriction and nuclear scope of a Q-adverb must not be known to have cardinality less than two. A set of situations is known to be a singleton set if:
1)   the predicate contained in the sentence satisfies the uniqueness presupposition on the Davidsonian argument, and
2)   there is no (in)definite NP in the sentence which allows indirect binding by means of quantification over assignments.

3.6   Conclusions

This chapter provides first evidence for a distinction between individual- and stage-level predicates in Navajo. This distinction does not appear to result in a contrast in grammaticality along the lines of the English existential construction, but contrasts are found where a predicate is used to restrict generic quantifiers; as in English, SLPs that are not once-only can restrict a generic quantifier without the help of an indefinite nominal, but ILPs cannot.

We have noted that there is some speaker variation with respect to whether a null generic operator is available with -*go* adjuncts and when it is available and have left the reasons for this as a subject of further research. For all speakers, *łeh* is an overt generic quantifier that is subject to the Plurality Condition

This chapter has also argued that sentences like (34b) require contextual information to be admitted into the restriction of a quantifier if the prohibition against vacuous quantification is to account for them. I have also considered a number of examples of adverbial quantifiers in simple clauses. Since all the overt material in the sentence is mapped to the nuclear scope, a modification of the Plurality Condition was needed in which the condition applies to the scope as well as the restriction.

In closing, it is worth noting something which will come as no surprise to linguists who believe that the semantics of natural language is universal, but which may come as a surprise to others: generalizations are formed according to the same principles of logic in Navajo as they are in English. We have seen that the grammars of both Navajo and English provide ways for generalizations to be stated. Moreover, the restrictions (and nuclear scopes) of generic quantifiers must delimit a plurality of cases in both languages. It is not simply the case that the same tools of logical analysis have been used for understanding English and Navajo. Theories of quantification have been useful in explicating the interpretations of sentences, but we have seen something more than that. A violation of the Plurality Condition sounds just as odd in Navajo as it does in English. The effects described here are thus due to the way speakers of Navajo and English think and are not mere by-products of the tools of analysis. The conclusion is that, although there are substantial differences between the grammars of English and Navajo, particularly with respect to clause structure and morphology, generalizations are formed according to the same principles of logic.

Notes

Except where otherwise indicated, the data in this paper were elicited by the author. I am grateful to Doreena Curley, Lorene Legah, Alyse Neundorf, Paul Platero, and Mary Willie for help with Navajo data. Thanks are also due to Eloise Jelinek for comments on an earlier draft, and to Bill Ladusaw, Barry Miller, Paul Platero, and the participants in the Athabaskan Conference on Syntax and Semantics for discussing with me the ideas in this paper. I alone am responsible for any errors.

    1. Verbs are glossed IO-DO-S-root, consistent with the order in which these morphemes occur. Numbers in the glosses indicate person; Pf stands for perfective, I for imperfective, and It for iterative. Postpositions are indicated by P and agree with the NPs they appear with. YM abbreviates Young and Morgan.

    2. Eloise Jelinek points out that the -*go* clause could simply be an adjoined modifier rather than a complement. If so, (17) would be interpreted as 'I saw Bill when he was chasing Baa''.

    3. See Krifka, et al. 1995 for arguments in favor of treating the generic as a binary operator rather than as a monadic operator.

    4. Chierchia (1992) points out that, in general, determining the restriction of an adverb of quantification is more complicated than this, requiring an analysis of information structure. This issue is not central to this paper, however.

    5. Thanks to Paul Platero for these.

    6. Certain speakers prefer *hastói* to appear at the beginning of the entire sentence in these examples.

    7. This is grammatical on the conjunction reading: 'Because Mary knows Navajo, men respect her.' In some dialects, the argument structure of the main verb in this sentence is reversed. For these speakers, the sentences in (36) and (37) should end with *yił nilį́ łeh* rather than *bił danilį́ łeh*.

    8. See also Schubert and Pelletier (1989), Krifka et al. (1995), and Fernald (1994, 1996) for a discussion of these considerations with the ILP/SLP distinction or the similar episodic/non-episodic distinction.

    9. The Coercion analysis would need to explain why the examples in (39) do not indicate that a SLP is present. The answer to this (following Fernald 1996) is that coercion does not happen automatically; it needs to be induced by something and the interpretations of the examples in (37) are not able to induce it.

    10. An alternative to relying on ambiguity we might say that coercion is itself a pragmatic inference that can be defeated by an overt statement, as in (45).

    11. This is similar to the strategy of Kratzer (1977, 1979) in assuming that conversational background contributes significantly to the restriction of modals. Rooth (1992) posits a pragmatically-bound variable for his analysis of quantificational focus constructions.

    12. It is controversial whether the existential quantifier should be taken to have a restriction and nuclear scope or just a scope. If the latter is the best course, to get the reading in (49b), we would need to allow contextual information to appear in nuclear scopes as well as restrictions. If we can avoid this, our theory will have more predictive power.

References

Carlson, Gregory N. 1977. *Reference to Kinds in English*. Ph.D. dissertation. University of Massachusetts, Amherst. [published 1980, New York: Garland].

Carlson, Gregory N., and Francis J. Pelletier. 1995. *The Generic Book.* Chicago: University of Chicago Press.

Chierchia, Gennaro. 1992. Anaphora and Dynamic Binding. *Linguistics and Philosophy* 15:111–183.

Diesing, Molly. 1992. *Indefinites*. Cambridge, Mass.: MIT Press.

Fernald, Theodore B. 1994. *On the Nonuniformity of the Individual- and Stage-level Effects*. Doctoral dissertation. University of California, Santa Cruz.

Fernald, Theodore B. 1999. Evidential Coercion: Using Individual-Level Predicates in Stage-Level Environments. *Studies in the Linguistic Sciences* 29:43-63.

Fernald, Theodore B. 2000. *Predicates and Temporal Arguments*. Oxford: Oxford University Press.

Hale, Kenneth. 1972. *Navajo Linguistics: Part I*. Massachusetts Institute of Technology manuscript.

Hale, Kenneth. 1976. The Adjoined Relative Clause in Australia. In R. M. W. Dixon (ed.), *Grammatical Categories in Australian Languages*, Canberra: Australian Institute of Aboriginal Studies.

Heim, Irene. 1982. The Semantics of Definite and Indefinite Noun Phrases. Ph.D. dissertation, University of Massachusetts, Amherst.

de Hoop, Helen and Henriette de Swart. 1989. Over indefinite objecten en de relatie tussen syntaxis en semantiek. *Glot* 12:19–35.

Jelinek, Eloise. 1989. Argument Type in Athapaskan: Evidence from Noun Incorporation. Paper presented at the Conference on American Indian Languages, Annual Meeting of the American Anthropological Association, Washington, DC.

Jelinek, Eloise, Sally Midgette, Keren Rice, and Leslie Saxon (eds.). 1996. *Athabaskan Language Studies: Essays in honor of Robert W. Young*. Albuquerque: University of New Mexico.

Jelinek, Eloise, and MaryAnn Willie. 1993. Pronoun Attachment to the Verb in Navajo. Paper presented at the Athapaskan Linguistics Conference, Santa Fe, New Mexico.

Kamp, Hans. 1981. A Theory of Truth and Semantic Interpretation.In J. Groenendijk et al. (eds.) *Truth Interpretation and Information*. Dordrecht: Foris.

Kratzer, Angelika. 1977. What 'Must' and 'Can' Must and Can Mean. *Linguistics and Philosophy* 1:337–355.

Kratzer, Angelika. 1979. Conditional Necessity and Possibility. In R. Bäuerle, U. Egli, A. von Stechow (eds.), *Semantics from Different Points of View*. Berlin: Springer-Verlag.

Kratzer, Angelika. 1988. Stage-level and Individual-level Predicates. In M. Krifka, ed., *Genericity in Natural Language,* 247-284, Univeristy of Tübingen. [Also in Carlson and Pelletier 1995.]

Krifka, Manfred, Francis Jeffry Pelletier, Gregory N. Carlson, Alice ter Meulen, Gennaro Chierchia, and Godehard Link. 1995. Genericity: An Introduction. In Carlson and Pelletier 1995.

Lewis, David. 1975. Adverbs of Quantification. In E. L. Keenan et al. (eds.), *Formal Semantics of Natural Language*. Cambridge: CambridgeUniversity Press.

Milsark, Gary L. 1974. Existential sentences in English. Ph.D. dissertation, Massachusetts Institute of Technology. [published 1979, New York: Garland].

Moens, Marc, and Mark Steedman. 1988. Temporal ontology and temporal reference. *Computational Linguistics* 14:15–28.

Perkins, Ellavina Tsosie. 1978. The Role of Word Order and Scope in the Interpretation of Navajo Sentences. Ph.D. dissertation, University of Arizona.

Platero, Paul. 1978. Missing Noun Phrases in Navajo. Ph.D. diss., Massachusetts Institute of Technology.

Platero, Paul. 1982. Missing Noun Phrases and Grammatical Relations in Navajo. *International Journal of American Linguistics* 48:286–305.

Rooth, Mats. 1992. A Theory of Focus Interpretation. *Natural Language Semantics* 1: 75–116.

Schauber, Ellen. 1975. *The Syntax and Semantics of Questions in Navajo.* Ph.D. diss., Massachusetts Institute of Technology. [Published 1979, New York: Garland].

Schubert, Lenhart K., and Francis Jeffry Pelletier. 1989. Generically Speaking: Or, Using Discourse Representation Theory to Interpret Generics. In G. Chierchia, B. Partee, and R. Turner (eds.), *Properties, Types and Meaning,* vol. 2: *Semantic Issues,* 193–268. Dordrecht: Kluwer.

Speas, Margaret J. 1990. *Phrase Structure in Natural Language.* Dordrecht: Kluwer.

Speas, Margaret, and Evangeline Parsons Yazzie. 1996. Quantifiers and the Position of Noun Phrases in Navajo. In Jelinek, et al. 1996.

Stump, Gregory T. 1985. *The Semantic Variability of Absolute Constructions.* Dordrecht: Reidel.

de Swart, Henriette E. 1991. *Adverbs of Quantification: A Generalized Quantifier Approach.* Ph.D. diss., Rijksuniversiteit Groningen. [published 1993, New York: Garland].

Willie, MaryAnn. 1989. Why There Is Nothing Missing in Navajo Relative Clauses. In Eung-Do Cook and Keren D. Rice (eds.), *Athapaskan Linguistics: Current Perspectives on a Language Family,* 407–437, Berlin: Mouton de Gruyter.

Willie, MaryAnn. 1991. Navajo Pronouns and Obviation. Ph.D. diss., University of Arizona.

Young, Robert, and William Morgan. 1987. *The Navajo Language.* Albuquerque: University of New Mexico.

4

NEGATIVE POLARITY EXPRESSIONS IN NAVAJO

Ken Hale and Paul Platero

The overt expression of negative polarity is achieved in Navajo by means of two constructions. The following sentences exemplify one of these:[1]

(1) a. *Doo háí-da níyáa-da.*
    NEG who-DA P.3.go-DA
    'No one has arrived.'

  b. *Shi-zhé'é doo ha'át'íí-da nayiisnii'-da.*
    my-father NEG what-DA 3.P.3.-DA
    'My father has not bought anything.'

  c. *Shi-zhé'é doo háágóó-da deeyáa-da.*
    my-father NEG where-AL-DA P.3.go-DA
    'My father is not going anywhere.'

  d. *Shi-zhé'é doo háágóó-da deesháál nízin-da.*
    my-father NEG where-AL-DA F.1s.go P.3.want-DA
    'My father does not want to go anywhere.'

The construction illustrated by the sentences of (1) involves the use of Navajo h-initial nominals, "h-words." These are indefinites which are close functional parallels of English wh-words. They are identical to the interrogative nominals used in content questions, as in (2), and in sentences containing positive indefinites, as in (3):

(2) a. *Háí-lá   níyá.*
         who-LA   P.3.go
         'Who has arrived?'

     b. *Shi-zhé'é   ha'át'íí-lá   nayiisnii'?*
         my-father   what-LA   3.P.3.buy
         'What did my father buy?'

     c. *Shi-zhé'é   háá-góó-lá   deeyá?*
         my-father   where-AL-LA   P.3.go
         'Where is my father going?'

     d. *Shi-zhé'é   háá-góó-lá   deesháál   nízin.*
         my-father   where-AL-LA   F.1s.go   P.3.want
         'Where does my father want to go?'

(3) a. *Háí-shíí   níyá.*
         who-INDEF   P.3.go
         'Someone arrived.'

     b. *Shi-zhé'é   ha'át'íí-shíí   nayiisnii'.*
         my-father   what-INDEF   3.P.3buy-DA
         'My father bought something.'

     c. *Shi-zhé'é   háá-góó-shíí   deeyá.*
         my-father   where-AL-INDEF   P.3.go
         'My father is going somewhere.'

     d. *Shi-zhé'é   háá-góó-shíí   deesháál   nízin.*
         my-father   where-AL-INDEF   F.1s.go   P.3.want-DA
         'My father wants to go somewhere.'

The sentences of (1)–(3) represent the prevailing pattern for overt quantifier-like expressions in Navajo. The "quantifier" is in situ—that is, in the same position where an ordinary NP or DP argument would appear, as in (4):

(4) a. *Si-tsilí   níyá.*
         my-YBro   P.3.go
         'My younger brother arrived.'

b. *Shi-zhé'é béégashii nayiisnii'.*
my-father cow 3.P.3.buy
'My father bought a cow.'

c. *Shi-zhé'é Kinłání-góó deeyá.*
my-father Flagstaff-AL P.3.go
'My father is going to Flagstaff.'

d. *Shi-zhé'é Kinłání-góó deesháał nízin.*
my-father Flagstaff-AL F.1s.go P.3.want
'My father wants to go to Flagstaff.'

The negative polarity constructions of (1) are characterized by the use of the negative particle *doo* immediately before the indefinite nominal, and the latter is followed immediately by the enclitic *-da* (glossed DA)—the same element that appears as the "scope-marker" at the end of the clause in negatives. What is essential here is that the negative particle *doo* must precede the indefinite, despite the fact that the unmarked position for this element in Navajo constructions of simple negative polarity is just before the verb, as illustrated in (5):

(5) a. *Si-tsilí doo níyáa-da.*
my-YBro NEG P.3.go-DA
'My younger brother did not arrive.'

b. *Shi-zhé'é béégashii doo nayiisnii'-da.*
my-father cow NEG 3.P.3.buy-DA
'My father did not buy a cow.'

c. *Shi-zhé'é Kinłání-góó doo deeyáa-da.*
my-father Flagstaff-AL NEG P.3.go-DA
'My father is not going to Flagstaff.'

d. *Shi-zhé'é Kinłání-góó deesháał doo nízin-da.*
my-father Flagstaff-AL F.1s.go NEG P.3.want-DA
'My father does not want to go to Flagstaff.'

This is not the only position in which the negative particle can appear; it is merely the position which is more or less neutral. It can also appear initially or following the subject. In the polarity construction, however, the negative particle must precede the indefinite. It is best to have the negative particle immediately before the indefinite, but a sentence like (6) is also possible:

(6) *Doo shi-zhé'é háá-góó-da deeyáa-da.*
NEG my-father where-AL-DA P.3.go-DA
'My father is not going anywhere.'

Now let us turn to the second construction which Navajo uses to express negative polarity. This is exemplified in the sentences of (7):

(7) a.   *Doo   níyá(h)-í-da.*
          NEG   P.3.go-PRN-DA
          'No one has arrived.'

     b.   *Shi-zhé'é   doo   nayiisnii'-í-da.*
          my-father   NEG   3.P.3.buy-PRN-DA
          'My father did not buy anything.'

     c.   *Shi-zhé'é   doo   deeyá(h)-í-góó-da.*
          my-father   NEG   P.3.go-PRN-AL-DA
          'My father is not going anywhere.'

     d.   *Shi-zhé'é   doo   deesháát nízin-í-góó-da.*
          my-father   NEG   F.1s.go   P.3.want-PRN-AL-DA
          'My father does not want to go anywhere.'

In these versions of the Navajo polarity construction, the indefinite portion is missing from its expected postnegative position. Instead, an as yet unidentified element appears following the verb—specifically, between the verb and the enclitic -*da*, the negative scope marker. This new, unidentified element, having the shape -*í*-, is identical to the morphological base of certain pronouns, determiners, and question words, as shown in (8):

(8)   *sh-í*   'first singular'
      b-í   'third'
      há-í   'who'
      é-í   'that'

These are perspicuous examples of determiners containing the element at issue, though its use is general in this class of words, if often obscured phonologically in less perspicuous cases. We will assume that the -*í*- of the polarity constructions is the very same element as that which functions as the morphological base of pronominals and determiners.[2] The question we must now face is this: what is this element doing after the verb, and what is the nature of the position in which it appears? We begin with the first part of this question.

It is clear that something is missing from the preverbal part of the sentences of (7), and the position of the missing element—that is, the "gap"—is at some point following the negative particle *doo*. In fact, we can show that the gap directly follows the negative particle, since a sentence like (9) below can only have the reading according to which the missing indefinite corresponds to the subject:

(9)   *Doo*   *béégashii*   *yizloh-í-da.*
      NEG   cow   3.P.3.rope-PRN-DA
      'Nobody roped the cow.'

This cannot have the meaning according to which the cow didn't rope anything, an idea which could only be rendered as in (10):

(10) *Béégashii*   *doo*   *yizloh-í-da.*
      cow   NEG   3.P.3.rope-PRN-DA
      'The cow didn't rope anything.'

We have reason to suppose, then, that the sentences of (7) and (9) have a gap—an empty category, possibly a trace of movement—immediately following the negative particle. Putting this observation together with that concerning the postverbal pronominal element -*í*- (glossed PRN), it is natural to suggest that the surface positioning of the latter is effected by rightward movement from the preverbal, and postnegative, position which we have identified with the gap. That is to say, the postverbal element -*í*- is a "clitic," more exactly "enclitic," variant of the indefinite item appearing in sentences of the type represented by the overt polarity constructions of (1) above. This clitic has the morphosyntactic property that it must attach to some word, and, further, it must attach to a particular word in the clause—namely, the verb. We leave aside for now the question of what forces it to move to the verb rather than to some other word. At this point, we are interested in establishing that a movement process is involved in this construction.

By assuming that the sentences of (7), say, are derived by movement from structures in which the clitic PRN originates in the position following the negative particle, we give a natural account of the paraphrase relation which holds between the sentences of (1) and (7). The two sets have essentially identical d-structures, and the entities involved in the negative polarity relations are essentially identical, abstractly speaking, in the two sets. Furthermore, movement is strongly suggested not only by the displacement of the PRN enclitic itself but also by the caselike locational and directional enclitics which are likewise displaced—pied-piped, so to speak—with the pronominal enclitic, as in (7c) and (11):

(11) a.   *Doo*   *naashá(h)-í-déé'-da.*
           NEG   I.1s.walk.around-PRN-AL-DA
           'I don't come from anywhere.'

      a'. *Kinłání-déé'*   *naashá.*
           Flagstaff-EL   I.1s.walk.around
           'I come from Flagstaff.'

b. *Awéé'   doo   si·dá(h)-í-gi-da.*
    baby   NEG   P.3.sit.sg-PRN-LOC-DA
    'The baby isn't sitting anywhere.'

b'. *Awéé'   ni'-gi   si·dá.*
    baby   ground-LOC   P.3.sit.sg
    'The baby is sitting on the ground.'

c. *Hastiin   doo   ni'nítbáz-í-jí'-da.*
    man   NEG   P.3.drive-PRN-EPT-DA
    'The man didn't drive up to anything.'

c'. *Hastiin   hooghan-jį'   ni'nítbą́ą́z.*
    man   house-EPT   P.3.drive
    'The man drove up to the house.'

In each of the sentences (11a') through (11c'), a locational or directional phrase appears with a verb which "selects" it, in an intuitively clear sense. These sentences conform to the natural or "basic" verb-final order of Navajo. Accordingly, the locational or directional phrase *precedes* the verb which selects it. The phrases at issue here consist of nominal expressions followed by one or another of the so-called "spatial enclitics" (AL 'allative', EL 'elative', EPT 'endpoint allative', LOC 'locative'). They correspond, clearly, to adpositional phrases in other languages. They belong, therefore, to the category commonly represented by the phrasal abbreviation PP. We will adopt this usage here, and, furthermore, we will refer to the spatial enclitics as "(enclitic) postpositions," departing to some extent from normal Athabaskanist usage, for the sake of general cross-linguistic reference. Accordingly, we will use the abbreviation P for the spatial enclitics for present purposes (reserving RN, relational noun, for the traditional Athabaskanist "postposition").

Consider now the sentences (11a–c), that is to say, the first in each of the pairs in (11) above. In those sentences, the PP constituent is missing from its putative base position, and the enclitic postposition (P) itself appears attached to the pronominal clitic element *-í-* (PRN) suffixed to the verb word. Here again, the semantic relation holding between the members of each pair in (11) is accounted for very naturally under the assumption that the first member is derived by movement from an underlying representation in which the pronominal element PRN (with P, if present) appears in the basic preverbal position, as depicted in (12):

(12) ... *doo* PRN(-P) ... V *-da*

We extend this analysis to all cases of the polarity construction involving displaced PRN. We can assume that PRN, being a bound element, must attach to some head. This requirement is satisfied by movement to a position from which it can attach to the verb word, although we must suppose also that the particular target or landing site is determined by more fundamental linguistic principles. Though a number of possibilities suggest themselves, we will be concerned here primarily with limitations on the movement process, assuming it to be real for now, and we will be concerned eventually with some of the implications the process has in relation to the position of Navajo in a theory of Pronominal Argument (Jelinek 1984; Jelinek and Demers 1994) and Polysynthetic (Baker 1996) languages.

The process involved in forming the polarity construction under consideration here exhibits behavior expected of an extraction operation. While "long extraction" is possible, it is not possible to extract over certain barriers or out of certain contexts. Putative long extraction is limited to movement out of direct discourse complements (cf. Kaufman 1974, Schauber 1979), as in (7d) above, repeated here as (13):

(13) *Shi-zhé'é   doo   deesháát   nízin-í-góó-da.*
      my-father   NEG   F.1s.go   P.3.want-PRN-AL-DA
      'My father does not want to go anywhere.'

The clausal complement here represents a type which can be selected by the members of a small set of verbs of saying and thinking. Sentences having the essential structure of (13) are characterized not only by "direct discourse" personal deixis but also by the absence of an overt complementizer. Additional examples of extractions from direct discourse complements are given in (14) and (15):

(14) a. *Shi-zhé'é   doo   naháłnii'   ní(n)-í-da.*
         my-father   NEG   P.1st.buy   3.say-PRN-DA
         'My father didn't say he bought anything.'
cf.

     b. *Shi-zhé'é   chidí   naháłnii'   ní.*
         my-father   car   P.1st.buy   3.say
         'My father said he bought a car.'

(15) a. *Shi-zhé'é   doo   ji-deeyá   shó'ní(n)-í-góó-da*
         my-father   NEG   4.P-go   1s.P.3.regard-PRN-AL-DA
         'My father doesn't think I'm going anywhere.'
cf.

     b. *Shi-zhé'é   Na'nízhoozhí-góó   ji-deeyá   shó'ní.*
         my-father   Gallup-AL   4.P-go   1sP.3.regard
         'My father thinks I'm going to Gallup.'

In the (a) sentences of (14) and (15), the gap which is construed with the verb-final dislocated pronominal enclitic clearly corresponds to a phrase selected by the embedded verb, not the main verb. That is to say, the gap in (14a) and (15a) corresponds to the overt phrases selected by the subordinate verbs in the sentences without extraction—that is, (14b) and (15b). Thus, it is reasonable to conclude that "long extraction" is involved here, as depicted in (16):

(16) XP *doo* [S . . . <u>PRN(-P)</u> . . . V] V -*da*

In this figure, we give the impression that the movement we have assumed is effected in one step, without interruption. This is not an impression we want to leave unchallenged. It could be, of course, that the extraction takes place in two stages—that is, successive cyclically—with the PRN moving first to a final (nonovert) complementizer position associated with the embedded clause and then to its eventual surface location, also possibly a complementizer associated with the main clause. The evidence for one thing or the other is not overwhelming. In any event, we will consider next the relationship between extraction and the appearance of an overt complementizer.

By far the greatest number and variety of dependent clause constructions in Navajo involve the use of postverbal subordinating morphology which, we suppose, occupies the complementizer position in the syntactic structure projected for the relevant sentences. This morphology includes the nominalizing, referentially definite, enclitic morphology involved in the Navajo internally headed relative clause, as in (17), and Navajo expressions corresponding to factive complements in English and other familiar languages, as in (18). On relative clauses, this enclitic morphology comes in two forms, one involving reference to past events, states, or mentionings (e.g., -*ę́ę* ~ -*ą́ą* in (17b, d)), the other to nonpast events, states, or mentionings (-*ígíí* in (17a, c)); factives generally bear the second of these (as in (18)):

(17) a. *Shi-zhé'é   bįįh   néíł'ah-ígíí   dadiidį́į́ł.*
          my-Fa   deer   I.3.butcher-REL   F.1ns.eat
          'We will eat the deer my father is butchering.'

      b. *Shi-zhé'é   bįįh   yiyiisxí(n)-ę́ę   nídeesh'ah.*
          my-Fa   deer   3.P.kill-REL   F.1s.butcher
          'I will butcher the deer my father killed.'

      c. *Bá'ólta'í   KinŁání-dę́ę́'   naaghá(h)-ígíí   'ayóo   sh-aa   jooba'.*
          teacher   Flagstaff-EL   I.3.come.from-REL   very   1-to   I.3.kind
          'The teacher who comes from Flagstaff is very nice to me.'

      d. *Hastiin   Na'nízhoozhí-góó   naayá(h)-ą́ą   bi-ł   naashnish.*
          man   Gallup-AL   P.3.go-REL   3-with   I.1s.work
          'I work with the man who went to Gallup (and returned).'

(18) a. *K'ad*   *'íínílta'-ígíí*   *b-aa*   *shi-ł*   *hózh,ó.*
      now   I.2s.sgo.school-REL   3-about   1-with   I.A.good
      'I'm glad that you are going to school.'

    b. *'Adą́ą́dą́ą́'*   *łį́į́'*   *naníílgo'-ígíí*   *yínii'.*
      yesterday   horse   2s.P.3.throw-REL   P.1s.hear
      'I heard that the horse threw you yesterday.'

By contrast with direct discourse complements of the type represented by (13), relative clauses and factives are "opaque," resisting extraction from a position internal to them—thus, the following patterns are observed (illustrating first the relative clause, in (19) and (20)):

(19) a. *Bee'eldǫǫh*   *nahínílnii'-ę́ę*   *n-ee*   *né'íí'.*
      gun   3.P.2s.buy-REL   2s-post   3.P.1s.steal
      'I stole (from you) the gun you bought.'

    b. *Doo*   *bee'eldǫǫh*   *nahínílnii'-ę́ę*   *n-ee*   *né'íí'-da.*
      NEG   gun   3.P.2s.buy-REL   2s-post   3.P.1s.steal-DA
      'I didn't steal (from you) the gun you bought.'

    c. *Doo*   *ha'át'íí-da*   *nahínílnii'-ę́ę*   *n-ee*   *né'íí'-da.*
      NEG   what-DA   3.P.2s.buy-REL   2s-post   3.P.1s.steal-DA
      'I didn't steal (from you) whatever you bought.'

    d. **Doo_____*   *nahínílnii'-ę́ę*   *n-ee*   *né'í'-í-da.*
      NEG _____   3.P.2s.buy-REL   2s-post   3.P.1s.steal-PRN-DA

(20) a. *Na'nízhoozhí-góó*   *naayá(h)-ą́ą*   *yiiłtsą́.*
      Gallug-AL   P.s.go.sg-REL   3.P.1s.see
      'I saw the one who went to Gallup.'

    b. *Doo*   *Na'nízhoozhí-góó*   *naayá(h)-ą́ą*   *yiiłtsą́ą-da.*
      NEG   Gallup-AL   P.s.go.sg-REL   3.P.1s.see-DA
      'I didn't see the one who went to Gallup.'

    c. *Doo*   *háá-góó-da*   *naayá(h)-ą́ą*   *yiiłtsą́ą-da.*
      NEG   where-AL-DA   P.s.go.sg-REL   3.P.1s.see-DA
      'I didn't see the one who went somewhere.'

    d. **Doo_____*   *naayá(h)-ą́ą*   *yiiłtsá(n)-í-da.*
      NEG _____   P.s.go.sg-REL   3.P.1s.see-PRN-DA

The relevant observation here, of course, is that the enclitic pronominal *-í-* (PRN) cannot be construed with the vacant position (symbolized _____) following the negative particle in the (d) sentences of (19) and (20). The hypothetical "gap," theoretically the trace of the extracted enclitic, is inside a relative clause here, while its putative antecedent, the enclitic PRN itself, is outside that clause.

The same restriction is observed in relation to factive nominalizations, formally identical to internally headed relatives:

(21) a. *Na'nízhoozhí-góó   nisíníyá(h)-ígíí   b-aa   shi-ł   hózhǫ́.*
         Gallup-AL   P.2s.go-REL   3-about   1s-with   A.P.good
         'I'm happy about the fact that you went to Gallup.'

   b. *Doo   N.-góó nisíníyá(h)-ígíí   b-aa   shi-ł   hózhǫ́ǫ-da.*
       NEG   G.-AL P.2.go-REL   3-about   1s-with   A.P.good.DA
       'I'm not happy about the fact that you went to Gallup.'

   c. *Doo   háá-góó-da   nisíníyá(h)-ígíí b-aa   shi-ł   hózhǫ́ǫ-da.*
       NEG   where-AL   P.2s.go-REL   3-about 1s-with   A.P.good.DA
       'I'm not happy about you having gone somewhere.'

   d. **Doo____   nisíníyá(h)-ígíí b-aa   shi-ł   hózhǫ́(n)-í-góó-da.*
       NEG ____   P.2s.go-REL   3-about   1s-with   A.P.good-PRN-AL-DA

Here again, a gap within the nominalized clause cannot be construed with an antecedent outside that clause.

This restriction is not limited to nominalized clauses, since it is also observed with adjoined (adverbial) clauses of the type represented by (22) below. In general, in strictly observational terms, a gap cannot be construed with an antecedent "across an overt complementizer":

(22) a. *Shi-ye' hastl'ishítlizh-go   hadeeshghaazh.*
         1s-son   mud.P.3.fall-COMP   P.1s.shout
         'I shouted out when my son fell into the mud.'

   b. *Doo   shi-ye' hashtl'ishítlizh-go   hadeeshghaazh-da.*
       NEG   1s-son mud.P.3.fall-COMP   P.1s.shout-DA
       'I didn't shout when my son fell into the mud.'

   c. *Doo   háí-da   hastl'ishítlizh-go   hadeeshghaazh-da.*
       NEG   who-DA   mud.P.3.fall-COMP   P.1s.shout-DA
       'I didn't shout out when someone fell into the mud.'

   d. **Doo____   hashtl'ishítlizh-go   hadeeshghaazh-í-da.*
       NEG ____   mud.P.3.fall-COMP   P.1s.shout-PRN-DA

We are left now with the question of how this constraint should be explained. What is the principle which prevents an gap-antecedent relation here? And how are the (d) sentences of (19)–(22) different in nature from the direct discourse complements of (13) and (14), where the hypothetical "long extraction" is allowed to relate a gap to an antecedent in a higher clause? There are two obvious possibilities: (i) the ill-formed sentences of (19)–(22) violate subjacency, the overt complementizer reflecting the presence of a barrier for extraction, absent in the complementizerless direct discourse complement; (ii) the ill-formed sentences are so because they violate the Condition on Extraction Domains (CED; Huang 1982)—nominalized clauses, like adverbials, are adjuncts, opaque to government and hence to extraction, while direct discourse complements are truly *complements*, transparent to government (ceteris paribus).

We will return to this question later. For now, however, we should point out, as an aside, that the slightly degraded (c) sentences of (19)–(22) suggest that the principles accounting for the ill-formedness of the (d) sentences, with apparent overt extraction, are also implicated in the semantics of Navajo in situ h-words in relation to negation. These elements do not have their usual polarity function, being interpreted rather as indefinites, in structures in which an overt complementizer separates them from the negative (NEG) particle. Again, depending on the answers to certain well-known theoretical questions, this could be a subjacency effect or a CED effect.

For present purposes, we will be content to point out that the facts surrounding the relation between the enclitic PRN element and the gap with which it is associated are consistent with the syntactic movement hypothesis suggested earlier. There is a dependency between an overt element (PRN) and a gap, hypothetically a trace, which is what we will take it to be henceforth. That is to say, there is the expected "displacement." An element appears in a position which it is reasonable to assume is different from its d-structure position; thus, for example, a postposition appears in a position removed from the preverbal position in which it is "selected"; and, by extension, a "bare PRN" is likewise found in an A-bar position, removed from the argument position in which it is governed and selected by the verb. Moreover, the observed gap-antecedent relation is limited by principles typically involved in blocking extraction. All of this smacks clearly of movement, and we will consider this issue essentially closed for the purposes of the present discussion (see also Kaufman 1974 and Schauber 1979, where the same conclusion is reached in relation to the identical gap-antecedent relation observed in certain Navajo indirect question constructions).

We turn now to a brief consideration of certain technical questions raised by the movement hypothesis. What is the nature of PRN? And what is the nature of the position to which it moves? These are related questions, since if PRN is a head, its landing site is presumably likewise a head; if it is a maximal projection, then its landing site is presumably a structural position (specifier, complement) to which a maximal projection may move. We know that PRN is morphologically enclitic at surface structure; but this does not, of course, preclude the possibility that it is a maximal projection at d- and s-structures. In favor of the idea that PRN is a maximal projection is the fact that it undergoes "long movement," leaving intermediate heads behind (e.g., V and various functional heads c-commanding V, as well as N, as we shall see presently). This, in and of itself, is enough to eliminate the alternative, since the Head Movement Constraint, precluding precisely this, is generally exceptionless in natural language (Travis

1984).[3] Thus, the appearance of PRN in a canonical "head position" (final in Navajo) is a purely morphological fact, essentially accidental in relation to strictly syntactic considerations. The "pied-piping" of spatial enclitics (P) is consistent with either hypothesis.

We will assume the analysis according to which PRN is a maximal (i.e., phrasal) projection and that it is motivated by the same factors that motivate overt syntactic movement of [+Wh]-phrases to the Spec position of a [+Wh] complementizer in linguistically well-known cases. We cannot explain why this movement is *nonovert* in the case of Navajo *h*-words (but see Schauber 1979 for optional overt leftward movement of h-words in questions in some Navajo speech). Be this as it may, PRN movement is overt and obligatory, and it is constrained in accordance with well-known limits on extraction.

What now can be said about this polarity construction and the question of the position of Navajo in relation to the typological distinction drawn around polysynthesis and nonconfigurationality in recent work (Baker 1996; Jelinek 1984)?

First, it is clear that the existence of a movement rule is perfectly consistent with the Polysynthesis Parameter of Baker (1996) which, while precluding the appearance of an overt nominal expression in an argument position, specifically permits the appearance there of an empty category, including the trace of movement. On the other hand, we have not considered the full range of structures in which PRN-movement applies. Specifically, we have not considered one class of cases in which movement directly confronts the issue of polysynthesis and the pronominal argument parameter.

Overt nominals, in particular the "thematic arguments" of verbs and other argument-taking heads, cannot appear in core argument positions at s-structure. Instead, they must appear in adjunct (A-bar) positions. We will assume, with Baker (1996), and without further comment, that this is to be explained in relation to the "licensing" function of Case. Core argument positions are not positions to which Case can be assigned; hence, empty categories (including traces of movement) are permitted there, while overt nominals are precluded. Overt nominals are permitted in adjunct positions, on the other hand, presumably because Case is not required there, and their thematic relations are satisfied through a "linking" relation with their associated core argument positions. Linking is accomplished in virtue of the antecedent-trace relation, in the case of movement, and in the case of basic adjuncts, through an inherent linking relation between argumental *pro* elements and base-generated adjunct nominals.

We now have a prediction. If a language is polysynthetic, then overt nominals in it are adjuncts, and extraction from a nominal expression is impossible, by the CED. If this is in fact the case in Navajo, then Navajo is possibly polysynthetic in Baker's sense. We have seen that extraction out of a nominalized clause is impossible (cf. the (d) sentences of (19)–(21)), but this is possibly due to subjacency and, hence, irrelevant to the issue at hand. Consider now the following examples:

(23) a.   *Doo   shi-zhé'é bi-łį́į́'   yiiłtsą́ą-da.*
          NEG   1s-father 3-horse   P.1s.see-DA
          'I didn't see my father's horse.'

   b.   *Doo   háí-da   bi-łį́į́'   yiiłtsą́ą-da.*
        NEG   who-DA   3-horse   P.1s.see-DA
        'I didn't see anyone's horse.'

   c.   *Doo ____ bi-łį́į́'   yiiłtsá(n)-í-da.*
        NEG ____ 3-horse   P.1s.see-PRN-DA
        'I didn't see anyone's horse.'

(24) a.   *Doo   si-tsilí   bi-łééchąą'í shishxash-da.*
          NEG   1s-YBro   3-dog   1s.P.3.bite-DA
          'My younger brother's dog didn't bite me.'

   b.   *Doo   háí-da   bi-łééchąą'í shishxash-da.*
        NEG   who-DA   3-dog   1s.P.3.bite-DA
        'No one's dog bit me.'

   c.   *Doo ____ bi-łééchąą'í shishxash-í-da.*
        NEG ____ 3-dog   1s.P.3.bite-PRN-DA
        'No one's dog bit me.'

(25) a.   *Doo   sh-ínaaí   bi-ye' Na'nízhoozhí-góó deeyáa-da.*
          NEG   1s-OBro   3-son   Gallup-AL   P.3.go-DA
          'My elder brother's son isn't going to Gallup.'

   b.   *Doo   háí-da   bi-ye' Na'nízhoozhí-góó deeyáa-da.*
        NEG   1s-OBro   3-son   Gallup-AL   P.3.go-DA
        'No one's son is going to Gallup.'

   c.   *Doo ____ bi-ye' Na'nízhoozhí-góó deeyá(h)-í-da.*
        NEG ____ 3-son   Gallup-AL   P.3.go-PRN-DA
        'No one's son is going to Gallup.'

The crucial cases here are the (c) sentences on the view that movement is involved in producing their s-structure forms. Of course, the central question is the nature, not of the landing site of PRN, unremarkable here, but of the point of origin—that is, the position of the gap, or trace. If, as is generally assumed, the trace (corresponding to the possessor argument in the possessive constructions) is *internal* to a nominal expression, then the status of Navajo as a polysynthetic language is in question. If the s-structures corresponding to the (c) sentences involve the profile depicted in (26), then we have extraction from a nominal constituent:

(26) ... *doo* [$_{DP}$ _____ N] ... V-PRN-*da*
      |_____↑

If overt nominals are adjuncts, then (26) is impossible, being a CED violation—PRN is extracted from DP, an adjunct, by hypothesis.[4] If (26) is the correct analysis of the (c) sentences of (23)–(25), which are grammatical, then Navajo is not a polysynthetic language in the sense of Baker.

This result might be seen as conflicting with evidence which has been cited from relative clause structures in Navajo. The evidence at issue includes data of the type represented in (27) below, originally pointed out by Ellavina Perkins (Hale et al. 1977; cf. Platero 1982 and Speas 1990 for discussions of analogous structures):

(27) [*Jįįdą́ą́'   shi-zhé'é   łįį'   nayiisnii'-ę́ę*]   *yí'didoołił.*
       day.past   1s-father   horse   3.P.3.buy-REL   3.F.3.brand.
       'My father$_i$ will brand the horse he$_i$ bought (earlier) today.'

Sentences of this type are subject to a number of interpretations, but the translation given corresponds to a prominent reading—the most prominent, for some speakers. Crucially, on this interpretation, the subject of the final verb is nonovert—that is, *pro* by hypothesis—and it is coreferential with the overt nominal argument *shi-zhé'é*, 'my father', appearing internal to the bracketed relative clause—that is, internal to the object of the final verb. This is theoretically possible under either of two conditions: (i) Navajo is a polysynthetic language, in which the relative clause (an overt nominal expression) is an adjunct, while the core arguments are nonovert pronominals (*pro*) occupying in the core subject and object position; or (ii) Navajo is a standard configurational language (cf. Speas 1990), with the usual null-pronominal possibilities of languages with rich agreement, and in which relative clauses have the *option* of appearing as adjuncts, as in standard dislocation constructions. In either case, a relative clause (symbolized N$_{rel}$ in (28) below), with overt nominals (NP$_i$ and NP$_j$), will occupy a position which is, in the relevant respects, external to the main clause and therefore outside the c-command domain of any of the arguments of the main verb (i.e., Pro$_i$, the subject, and Pro$_j$, the object):

(28)

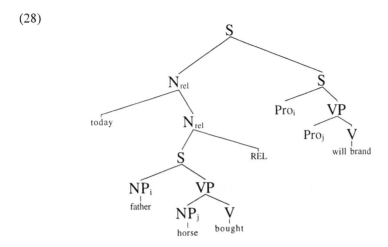

It follows, then, that there can be no Condition C violation in this situation (cf. Baker 1996; Chomsky 1981). On the other hand, if the relative clause of (28) occupied the object position within the main clause (i.e., if it appeared in place of Pro$_j$), then the main clause subject (Pro$_i$) would c-command an R-expression with which it is coindexed (the overt nominal NP$_i$)—this would be a clear Condition C violation. There is more to this than meets the eye, however.

So far as we can tell, the "problem" illustrated by (27) is specific to internally headed relative clauses, and especially sentences which, like (27), consist of main and subordinate clauses that are "GF-parallel"—that is, in which the main and subordinate clauses share arguments of the same grammatical function.

Where such parallelism is not present, as in the following sentences with (bracketed) factive complements (ignoring for present purposes the problem of identifying true parallelism in the relevant sense), a *pro* subject in the main clause cannot be interpreted as coreferential with an overt nominal in the embedded factive clause, hence:

(29) a. [*Yiskággo ni-tsilí nih-aa doogáł-ígíí*] *y-ee shi-ł hoolne'.*
   tomorrow 2s-YBr 1ns-to FUT.3.go-REL 3-of 1s-with 3.P.tell
   '(S)he$_i$ told me about your younger brother$_j$ coming to us tomorrow.'

b. [*Yiskággo ni-tsilí nih-aa doogáł-ígíí*] *b-aa bi-ł*
   tomorrow 2s-YBr 1ns-to FUT.3.go-REL 3-about 3-with
   hózhǫ.
   A.P.good
   '(S)he$_i$ is happy about your younger brother$_j$ coming to us tomorrow.'

The factive complements here exhibit the behavior expected of core arguments, not that of adjuncts. This is clear immediately for (29a), whose main verb takes a standard subject argument which, whether overt or nonovert, would c-command the embedded factive clause—the latter is the grammatical object of the relational noun expression *y-ee* 'about it'. The same c-command relation holds in (29b), though less obviously so, since this is an inverse construction—the experiencer is raised from the complement position within the relational noun expression *bi-ł*, 'with him/her'. Since coreference between *ni-tsilí* 'your younger brother' and the relevant nonovert main clause argument is not possible, we must assume that the option available for relative clauses like (27) is not available for factive clauses, despite their nominal morphology. In this respect, these factives behave like the possessive nominal constructions of (23)–(25). But this is not a property of factives, per se; it has to do rather with GF-parallelism. Thus, where the GF relations are parallel, as in (30) below, the relevant cross-clausal coreference is possible:

(30) [*Yiską́ągo   shi-zhé'é   shi-má y-íká-'adoolwoł-ígíí*] *y-ee   yi-ł   hoolne'.*
       tomorrow   1s-Fa   1s-Mo 3-for-FUT.3.run-REL 3-of   3-with P.3.tell
       'My father$_i$ told my mother he$_i$ would help (lit. about his$_i$ helping) her to-
       morrow.'

As in the case of (27), so also here on the reading given, the subject of the main verb is nonovert and coreferential with the overt subject of the embedded factive clause.

     Speas (1990) has argued that parallelism is the factor which is relevant in complex sentences of the type represented by (27) and (30), and in other comparable cases in which nonovert arguments are construed with heteroclausal overt arguments. She proposes the following Parallel Function Constraint on interpretation (Speas 1990:232):

(31) In a construction in which an embedded clause is dislocated and adjoined
      to the matrix clause, interpret *pro* in a given clause as coreferent with the
      NP that bears the same GF in the other clause.

This will account for the relevant interpretation of (27), and assuming that the relative clause there is dislocated, i.e., an adjunct, there is no Condition C violation. However, GF parallelism is logically independent of dislocation or adjunction. Consider the parallelism constraint autonomously, as in (32):

(32) In a complex construction, interpret *pro* in a given clause as coreferent
      with the NP that bears the same GF in the other clause.[5]

This version will apply to give the relevant interpretation of (27) whether the relative clause is adjoined, as in (28), or in the core object position (i.e., the position occupied by Pro$_j$ in that structure). In the second case, of course, a

Condition C violation results. But the parallelism principle could, in fact, be "strong enough" or override the otherwise inviolate Binding Theory principle.

In relation to our basic question—polysynthesis versus standard configurationality—we are left with the following logical possibilities:

(33) a.   All overt nominal arguments occupy core argument positions.
     b.   All overt nominal arguments are adjuncts (linked to *pro*s in core argument positions).
     c.   Some overt nominal arguments (e.g., certain clausal ones) are adjuncts; all others are in core argument positions.

If (33a) is correct, then (32) operates in some cases *in spite of* Condition C. If (33b) is correct, then Condition C is never obtruded by (32). If (33c) is correct, (32) may operate without violating Condition C.

If the Parallel Function Constraint is correct, and we believe it is (in some form or other; cf. Platero 1978, 1982 for discussion of certain interpretive strategies), then, with the possible exception of the extraction of possessors (as in (23)–(25)), the evidence we have considered in this paper does little to decide the issue of Navajo polysynthesis and standard configurationality. It will be necessary to determine the correctness of one or another of the structural arrangements in (33); and to do that, we must look elsewhere—for example, the kinds of arguments presented by Speas (1990:237–240 and elsewhere) in favor of (33a, c), and the kinds of arguments presented by Jelinek (1984, 1995, and elsewhere) in favor of (33b) and pronominal argument grammar.

Notes

We are very much indebted to Linda Platero for her judgments on many of the Navajo sentences in this article. She is not responsible for errors which undoubtedly remain. We are indebted to Maria Bittner, Leonard Faltz, and Irene Heim for valuable comments on aspects of this article, and we are grateful to members of the Navajo Language Seminar, MIT fall 1995, and the Swarthmore Conference on Athabaskan Syntax and Semantics, spring 1996, for many helpful comments on this and other aspects of Navajo syntax and semantics.

1. The construction exemplified in (1) has an alternative interpretation, the existential, in which the h-word has wide scope. Thus, (1a) 'Someone has not arrived.'

2. This element is also the basic component in derived nominals, appearing in its "pure" form in lexicalized expressions like *yadiizí(n)-í* 'tin can' (lit. 'that which stands upright') and *dzi'iz-í* 'bicycle' (lit. 'that which one pedals'). And we assume that it is also a subpart of the more complex element *-ígíí* appearing with unbridled productivity in relative clauses and factive nominalizations (cf. the sentences of (29) and (30)). As Leonard Faltz points out (personal communication), it is relevant to point out that neither

the element -*í,* which we gloss PRN (suggesting "pronominal"), nor the "scope marker" -*da* is a polarity item. Rather, we maintain that, in sentences of the type appearing in (7), the polarity item is an empty category (a trace) immediately following the negative particle *doo*—that is, an empty category occupying the same position as the h-words (overt polarity items) in the sentences of (1).

3. We are especially grateful to Maria Bittner (personal communication) for correcting a conceptual error which we made in our initial account of this construction, an account which assumed Head Movement. We were misled by the final position of -*í* and its suffixal appearance, suggesting movement to the prevailing head-final position in Navajo. It is, of course, perfectly possible that movement is actually to Specifier position, in keeping with the usual cross-linguistic behavior in A-bar movement of quantifiers and quantifier-like elements (cf. Schauber, 1979 for discussion of overt leftward movement in Navajo). The suffixal, or enclitic, character of -*í* is responsible for its ultimate positioning enclitic to the verb, a fact of Phonological Form, not of syntax.

4. Leonard Faltz points out correctly (personal communication) that (26) might not be the actual structure of sentences such as (23) through (25). Rather, the possessor phrase might in fact be external to the DP expression containing the possessum. We are assuming that the possessor is internal and that the extracted PRN originates there, a proposal which is perfectly consonant with the Polysynthesis Hypothesis, which permits the trace of extraction to occupy an argument position, as suggested in (26). It is a fact, however, that Navajo permits the parts of a possessive construction to be separated, the possessor and possessum appearing as structurally separate constituents. There is the possibility, which we cannot pursue here, that movement of the possessor under this condition would not involve extraction from a DP at all (see Willie 1991, chapter 7, for a discussion of Possessor Raising).

5. This is sufficient for the direct construction. An adjustment will have to be made for the inverse (Subject-Object-Inversion) construction, however (cf. Platero 1978, 1982). Consider, for example, the interpretation which results if the verb of the factive clause in (30) is changed to the *bi*-form (the inverse), giving *b-íká-'adoolwoł,* 'x will help y$_i$, y$_i$ will be helped by x'. In this case, the non-overt subject of the main clause is coindexed with the overt (fronted) object of the factive clause—that is, *shi-shé'é$_i$* 'my father'. Here 'my father', not 'my mother', is the person to be helped; but it is still 'my father' who communicates the content of the factive clause to 'my mother'.

References

Baker, Mark. 1996. *The Polysynthesis Parameter.* New York: Oxford University Press.
Chomsky, Noam. 1981. *Lectures on Government and Binding.* Dordrecht: Foris.
Hale, Kenneth, Ellavina Tsosie-Perkins, Richard Demers, and Dorothy Shank. 1977. The Structure of Navajo (Course Notes). University of Arizona. Unpublished manuscript.
Huang, C.-T. James (1982) Logical Relations in Chinese and the Theory of Grammar Ph.D. dissertation, Massachusetts Institute of Technology.
Jelinek, Eloise. 1984. Empty Categories, Case, and Configurationality. *Natural Language and Linguistic Theory* 2:39–76.
Jelinek, Eloise. 1995. Pronoun Classes and Focus. University of Arizona. Unpublished manuscript.
Jelinek, Eloise, and Richard Demers. 1994. Predicates and Pronominal Arguments in Straits Salish. *Language* 70:697–736.

Kaufman, Ellen. 1974. Navajo Spatial Enclitics: A Case for Unbounded Rightward Movement. *Linguistic Inquiry* 5:507–33.

Platero, Paul. 1978. Missing Noun Phrases in Navajo. Ph.D. dissertation, Massachusetts Institute of Technology.

Platero, Paul. 1982. Missing Noun Phrases and Grammatical Relations in Navajo. *International Journal of American Linguistics.* 48:286–305.

Schauber, Ellen. 1979. *The Syntax and Semantics of Questions in Navajo.* New York: Garland.

Speas, Margaret J. 1990. *Phrase Structure in Natural Language.* Dordrecht: Kluwer.

Travis, Lisa. 1984. Parameters and Effects of Word Order Variation. Ph.D. dissertation, Massachusetts Institute of Technology.

Willie, MaryAnn. 1991. Navajo Pronouns and Obviation. Ph.D. dissertation, University of Arizona, Tucson.

5

WORD ORDER IN APACHE NARRATIVES

Dagmar Jung

The following text-based study investigates the relationship between word order and bound pronominal expressions exemplified by two closely related languages of the southern Athabaskan language group, Jicarilla Apache and Lipan Apache.

Athabaskan languages are usually analyzed as exhibiting the word order Subject-Object-Verb in the unmarked case (cf. e.g., Young and Morgan 1987:205). Saxon and Rice (1993) present an exception to this analysis by suggesting an underlying OSV as the underived order, at least for the Northern Athabaskan languages Ahtna and Koyukon. The very frequent SOV surface order is then explained by a process of raising of topical subjects.

These analyses raise the following two questions: (1) What is the unmarked word order in Athabaskan languages (or subgroups of Athabaskan languages)? and (2) How 'free' is this word order? A prominent characteristic of Athabaskan verbs is their pronominal inflection: the participants in a clause do not have to be expressed as free noun phrases but can be marked just by pronominal expressions in the verb. This trait has been described by various linguists, especially in relationship to the polysynthetic language type (Jelinek 1984, Hale 1992). Mithun (1992) analyzes three languages with a similar obligatory expression of pronominal marking in the verb (i.e., Cayuga, Coos, and Ngandi). She shows that noun phrases in these languages function as appositives rather than as grammatical arguments. The arguments of the verb are the pronominal expressions in the verb which are not merely agreement markers in these languages. This structure allows for a pragmatically based word order instead of a grammatically based one—that is, the information flow determines the order of noun phrases.

This characteristic of free word order made possible by obligatory pronominal inflection is considered by Baker (1996) as one of the defining traits of a polysynthetic language (besides, for example, syntactic noun incorporation and lack of true quantification).

If Athabaskan languages exhibit pronominal inflection, it can be expected that they also exhibit free word order—that is, subject NPs and object NPs should occur in alternative orders relative to each other and/or relative to the verb. But Jelinek (1989) shows that it is necessary to make a distinction between the Northern Athabaskan (NA) and the Southern Athabaskan (SA) language groups with respect to their overall structure: although pronominal inflection for subject and object is obligatory in Southern Athabaskan, this is not the case in Northern Athabaskan. In most languages of the latter group, pronominal inflection for the object is only present if there is no object noun phrase in the clause. If the noun phrase is present, the object is not pronominally expressed on the verb, but an alternating structure is exhibited, as in the following example from Slave (NA) (Rice 1989:1016):[1]

(1) a. *golǫ*   *thehk'éh*
         Moose **3S**.shoot
         'S/he shot a moose.'

     b. *yéhk'é*
         3S.3O.shoot
         'S/he shot it'.

In the first example, the object noun phrase is expressed and the verb is not marked for the object, while in the second example the transitive relationship involving two third persons is overtly marked.

Noun phrases as in (1a) have therefore to be considered to occur in an argument position. The case is different in Southern Athabaskan, where pronominal inflection is obligatory and the noun phrases are always in adjunct position.

(2) a. *łį*   *yiłnaasdee*
         Horse **3S.3O**.chase
         'S/he chased the horse around.'

     b. *yiłnaasdee*
         3S.3O.chase
         'S/he chased the horse around.'

In this Jicarilla Apache example, the verbal morphology is not changed by the presence or absence of overt noun phrases, but it always shows full paradigmatic inflection (in the above example the prefix *yi-*, which is coreferential with the noun phrase *łį* 'horse,' is constructed as an indirect object). The status of the noun phrase in example (2) differs from the one in example (1) in that there is no alternation in the verbal marking.

Since the function of noun phrases as either arguments or adjuncts is an important distinction between the language groups, the relative freedom of word order would be expected to be greater in the Southern group (noun phrases being adjuncts, obligatory pronominal inflection), and more restricted in the Northern group (noun phrases being arguments, no obligatory pronominal inflection).

In the following sections I will consider the word order data in narrative texts in two Southern Athabaskan languages and evaluate if there is indeed a connection between obligatory pronominal marking and freedom of word order.

5.1   Word Order in Jicarilla Apache

If transitive clauses contain both subject and object noun phrases, the most frequent order in Jicarilla Apache is SOV, as in example (3):[2]

(3)   *Į́ís'ádą   Higalį́íya Abáachi   ke'dzidéé   nádaiłka.*
       long ago   Jicarilla   Apache   moccasin   3p.sew
       'A long time ago, the Jicarilla Apache used to make moccasins.'

(4)   *Bí łį   naamiyéh   da'ko shigo   łį   naashiyéh.*
       3   horse   **3S.3O**.carry   then   1s.EMPH   horse   3S.1sO.carry
       'She was riding a horse, and I was riding, too.'

Example (4) shows a marked construction, the voice-related subject/object-inversion, in which the object of a clause occurs before the subject if the animacy of the object is on a higher scale than the animacy of the subject (prototypically this occurs in the interaction between humans and animals).[3] In this example, the independent third-person pronoun occurs before the actual agent of the action (the horse)—the literal meaning of the verb in (4) is 'it carried her.' The verb is marked for this voice inversion by the pronominal prefix *mi-* (varies with *bi-*, cognate with Navajo *bi-*). The following example shows that the interpretation of the verbal semantics depends crucially on the *yi-/mi-* distinction:

(5)   a.   *łį   yił-naasdee*
            horse   3S3O.chase
            'S/he chased the horse around.' (= 2a)

      b.   *łį   bił-naasdee*
            Horse   3S3O.chase
            'The horse chased him/her around.'

The noun phrase is understood in the first example as the patient, in the second example as the agent of the action. Although this subject-object inversion occurs in texts (as in example 4), its usage with two noun phrases in inverted positions is very rare and will not be further considered here. But the fact that this kind of transitive construction occurs should be kept in mind in the following discussion.

To be able to determine the conditions of use of word order, it is necessary to analyze word order in situ—that is, how speakers in natural discourse make use of word order. The following example is taken out of a Jicarilla Apache story about the search for a man with big feet in order to sew the right moccasin:

(6) *Mikee   yeemándeenłees   náałtsoosi yika'éé.*
     3POSS.foot   3S.3O.3BEN.put down   paper   on top of
     'He put his foot down on top of the paper for them.'

     Adą   yina'iiszo.
     Then   3S.3O.circle
     'And then he circled it.'

     Adą   da'kwéé   inaayíí'įį.
     Then there   3S.3O.take
     'And then they took it (back) over there again.'

     Mika'éé   miłhagǫ́ǫ́tso.
     3POSS.father   3S.3O.surprised
     'His father was surprised.' (lit. 'It surprised his father.')

     Adą   ihagoołninéh: iyáhna'   me'naał'ąą?
     Then   3.told.thus: what   2sS.3O.measure
     'And then he said this to him: What did you measure?'

This sequence is typical for the narrative style in stories: there are hardly any subject or object noun phrases in example (6). Clauses containing subject and direct object expressions are very rare in natural discourse. If a noun phrase is used at all in subject or object position, it will generally be only one per clause, not two noun phrases in one clause. This discourse pattern makes the search for natural occurring word order data more difficult, and also poses the question of whether the assumption of an unmarked word order relating to subject and direct object noun phrases can be justified at all.

5.2 Alternative Word Orders

Although SOV order is prevalent in (the few) clauses expressing both noun phrases, variation in word order can be found in some examples. Postverbal and preverbal domains are considered in the following.

5.2.1 *Postverbal Domain*

Clauses are not consistently verb-final: adpositional phrases may follow the verb, as in the following example (Hoijer n.d.:3(1)):

(7) ashį́į́' nkeenáánádzá-ná **dagi ts'ę́tso'yé**.
     Then   3.INC.walk-NARR up   meadow.ALL
     'Then he started to walk up to the meadow.'

Object noun phrases are also found to occur postverbally instead of right before the verb in the clause.

(8) adą   ha'dééshį ayį́įla-**ná**   **łį**.
     Then   something 3S.3O.made-NARR horse
     'Then he did something to the horse.'

(9) k'aadaanagésh biké'híí   yiiłni-**ná**   **dindéí**.
     2pS.look at   3.POSS.track.DEF 3S.3O.tell-NARR men.DEF
     '"Look at her tracks," he told the men.' (Hoijer n.d.:8(102))

(10) binádaaskah **ibąą   daagókii**. (LIPAN)
     3S.3O.p.sew   buckskin 3p.POSS.shoe
     'They sew their shoes with buckskin.' (Hoijer 1975:10)

Examples (8) and (9) (Jicarilla Apache) exhibit postposed indirect objects. Interestingly, both clauses contain the narrative particle *ná* directly following the verb. This particle occurs only in texts and seems to be related to an evidential function. It is most commonly used clause-finally, attached to the verb. The occurrence of the narrative particle before the object noun phrases in the examples above indicates that these noun phrases are not integrated into the clause but that they are additional information. The postverbal noun phrases cannot be analyzed as right-dislocation within the clause, but must be seen as a kind of appositive attached to the clause.[4]

     Example (10) (Lipan Apache) is different from the other two examples in that both the direct object of the verb ('shoes') as well as the instrumental expression are expressed postverbally and the verb is not marked by a narrative particle. Although it is the only example found, it still demands explanation, since the word order in this example seems to be a true VO ordering within a single clause.

     But even more interesting than postverbal alternations are the preverbal alternations, since the preverbal occurrences of noun phrases might be more clearly integrated into the clause and still not show SO order.

5.2.2 Preverbal Domain

Alternative word order in the preverbal domain—that is, OS order instead of SO order—is also very rare (except in the form of the voice-related inversion, as discussed in chapter 2, this volume). A Lipan Apache example is the following (Hoijer 1975:11):

(11) *áshị* *diłkałí* *biniist'ạ'íí* *diłkałíłbaihii* *áshị* *chíshzhinii* . . . .
    Then   cedar   3.POSS.fruit juniper   and   blackwood
        áí   **kónitsạạhịị** *yiłda'gooyạ.*
        those Lipan   3S.3O.p.eat
    'The Lipan ate the fruits of the cedar, the juniper and the blackwood . . . .'

In this Lipan example, the clause starts out with a sequence of object noun
phrases, followed by the subject noun phrase *áí kónitsạạhịị* 'those Lipan,' resulting in an OSV order (the pronominal object marking is exactly the same as to
be expected in a SOV clause). The only other examples of OSV order exhibit
the same clausal structure as example (11): heavy coordinated object noun
phrases—that is, several noun phrases, all in object function—are conjoined by
an enumeration. This suggests that there is a constraint against heavy object
noun phrases in the nuclear SOV construction, with an obligatory left dislocation of the conjoined expression.

5.3 Particles

The rigidity of SO order might still be sensitive to topicalizing or emphatic
particles. It is conceivable that by an explicit marking of a constituent in question an alternation in order should be possible. Jicarilla and Lipan make extensive use of such topicalizing particles in conversation, but they are less frequent
in narratives.

(12) *dáá'ko'a* *bí-'a* *dághe'iikaas-na*[5]
    then   3-PART   3S.run-NARR
    'Then he ran in.' (Hoijer n.d.:3(24))

(13) *Shọ́di* *shạ́ạ́yá-'a*   *gołni-na.*
    Shọ́di 1sBEN.2sS.come-PART 3S.4O.said.NARR
    '"Friend, come visit me!" he said to him.' (Hoijer n.d.:4(11))

(14) *Da'ya'déé* *gọnị-'ạạ:*   *go'é*   *yenách'ijish'í* *go'é*   *daoda*
    Things   3.have-PART clothes 4S3O.put in clothes up
    naach'ijish'í-shị   *kooshk'e-go.*
    4S.3Oput-and   bed-PART
    'There is furniture: a closet to put your clothes up, and also a bed for each
    one.'

The emphatic particle *'ạạ* can attach to every constituent in the clause. But surprisingly there are no examples in the narratives in which the use of the emphatic, or topicalizing, particle can be shown to have any effect on a change in
word order when compared to the basic SOV order.

5.4   Stylistic Means

Although in narratives usually only one noun phrase occurs in the clause, this preference can be overridden by stylistic considerations of the narrator, as in the following example from Lipan Apache:

(15) **Kónitsąą-hįį** *dá'á'ii*   *ghánádaagodisíí.*
     Lipan-DEF   right.there   3S.travel
     'The Lipan traveled about just there.'

   Kónitsąą-hįį *áshį chishįįhįį   áshį gołgahįį   áníí*
   Lipan-DEF   then forest.people and plains.people they
                    gołdini ch'íłį-ná.
                    with.4   3.be-narr
   'The Lipan—then the Forest Lipan and the Plains Lipan were with them.'

   Kónitsąą-hįį *áshį'aa łi'   inaashii'įį bikíyaa   łi'   naanádaazą́.*
   Lipan-DEF   then   some Comanche 3.POSS.land some 3p.go again
   'Then some of the Lipan traveled to the country of the Comanche.'

   Kónitsąą-hįį *áko'a   doo-diłdaagooghí.*
   Lipan-DEF   then   NEG-3p.like
   'The Lipan did not like it.'

   Áko'aa   t'ą́ą́'shį kikíyaa'-ii   nádaajiiskah   kįłą́ii.
   Then   back   3.POSS.country-DEF   4.come again   Many.Houses
   'And then they returned back to their country, to Many Houses.' (Hoijer 1975:8)

This paragraph out of a longer narrative tells us about the customs and life of the Lipan Apache, who figure prominently at the beginning of several clauses above: *kónitsąąhįį* is repeated at the beginning of each clause. The clauses show a parallel construction with the subject (which in this case is also the topic) mentioned at the beginning, and then the comment—their specific doings—follows. But these expressions are not fully part of the core clause (as the postposed objects in 5.2.1): the clause combining conjunctions expressing subsequent events such as *áshį'aa* or *áko'aa* 'then' actually follow the initial noun phrase *kónitsąąhįį*.

Stylistic usages such as repetition and parallel construction—as exemplified in (15) above—must be considered a driving force in shaping discourse, and in turn shaping the structure of single clauses. Although no 'ungrammatical' constructions are used, the stylistic play still welcomes new formal collocations and may lead to new obligatory uses in the long run.

5.5   Conclusions

Although a language exhibiting obligatory pronominal inflection of subject and object is expected to have a pragmatically and not grammatically determined word order, Jicarilla Apache and Lipan Apache do not follow this constraint.

These Athabaskan languages show a quite robust SO order. Although there exists some variation within the preverbal and postverbal domain, these alternative orders are marked as being outside the core clause. Even topicalizing constructions do not break up this SO pattern.

The subject and object noun phrases can be analyzed as adjuncts to the pronominally inflected verb in Southern Athabaskan, but this does not enable a more flexible word order in discourse. This indicates that the relationship between pronominal inflection in the verb and word order is not as straightforward as it has been assumed. Further investigation of pragmatic structuring of naturally occurring data in Northern as well as in Southern Athabaskan will be necessary to establish deeper links between word order alternations and verbal structure.

Notes

I am very grateful to Mrs. Patricia Trivio, Mrs. Wilma Phone, and Mrs. Charlotte Vigil for sharing their expertise on the Jicarilla Apache language. The Lipan Apache language data are presented in Hoijer (1975). Initial research was supported by a grant from the Deutscher Akademischer Austauschdienst. Further research was supported by a grant from the American Philosophical Society. I would also like to thank the Library of the American Philosophical Society for kindly supporting my research.

1. The following abbreviations are used throughout the examples: s = singular, p = plural, 1, 2, 3, 4 = first, second, third, fourth/distant person, ALL = allative, BEN = benefactive, DEF = definite, DIST = distributive, EMPH = emphatic, INC = inceptive, NARR = narrative, NEG = negative, O = object, PART = particle, POSS = possessive, S = subject. Throughout the examples, the practical orthography is used.

2. Unless otherwise marked, the example sentences are taken out of Jicarilla Apache narratives collected on various fieldwork occasions (1993–96).

3. This ranking according to an animacy hierarchy (humans precede nonhumans, living beings precede objects) has been described for Navajo (Young and Morgan 1987:205a). The detailed semantics triggering the inversion must be investigated language-specifically (cf. Shayne 1982).

4. See Thompson (Chapter 10, this volume) for an in-depth discussion of the function of postposed noun phrases in Koyukon Athabaskan.

5. Hoijer transcribed this particle consistently as 'a, but it seems to correspond exactly to the modern particle 'ąą.

References

Baker, Mark C. 1996. *The Polysynthesis Parameter*. New York: Oxford University Press.

Hale, Kenneth. 1992. Basic Word Order in Two Free Word Order Languages. In Doris L. Payne (ed.), *Pragmatics of Word Order Flexibility*, pp. 63–82. Amsterdam: Benjamins.

Hoijer, Harry. n.d. Jicarilla Texts. American Philosophical Society Library, Philadelphia. Unpublished manuscript.

Hoijer, Harry. 1975. The History and Customs of the Lipan, as Told by Augustina Zua-
  zua. *Linguistics* 161:5–38.
Jelinek, Eloise. 1984. Empty Categories, Case and Configurationality. *Natural Lan-
  guage and Linguistic Theory* 2:39–76.
Jelinek, Eloise. 1989. Argument Type in Athabaskan: Evidence from Noun Incorpora-
  tion. Unpublished manuscript, University of Arizona.
Mithun, Marianne. 1992. Is Basic Word Order Universal? In Doris L. Payne (ed.),
  Pragmatics of Word Order Flexibility, pp. 15–62. Amsterdam: Benjamins.
Rice, Keren. 1989. *A Grammar of Slave*. Berlin: Mouton de Gruyter.
Saxon, Leslie and Keren Rice. 1993. On Subject-Verb Constituency: Evidence from
  Athapaskan languages. In *Proceedings of the West Coast Conference on Formal
  Linguistics,* 11:434–50
Shayne, Joanne. 1982. Some Semantic Aspects of yi- and bi- in San Carlos Apache. In
  Paul Hopper and Sandra A. Thompson (eds.), *Studies in Transitivity*, pp. 379–407.
  New York: Academic Press.
Young, Robert W., and William Morgan. 1987. *The Navajo Language: a Grammar and
  Colloquial Dictionary*. Albuquerque: University of New Mexico Press.

6

THE NEGATIVE/IRREALIS CATEGORY
IN ATHABASKAN-EYAK-TLINGIT

Jeff Leer

In this chapter I survey the morphology and semantics of the Athabaskan-Eyak negative and the Tlingit irrealis. Sections 6.1-6.3 describe the morphology of these verbal categories and describe the salient features of their syntax and/or semantics. Section 6.4 presents a morphological comparison of the verbal morphology in Athabaskan-Eyak-Tlingit (AET). Sample verb conjugations are given in section 6.5. Section 6.6 addresses the problem of how to reconstruct the Athabaskan negative imperfective stem of open roots. In section 6.7, I reconstruct a PAET negative particle *(ʔ-)łeʔ, arguing that it is by origin a negative form of the verb 'to be.' In section 6.8, I discuss briefly the PAET perfective/stative suffix and its lack in the negative/irrealis categories and verbal nouns. Sections 6.9 and 6.10 argue that the Tlingit "nonassertive" verbal categories (gerundive, subordinative, and decessive) are by origin nominalized verb forms and discuss the semantic connection between the Tlingit irrealis and the non-assertive verbal categories. In section 6.11, I comment on the connection between perfectivity and the negative/irrealis morphology in AET.

6.1 The Athabaskan Negative

The original Athabaskan negative is reconstructible from Northern Athabaskan languages in Alaska (Ahtna, Dena'ina, Ingalik, Holikachuk, Koyukon, Upper

Kuskokwim, Lower Tanana, Tanacross, Upper Tanana, and Biblical Canadian Gwich'in) and British Columbia (Witsuwit'en, Carrier, Chilcotin). Fossilized negative stative verb forms occur also in Chipewyan and the Slave dialect complex. Morphologically, the negative is marked by a combination of

1. One of two prefixes, which I will call the glottal-negative prefix and the s-negative prefix, respectively.
2. Lack of the perfective/stative prefix PA *$(\eta^y)\vartheta$- < Pre-PA *$(\eta)i$- (~I-element of D-type classifiers, see section 6.4).[1]
3. Lack of the perfective/stative suffix PA *$(-\eta^y)$ < Pre-PA *$-(\eta)i$ (see sections 6.8).
4. The suffix PA *$-l$ < Pre-PA *$-l$, in the negative perfective only.
5. The negative suffix PA *$-(h)e\cdot$, originally an enclitic.[2]

In some languages an independent negative particle (Ahtna *?ele?* and Biblical Canadian Gwich'in *?əlìt*, Tanacross *k'á*, and Upper Tanana *k'à·*) or preverbal proclitic (e.g. Witsuwit'en *we=*, Carrier *ł(ə)=*, and Chilcotin *ła=*) occurs in addition to the negative morphological marking on the verb.

The two negative prefixes are in complementary distribution with each other: the glottal-negative prefix occurs in the perfective and stative imperfective: PA *$i'\cdot$-/*ϑ'- < Pre-PA *$?i$- ~ *$i?$- (postvocalic allomorph); and the s-negative prefix occurs elsewhere: PA *$z\vartheta$-/$s\vartheta$- ~ *s- (allomorph with Ø subject prefix) < Pre-PA *$s\vartheta$- ~ *s- (allomorph with Ø subject prefix).

6.1.1 Complementary Distribution of the Negative Prefixes

Both the negative prefixes are in complementary distribution with the perfective/stative prefix PA *$(\eta^y)\vartheta$ - < Pre-PA *$(\eta)i$-. Furthermore, the glottal-negative prefix is in complementary distribution with the perfective/stative suffix PA *$(-\eta^y)$ < Pre-PA *$-(\eta)i$, i.e. PA *$-\eta^y$ ~ Ø (postconsonantal allomorph) < Pre-PA *$-\eta i$ ~ *$-i$ (postconsonantal allomorph). It is worth emphasizing that the perfective/stative prefix and the perfective/stative suffix are identically reconstructible in Pre-PA and PAET—namely as *$(\eta)i$—and that both the prefix and the suffix are in complementary distribution with the glottal-negative prefix.

The negative prefixes are also in complementary distribution with the 'conjugation markers'; that is, the prefixes that mark perfective and imperfective type, namely the s-perfective/imperfective prefix (PA *$z\vartheta$-/$s\vartheta$- ~ s- < Pre-PA *$s\vartheta$- ~ *s-), the n-perfective/imperfective prefix (PA *$n\vartheta$- < Pre-PA *$n\vartheta$-), and the γ-perfective prefix (PA *$\varkappa\vartheta$- < Pre-PA *$\varepsilon\vartheta$-). The choice of conjugation marker that the verb takes in the affirmative perfective and imperfective is therefore not reflected in the negative perfective and imperfective. For example, the affirmative forms of the following pair of verbs are distinguished solely by choice of conjugation marker (γ-perfective for 'to go up out' vs. s-perfective for 'to climb up'); this distinction is neutralized in the negative forms.

AFFIRMATIVE	NEGATIVE
qa'·=ʁə-ŋ^y^{ə}-ya·	*qa'·=hi'·-ha·l-e·*
'he/she went up out'	'he/she didn't go up out'
qa'·=sə-ya·	*qa'·=hi'·-ha·l-e·*
'he/she climbed up'	'he/she didn't climb up'

The negative prefixes do not occur at all with the s-perfective/imperfective prefix nor with the n-perfective/imperfective prefix. Although they do not occur with the γ-perfective prefix (PA *ʁə- < Pre-PA *ɢə-), the s-negative prefix does cooccur with the progressive prefix (also PA *ʁə- < Pre-PA *ɢə-). The only schetic (tense-mode-aspect) prefixes that can cooccur with a negative prefix are the progressive prefix (PA *ʁə- < Pre-PA *ɢə-), the optative prefix (PA *ʁʊ- <Pre-PA *ɢu-), and the inceptive prefix (PA *tə -). Tables 6.1 and 6.2 sum up the

TABLE 6.1. *Affirmative and Negative Prefixes*

	Affirmative		Negative
	Conjugation (Marker)	Perfective/Stative (Prefix)	Negative (Prefix)
s- perfective	*zə/s(ə)-	*(ŋ^y)ə-	*i'·-
n- perfective	*nə-	*(ŋ^y)ə-	*i'·-
γ-perfective	*ʁə-	*(ŋ^y)ə-	*i'·-
Ø- stative imperfective	*(ŋ^y)ə-	*(ŋ^y)ə-	*i'·-
s- stative imperfective	*zə/s(ə)-	*(ŋ^y)ə-	*i'·-
s- active imperfective	*zə/s(ə)-	—	*zə/s(ə)-
n- active imperfective	*nə-	—	*zə/s(ə)-
Ø- active imperfective	—	—	*zə/s(ə)-

TABLE 6.2. *Optative and Progressive Prefixes*

	Schetic (Prefix)	Negative (Prefix)	Schetic (Prefix)
Optative	*ʁʊ-	*zə/s(ə)-	*ʁʊ-
Progressive	*ʁə-	*zə/s(ə)-	*ʁə-

correspondences between the affirmative and negative prefix combinations for the various PA tense-mode-schetic-aspect categories.

The future is formed by adding the inceptive prefix *tə - to the progressive forms given above, so that the affirmative future is marked with the prefixes *tə - plus *ʁə-, and the negative future is marked with the prefixes *tə - plus *zə/s(ə)- plus *ʁə -.

6.1.2 Person-Marked Forms of Negative Paradigms

Tables 6.3 through 6.6 summarize the person-marked forms of the negative paradigms in most of the languages that have preserved the original negative paradigms.[3] The forms cited are with Ø-classifier, and without conjunct prefix. In most languages, the voicing alternation posited for the PA prefix *zə/sə - has disappeared—as in the s-perfective—with the reflex of the voiced allomorph *zə - being generalized, but in Witsuwit'en and Chilcotin the voicing alternation is preserved so that the nonperfective negative prefix combinations with first- or second-person subject are voiced where preceded by a conjunct prefix.

In Tanacross and Upper Tanana, the negative perfective/stative imperfective paradigm is comparable with that of the rest of the languages, but the negative nonperfective paradigms have been restructured in a striking fashion. The prefixes used are the same as those for the affirmative paradigms except that they are tonally marked. There is no trace of the s-negative prefix. The Biblical Canadian Gwich'in forms are not well enough attested to provide complete paradigms, although the forms that have been found appear comparable with those given in Table 6.3.

TABLE 6.3. *Negative Perfective and Negative Stative Imperfective*

	3.	1.sg.	2.sg.	1.pl.	2.pl.
PA	*i'·-	*ə'$-	*ə'ŋʸə- (or *i'·ŋʸə-?)	*i'·+D-	*ə'χʷ- = *ʋ'χ-
Ahtna	i-	es-	i-	—	oh-
Deg Hit'an	e-	əs-	en-	—	əχ-
Koyukon	i-	əs-	in-	—	αχ-
L. Tanana	i-	əs-	i-	—	ʋχ-
Tanacross	í·-	ìh-	ín·-	—	áh-
Biblical Can. Gwich'in	ì·-	ìh-	ìn-	?	òh-
Witsuwit'en	i-	is-	in-	idə+D-	ixʷ-
Carrier	i-	əs-	in-	í+D-	əh-
Chilcotin	i-	es-	en-	í+D-	eh-
Chipwyan	í-	és-	ín-	í+D-	úh-

TABLE 6.4. *Negative Active Imperfective*

	3.	1.sg.	2.sg.	1.pl.	2.pl.
PA	*əs-	*sə$-	*səŋʸə-	*si'·-D-	*səχʷ-
Ahtna	s-	His-[4]	zis-	—	Huh-
Deg Hit'an	əθ-	ðəs-	ðe-	—	ðəχ-
Koyukon	əɬ-	ləs-	li-	—	lαχ-
L. Tanana	əθ-	ðəs-	ði-	—	ðʋx-
Witsuwit'en	əs-	səs-	sen-	sdə+D-	səxʷ-
Carrier	əs-	zəs-	zin-	zi+D-	zəh-
Chilcotin	eŝ-	ses-	ŝin-	ŝi+D-	ŝeh-

TABLE 6.5. *Negative Optative*

	3.	1.sg.	2.sg.	1.pl.	2.pl.
PA	*ʁʊs-	*səʁʊ$-	*səʁʊŋ^yə-	*səʁu'·-	*səʁʊχ-
Ahtna	Hos-[5]	zʁos-	zʁus-	—	zuh-
Koyukon	ʁʊł-	ləʁʊs-	ləʁu-	—	luχ-
L. Tanana	ʁʊθ-	ðəʁʊs-	ðəʁu-	—	ðuχ-
Witsuwit'en	us-	sos-	son-	s(o)də+D-	soh-
Carrier	us-	zus-	zon-	zo-	zuh-
Chilcotin	ŵeŝ-	sus-	ŝeɣun-	ŝeɣú+D-	ŝuh-

TABLE 6.6. *Negative Progressive*

	3.	1.sg.	2.sg.	1.pl.	2.pl.
PA	*ʁəs-	*səʁə$-	*səʁəŋ^yə-	*səʁi'·-	*səʁəχ^w-
Ahtna	Has-	zʁas-	zʁis-	—	zuh-
Koyukon	ʁəł-	ləʁəs-	ləʁi-	—	luχ-
L. Tanana	ʁəθ-	ðəʁəs-	ðəʁi-	—	ðuχ-
Witsuwit'en	is-	sɛs-	sɛn-	s(ɛ)də+D-	sɛx^w-
Carrier	əs-	zis-	zan-	za-	zih-
Chilcotin	ɣeŝ-	sas-	ŝeɣin-	ŝeɣí+D-	ŝeh-

6.1.3 The Athabaskan Negative Prefixes

The s-negative prefix is formally similar to the s-perfective prefix, but there are several important differences between them:

1. The s-negative prefix always has the allomorph *s- in the third person, whereas the s-perfective prefix has the allomorph *s- in the third person (a) before the D-type classifiers (*də- and *lə-/łə-) and (b) following a conjunct prefix and before the classifier *ł-. Elsewhere the s-perfective prefix is PA *zə-/sə- < Pre-PA *sə-.

2. The s-perfective (as well as the n-perfective) requires PA constriction (which develops into tonal marking in those Athabaskan languages that have tone) and/or lengthening of the vowel of most conjunct prefixes immediately preceding the perfective prefix. Neither constriction nor lengthening occur after the 'peg' prefix *hə-[6] and the 'deictic subject' prefixes *qə- (third person human plural), *tš"ə- (human indefinite), and *k"ə- ~ *ʔə- (nonhuman indefinite, also an object prefix). Other object prefixes require constriction, but in most languages there is no evidence of lengthening.[7] Other conjunct prefixes require both constriction and lengthening: prefixal *Cə > *Ceʼ· (rather than *Ciʼ·). The s-negative prefix requires neither constriction nor lengthening of the vowel of any preceding prefix. For further discussion and useful data relative to this extremely complex phenomenon, see Rice (1983), Rice (1985), Rice and Hargus (1989), and Hargus (1989).

   The differences between these prefixes are rather complex and subtle, especially in the third person forms. Table 6.7 provides reconstructions for the PA third- person forms for each of the four classifiers, both without a conjunct prefix and with the conjunct prefix *tə- (inceptive).

TABLE 6.7. *Proto-Athabaskan Third-Person Forms*

	S-perfective		S-negative	
	No conjunct prefix	Inceptive prefix *tə-	No conjunct prefix	Inceptive prefix *tə-
*Ø-	*sə-	*teʼ·zə-	*həs-	*təs-
*ł-	*səł-	*teʼ·sł-	*həsł-	*təsł -
*də-	*həsdə-	*teʼ·sdə-	*həsdə-	*təsdə-
*lə-~łə-	*həsłə-	*teʼ·słə-	*həsłə-	*təsłə-

3. The s-negative prefix has the added peculiarity that the third-person allomorph **s-* follows a progressive or optative prefix, thus always occurring immediately before the classifier; whereas the non-third-person allomorph PA **zə-/sə-* < Pre-PA **sə-* precedes a progressive or optative prefix. The s-perfective prefix cannot co-occur with a progressive or optative prefix, and therefore has no such distributional peculiarity; it always precedes the subject prefix.

In all known languages that retain the original Athabaskan negative morphology, the glottal-negative prefix is formally identical with the transitional prefix and the semelfactive non-perfective prefix. In Northern Athabaskan, these prefixes share the peculiarity that in the absence of other schetic prefixes, the full vowel allomorph **i'·-* occurs only where the subject prefix is zero. Where there is a non-zero prefix, these prefixes take the form of constriction on the vowel preceding the subject prefix; there is no difference in vowel length. As seen in table 6.3, for example, the form with 1.sg. subject and zero classifier appears as **ə'$-* rather than **i·$-*. At present I have no explanation for this fact.

6.2 The Eyak Negative

The Eyak negative is morphologically a combination of the following:

1. The schwa-negative prefix *ə-* (Krauss' prefix position 6, before the subject prefix), in the negative active perfective.
2. The glottal-negative prefix *ʔ-* (Krauss' prefix position 8, but always occurring before the subject prefix),[8] in the negative neuter imperfective and perfective.
3. Lack of the neuter prefix *yi-* (Krauss' prefix position 8, after the subject prefix).
4. The variant s- of the perfective prefix (Krauss' prefix position 8, after the subject prefix), in the negative perfective active.
5. A negative circumfix consisting of the negative particle *dik'* 'not' or other negative word plus the negative suffix *-ɢ* (Krauss' suffix position 3, after the derivational and aspectival suffixes).

6.2.1 Affirmative and Negative Verb Prefix Paradigms

The Eyak affirmative and negative verb prefix paradigms are distinguished only in the active perfective and in the neuter imperfective and perfective; these paradigms are shown in Tables 6.8 and 6.9. Otherwise, negative forms are indistinguishable from affirmative forms except for the fact that they have the suffix *-ɢ*; however, this suffix can conveniently be regarded as part of the negative circumfix and hence

TABLE 6.8. *Active Perfective, Neuter Imperfective, and Perfective*

	Classifier		$\emptyset$-	də-
Neuter Imperf. & Perf.	Affirmative	3.&2.sg.	(ʔi)yi-[9]	(ʔi)di-
		1.sg.	(ʔi)xi-	(ʔi)xdi-
		2.pl.	(ʔi)ləχi-	(ʔi)ləχdi-
	Negative	3.&2.sg.	(ʔa)ʔ-	(ʔa)ʔdə-
		1.sg.	(ʔa)ʔx-	(ʔa)ʔxdə-
		2.pl.	(ʔa)ʔləχ-	(ʔa)ʔləχdə-
Active Perfective	Affirmative	3.&2.sg.	sə-	sdi-
		1.sg.	si-	xsdi-
		2.pl.	ləχsə-	ləχsdi-
	Negative	3.&2.sg.	(ʔə)s-	(ʔə)sdə-
		1.sg.	(ʔə)xs-	(ʔə)xsdə-
		2.pl.	ləχs-	ləχsdə-

TABLE 6.9. *Realis and Irrealis Stems*

		Realis	Irrealis
Stative imperfective and telic perfective	open	/ÿ/	/ʔ/
	closed	/ÿ/	/ˀ/
Active imperfective and future	/·/	/ˀ/

syntactically extraneous to the verb (see the following section for further discussion).

Table 6.8 gives forms for the $\emptyset$- and *də* -classifiers. Forms for the *ł*-classifier are obtained simply by adding this classifier to the right of the prefix combinations for the $\emptyset$-classifier, and forms for the *łə* -classifier are obtained by substituting *ł* for the d of the *də* -classifier.

6.2.2 *Negative Particles and Pronouns*

Eyak negative verb forms occur primarily in conjunction with the following negative particles and pronouns:

(dǝ=)k'udǝχ   'no way; can't'
(dǝ=)k'udu·   'nobody'
(dǝ=)k'ude·   'nothing'
dik'   'no; not' (apparently < *dǝ=k'u, according to Krauss, personal communication)

The negative particle *dik'* occurs either before a focused phrase (NP or PP) in initial position, in which case it negates the focused phrase, or in core-clause-initial position,[10] in which case the scope of negation is the entire clause. In the former case, the focused phrase is preceded by *dik'* and followed by *-G*. In this case the verb of the core clause takes affirmative rather than negative morphology. This fact can be explained as follows. First, the combination *dik'* plus *-G* constitute a negative circumfix which may bracket either a focused phrase or the core clause.It follows that *-G* cannot occur unpaired with *dik'*. Therefore, if a focused phrase is negated with *dik'* plus *-G*, the verb of the core clause cannot take *-G*, since this extra *-G* would be unpaired. Furthermore, *-G* is an integral part of the formal marking of the negative verb. Verbs that cannot be marked with *-G* are thus prohibited from taking any negative marking and thus appear in their affirmative form.

6.3   The Tlingit Irrealis

The Tlingit irrealis is both semantically and morphosyntactically more complex than the Athabaskan and Eyak negatives. Semantically, the primary use of the irrealis is to form negatives, but irrealis morphology is also required in dubitative and optative constructions.

The Tlingit irrealis is morphologically a combination of

1. The irrealis prefix *ʔu-* ~ *(u)`-* (postvocalic allomorph) (Leer's order +4).
2. Lack of the I-element of the classifier except in the potential mode and in attributive verb forms (used as the heads of relative clauses).
3. With both open and closed verb stems, a variety of patterns of distinctive stigmatic marking in various schetic categories (see Table 6.9.).

In the prohibitive and optative constructions, the optative suffix *-((ÿ)i`)G* (Leer's order -5) occurs. This is cognate with the Eyak negative suffix *-ǝ*, but is not part of the irrealis morphology in Tlingit. The cases where irrealis stems differ from realis stems as mentioned in (b) above are summarized in the table 6.9.

The realis stative imperfective and telic perfective suffix /ÿ/ is manifested as (1) -· (lengthening of the vowel) in open stems; (2) Ø with stem vowel reduction, in closed stems. The irrealis stative imperfective and telic perfective suffix for open stems /ʔ/ is manifested as: (1) Ø (i.e. lack of a stigma, which means that the stem-final vowel is short) word-finally; (2) the stigma ' before the decessive suffix *-(ÿ)i`n*; (3) the stigma ' before other suffixes of the form *-(ÿ)i`(C)*; (4) the stigma · before the optative suffix *-G*. See Leer (1991) for details.

The irrealis prefix, henceforth to be referred to as /u-/, is subject to a number of important co-occurrence restrictions, which seem to be phonologically conditioned. It therefore does not occur with subject pronominal prefixes containing high vowels, namely 2.sg. /i(·)-/, 2.pl. /ÿi-/, 1.pl. /tu(·)-/, and indefinite human /du-/. It zeroes out with all subject pronominal prefixes except for 3. Ø- and 1.sg. /χa-/. The irrealis prefix is also zeroed out in the perfective mode, which is characterized by the perfective prefix /ÿu-/, and in the future mode, which is characterized by the prefix string /ga-ŭ-ɢa-/; both these modes contain prefixes with the high vowel *u*.[11] However, /u-/ does not zero out following prefixes with high vowels further to the left in the verb template, such as *dži-* 'hand', *tu-* 'inside; inner being, mind', and the areal prefix *qu-*.

6.3.1 Irrealis Forms in Tlingit

Morphologically irrealis verb forms occur in a variety of constructions in Tlingit, most of which require the negative particle *ł*.

6.3.1.1 Negative Clauses

The most common use of the Tlingit irrealis is in negative clauses, in conjunction with the negative particle *ł*; this particle occurs as

1. A preverbal proclitic *ł=* in dependent clauses.
2. Cliticized to the interjectional particle *tłé·k'* 'no' in independent clauses, resulting in the combination *tłé·k'=ł* (archaic, found in early sources and in songs) > *tłé·ł* ~ *tłéł* (standard) ~ *hé·ł* ~ *héł* (innovative, in Northern Tlingit) 'not'; this is an independent particle which occurs either preceding a focused phrase or in core-clause-initial position, like Eyak *dik'*.[12]

Compare:

yé· yati· 'it is so'
/ÿa-ti~-`/ CL[Ø, +I]-be-`[13]

tłé·ł yé· ʔu-tí 'it isn't so'
/ʔu-Ø-ti~-ʔ/ IRR-CL[Ø, -I]-be-ʔ

ʔawsikú· 'he/she knows him/her/it'
/ʔa-ÿu-si-ku~-ÿ/ 3.OBJ-PERF-CL[s, +I]-know-ÿ

tłé·ł ʔawuskú 'he/she doesn't know him/her/it'
/ʔa-ÿu-sa-ku~-ʔ/ 3.OBJ-PERF-CL[s, -I]-know-ʔ[14]

ʔas ʔí· 'he/she is cooking it'
/ʔa-sa-ʔi~-·/ 3.OBJ-CL[s, -I]-cook-·

tłé·ł ʔu`s ʔí` 'he/she is not cooking it'
/ʔa-u-sa-i~-`/ not 3.OBJ-IRR-CL[s, -I]-cook-`

6.3.1.2 Dubative Independent Clauses

Irrealis verb forms occur also in dubative independent clauses, in conjunction with

1. The independent particle *gʷáł* 'maybe, perhaps', to be analyzed *gʷá=ł*,
   where *=ł* is the negative particle cliticized to the particle *gʷá* (perhaps 'How
   could it be?', probably an allomorph of the interjection and enclitic *gʷá·*
   'Wow!; is that so?!'); like *tłé·ł* (etc.) 'not', this occurs in main-clause-initial
   position.

gʷáł yé· ʔutí 'maybe it is so'
gʷáł ʔawuskú 'maybe he/she knows him/her/it'

2. A family of compound enclitics composed of the yes/no-interrogative clitic
   =gí followed by a demonstrative clitic such as *=wé* 'that' or *=yá* 'this'. Such
   compound enclitics have the meaning 'I guess . . . ; I suppose; it must be that
   . . .'. Note that this is the only irrealis construction that does not contain the
   negative particle *ł*. Furthermore, the irrealis form of the verb is used only
   where the enclitic precedes the verb.

yé·=gíwé ʔutí 'I guess it is so'
ʔawsikú·=gíwé 'I guess he/she knows him/her/it'
wé ša·wád=gíwé ʔawuskú 'I guess he/she knows the woman'

3. In a few rare constructions with the particle *gʷá*, with or without the particle
   ł. The only examples I have to date are

gʷá tš'a=du+ʔí`n kaχʷani`g 'I shouldn't have told her'
how.could.it.be ipse=3.ANIM+with I.told.3.[IRR]
(from Elizabeth Nyman notes)
ł=yé·=gʷá ʔad+ʔuhá·yi 'Such a thing has never happened before.'
NEG=thus=how.could.it.be
INDEF.INAN+3.came.to.be.situated.[IRR].[DEC].[ATTRIB]
(from a song transcribed from Charlie Joseph by his daughter Ethel Makinen
for the Sitka Native Education Program).

For many Tlingit speakers, however, realis verb forms can be used instead of irrealis forms in the case of 1 and 2. Nevertheless, the use of irrealis forms is clearly the older and more conservative practice.

6.3.1.3 Prohibitive and Optative Constructions

The irrealis occurs also in the prohibitive and optative constructions, in conjunction with the suffix *-((ÿ)i`)G* and the negative particle *ł* cliticized to a particle in main-clause-initial position:

1. *(ʔi)ḱ* 'don't!' plus *=ł* yields *(ʔi)ḱ=ł* 'don't . . .!', the mark of the prohibitive construction.

2. *guʔa*[15] plus *=ł* plus optional *=gušé ~ =gʷšé* 'I wonder' yields *guʔa'=ḱ=gʷšé)* 'Would that S; I wish that SUBJECT would VP', the mark of the optative construction. It appears that the optative construction is historically derived from a rhetorical question construction meaning 'I wonder how it could be the case that SUBJECT not VP?'

ḱ=ł yé· ʔutí·G 'let it not be so'
guʔa'=ḱ=gʷšé) yé· ʔutí·G 'I hope it is so'

Note in connection with this construction two Eyak optative constructions. First is the Eyak optative construction *tłaʔh-kih k'aʔ* (plus optative verb form) 'would that...', as in *tłaʔh-kih k'aʔ ʔixiʔeh* 'I wish I were married'. Here *-kih* is the diminutive suffix and *k'aʔ* is a particle meaning 'It would be a good thing that...; please do...'. Second is the Eyak construction *tła·qiʔ-P* (plus optative verb form, and where -P is a postposition) 'if indeed such a place does exist', as in *tła·qiʔ-tš' da·ʔi·ʔaʔtš'* 'let's go at least <u>somewhere</u>' and *tla·qiʔ-tš'ahd giyah ʔixdilah* 'where ever would I get any water to drink?' (lit. 'whence if such a place does indeed exist, would I drink water?'). Here *qiʔ(-P)* is a proclitic particle meaning 'place where ...'.[16] The morphemes *tłaʔh* and *tła·* are evidently related to each other, and are two of only four basic morphemes in Eyak with the phoneme *tł*. In the two remaining morphemes we find clues that Eyak *tł* comes from earlier **ł*: (1) *(dǝ -)tłi· ~ łi·* 'already, by then', and (2) *Ø-tłeʔχ* '(fish) swims rapidly, slithers', comparable with PA **Ø-le'·ʁ* '(fish) swims' (< Pre-PA **Ø-łeʔχ*). It thus seems within the realm of possibility that Eyak *tłaʔh* and *tła·* could ultimately be (at least in part) comparable with Tlingit *ł=*. However, these optative constructions in Tlingit and Eyak are by no means directly comparable, and no such conclusion can be drawn without first clarifying the historical evolution of these constructions.[17]

6.3.1.4 The irrealis prefix /u-/

The irrealis prefix /u-/ is also required in certain of the schetic categories called 'modes' in Tlingit, namely the potential and the admonitive. The potential typically translates as 'might, could' in English, and the admonitive occurs in constructions translating 'be careful/watch out or SUBJECT might VP; be careful not to let SUBJECT VP' and 'lest . . .' in English.

   1. Potential:
     yé· ʔunɢati`* or *yé·nɢʷati` 'it might/could be so'
     /u-na-ɢa-ti~-`/ IRREALIS-ASPECT-ɢa-be-`

   2. Admonitive:
     yé·=tsé ʔunatí· 'be careful not to let it be so' (with enclitic *=tsé*)
     yé· ʔunatí·ɢa`* 'lest it be so' (with postposition *-ɢa`)
     /u-na-ti~-·/ IRREALIS-ASPECT-be-·

6.3.1.5   General Remarks

In general, then, the irrealis category in Tlingit is used in negative and dubitative constructions.[18] Note, however, that at least some enclitics with what could be considered dubitative meanings such as *=šágdé·* 'perhaps, probably' and *=gʷšé* 'isn't that so?; huh?', do not require irrealis marking on the verb. Nor, for that matter, does the yes/no question enclitic *=gí ~ =gé*. This fact seems to imply that 'dubitative' is not a fixed semantic category but rather that there is a semantic gradient with respect to forms with meanings that semanticians may be tempted to class together as dubitatives. Apparently, then, Tlingit *gʷá=ł* 'maybe, perhaps' and *=gí=DEM* 'I guess . . .; I suppose . . .; it must be that . . .' fall on the more strongly dubitative end of this gradient and therefore require irrealis marking, whereas the aforementioned enclitics are only weakly dubitative and do not require irrealis marking. It would be an interesting challenge for semanticians interested in categories that have been characterized as 'irrealis' to see if it is possible to find a system of logical operators that can account for the attested distributions of meanings and semantic functions associated with irrealis marking among the languages of the world.

6.3.2   Irrealis Verb Morphology

In Tlingit as in Eyak, particles requiring irrealis verb morphology, such as *tłé·ł* 'not' and *gʷáł* 'perhaps', may precede focused phrases, in which case the scope of negation is the negated phrase. Unlike Eyak, however, Tlingit requires irrealis marking of the verb of the core clause even if only the focused phrase is negated. Compare, for example:

Tlingit:
     tłé·ł ša·wád ʔawuskú [not woman 3.knows.3.irrealis]
     'He doesn't know a woman.', 'He has never experienced a woman.'

tlé·ɬ ʔawuskú wé ša·wád [not 3.knows.3.irrealis that woman]
'He doesn't know the woman.'

tlé·ɬ wé ša·wád= ʔáwé ʔawuskú. [not that woman=FOCUS 3.knows.3.
IRREALIS]
'It's not that woman that he knows.'

Eyak:
dik' qe ʔɬ ʔu ʔla ʔɬga·-G-iʰ [not woman 3.knows.3-NEG-HUMAN.SING]
'He doesn't know a woman.'

dik' ʔəv qe ʔɬ ʔu ʔla ʔɬga·-G-iʰ [not that woman 3.knows.3-NEG-
HUMAN.SING]
'He doesn't know the woman.'

dik' ʔəv qe ʔɬ-G-q'uʰ ʔu ʔli·ɬgah [not that woman-NEG-
FOCUS.HUMAN.SING 3.knows.3]
'It's not that woman that he knows.'

6.4 The Athabaskan-Eyak-Tlingit Negative

The Athabaskan-Eyak negative and the Tlingit irrealis are morphologically comparable, as shown by Table 6.10.

A striking feature of the AET negative/irrealis perfective/stative forms is the lack of both the PAET perfective/stative prefix and the PAET perfective/stative suffix. The PAET perfective/stative prefix is reflected in Tlingit as the I-element of the classifier. In Athabaskan-Eyak, it manifests itself as the I-element of classifiers having the D-element, but as the perfective/stative prefix PA *(ŋʸ)ə -, Eyak *(y)i-* before classifiers lacking the D-element (see Krauss 1969 for the analysis of the Athabaskan-Eyak-Tlingit classifier system).[19] The PAET perfective/stative suffix will be discussed further in section 6.8.

Note also that the Tlingit irrealis prefix /u-/ occurs in all modes except for the perfective and future (where it is apparently deleted for phonological reasons, as mentioned in section 6.3). On the other hand, Pre-PA *ñ- ~ *-iʔ- and Eyak ʔ-, which appear to be cognate to the Tlingit irrealis prefix /u-/, occur only in the negative stative imperfective (in both Athabaskan and Eyak) and in the negative perfective (in Athabaskan). It is difficult to draw conclusions from this disparity in distribution, but one possibility is that the PAET glottal-negative prefix was originally confined to the negative perfective/stative, as in Athabaskan(-Eyak), but was generalized as an irrealis marker in Tlingit.

The origin and synchronic function of the Eyak negative perfective prefix *ə -* presents a real challenge. First, note that this prefix occurs only word-initially and zeroes out after a prefix. A homomorphic prefix *ə -* occurs also in negative neuter imperfectives, in neuter perfectives, optatives, and imperatives, and in a subset of

TABLE 6.10.   *Comparison of Negative/Irrealis Morphology in AET*

	Pre-PA	Eyak	Tlingit
	*ʔi- ~ *iʔ-	ʔ-	/u-/ ʔu- ~ (u)ʻ- (irrealis)
Prefix	—	ə-	—
	*s(ə)-	—	—
Lack of perfective/ stative prefix	Yes	Yes	Yes, except in attributive verb forms
Stem Stigma			
Neuter Imperfect	*Ø	—	/ʔ/
Perfect	*Ø	—	`
Perfective Suffix	*-ł	—	—
Suffix	—	-ɢ	-((ÿ)iˋ)ɢ (prohibitive/optative)
Enclitic	*=he·	—	—
Particle	*(ʔi)łeʔ	—	ł (negative)

affirmative neuter imperfectives. A similar prefix *i-* (which also zeroes out after a prefix) occurs in the Eyak gerundive, a nonproductive type of verbal noun that takes the unique suffix *-l* after open roots. A subset of the gerundives also takes the prefix *s-*, which appears to be an allomorph of the s-perfective prefix–the same allomorph, in fact, that occurs in the third person and second person singular negative perfective. Compare, for example:

Affirmative perfective:	*sə -dah-ł* 'it is sitting'
Negative perfective:	*dik' ʔə -s-dah-ł-ɢ* 'it is not sitting'; 'you are not sitting'
Gerundive:	*ñ-s-da·-l* 'sitting', e.g. in *ʔisda·l ɢəłəde ʔłiʰh* 'he (baby) is learning to sit'

The striking similarity between the prefix combinations found in the third person negative perfective *ʔə -s-* and the gerundive *ñ-s-* suggests that they might have a common origin. Perhaps the negative perfective prefix /ə-/ (word-initially appearing as *ʔə -*) was originally */i-/ (word-initially appearing as *ñ-*), identical with the gerundive prefix. If so, this prefix might have been identical with Pre-PA

ʔi- (the word-initial variant of the Pre-PA glottal-negative prefix *ʔi- ~ *(i)ʔ-). An important question remains, however. If both the Eyak schwa-negative prefix (in the negative perfective) and the glottal-negative prefix (in the negative neuter imperfective and perfective) are cognate with the Athabaskan glottal-negative prefix, why is there no trace of a glottal stop prefix in the negative perfective? In other words, if the original negative neuter had *ʔə- ~ *-ʔ-, why does the negative perfective show up as *ʔə-s-* word-initially but not as *ʔ-s-* after a *Cə-* prefix? I can offer no compelling answer to this question, and must therefore conclude that these two Eyak negative prefixes probably have different origins.

I recently discovered what is undoubtedly a rare survival of the original Athabaskan gerundive. This is the Navajo form *yisdá* 'sitting', which is found to my knowledge only in *yisdá nissin* 'to like to sit up (as a baby)' (Young and Morgan 1992, p. 756). The verb *nissin*, from PA *yəni·-Ø-zən* 'to have one's mind set (thus, on something)', occurs with other verbal nouns as well, e.g. Navajo *tša nissin* 'to feel like crying' with *tša* 'weeping', and *dlo nissin* 'to be jolly' with *dlo* 'laughter'; there are similar constructions in other languages. By comparing this one form *yisdá* with the Eyak cognate *ʔisda·l*, we can see that the PA gerundive was virtually identical in formation with that of Eyak (see Table 6.11).

Note that the initial *yi-* of *yisdá* is identical with the 'peg' prefix, from PA *hə-*. Note also that the reconstructed PA prefix *hə-s-* is exactly identical with the reconstructed third person negative prefix (not attested in Navajo). This evidence thus suggests that the prefix *ʔi-* in Eyak gerundives like *ʔisda·l* is not by origin a negative/irrealis prefix, but rather cognate with the Athabaskan 'peg' prefix. Note also in this connection that the Tlingit 'peg' prefix is *ʔi-*.[20] It further suggests that the prefix *ʔə-* in Eyak third person negative perfective (*ʔə-)s-*, like the prefix *hə-* of the PA third person negative imperfective *(hə-)s-*, is also the 'peg' prefix by origin. However, we are still confronted with the glaring paradox that the Eyak third person negative perfective prefix string looks just like the PA third person negative imperfective prefix string.

TABLE 6.11. *Comparison of Gerundives*

	Navajo	PA	Eyak
Affirmative perfective	sidá	*sə-da·	sə-dah-ł
Negative perfective	—	*h-i'·-da-he·	ʔə-s-dah-ł-ɢ
Gerundive	yisdá	*hə-s-da·	ʔi-s-da·-l

6.5   Affirmative/Realis and Negative/Irrealis Forms in AET

The formal differences between affirmative/realis and negative/irrealis forms in the AET languages is illustrated in the following selected paradigms of the active verb 'to say' and the stative verb 'to be lying (down)'. The verb 'to say' in Athabaskan-Eyak is based on the verb 'to have happen to one, to do', with the addition of the thematic prefix *də -*, which in this case refers to oral activity. The theme for 'to say' is (Pre-)PA *də -Ø-ni·*, Eyak *də -Ø-le~*. Tlingit has no cognate for this verb, but does have a cognate for 'to have happen to one', namely *Ø-ni~`*, cf. Eyak *Ø-le~*. All these verbs usually occur with one of a number of (often proclitic) adverbs of manner meaning, for example, 'thus' or 'how?'.

The Tlingit verb forms in Table 6.12 are not comparable with the corresponding Eyak forms for 'to happen' or 'to have happened to one' in several respects. First, the Tlingit verb theme belongs to the 'eventive' theme category and thus lacks a primary (i.e. simple) imperfective (see Leer 1991, chapter 7); the repetitive/customary imperfective is used to illustrate the irrealis morphology. Second, this theme, like all eventive themes, takes object (patient) inflection rather than subject (agent) inflection, so that the pronominal prefixes occur to the left of the schetic prefixes. Table 6.13 shows the Active/Perfective forms.

The Athabaskan stative imperfective forms illustrated by the verb 'to be lying' (Table 6.14) are by origin s-perfective forms. The Eyak cognate forms are still analyzable as perfective forms, but in most Northern Athabaskan languages, stative verbs such as this take the full array of modes (imperfective, perfective, optative, future), where the original s-perfective form assumes the role of the imperfective mode meaning 'is lying', and the perfective mode is supplied a γ-perfective form meaning 'was lying'.

The Tlingit forms in Table 6.15 are positional imperfectives (a subclass of active imperfectives; see Leer (1991), section 7.2.4) rather than stative imperfectives, and are therefore only partly comparable with the Athabaskan-Eyak forms. The Tlingit theme *Ø-ta~`* 'to sleep' is cognate with Eyak *Ø-te~* and (Pre-)PA *\*Ø-te·* 'to lie [conscious animate]', and the Tlingit theme *s-ta~`* is cognate with Eyak *ɬ-te~* and (Pre-)PA **ɬ-te·*, all of which mean 'to lie [dead or unconscious animate]' in their intransitive (AE stative, Tlingit positional) paradigms and 'to move [dead or unconscious animate]' in their transitive active paradigms.[21] I am a loss to explain the fact that these two themes assume different patterns of stem variation in Tlingit. The Eyak and Tlingit forms here are active forms meaning 'let me lie down', etc. in Eyak; and 'let me sleep', etc. (hortative), 'I might sleep', etc. (potential) in Tlingit. These are thus not comparable with the Athabaskan forms, which are stative, meaning 'let me be lying', etc.

TABLE 6.12. *Active Imperfective 'To Say'*

	Affirmative/Realis			Negative/Irrealis		
	1.sg.	2.sg.	3.sg.	1.sg.	2.sg.	3.sg.
PA	*dəʂniˑ	*dəŋ^yəniˑ	*(də)niˑ	*dəzəʂni-heˑ	*dəzəŋ^yəni-heˑ	*dəsni-heˑ
Ahtna	desniˑ	diniˑ	niˑ	diˑsneh	dizisneh	desneh
Deg Hit'an	dəsne	dene	ne	dəðəsneʔ	dəðeneʔ	dəθeneʔ
Koyukon	dəsni	dini	ni	dəlˀsneʔæ	delineʔæ	dəθneʔæ
Lower Tanana	dəsni	dini	ni	dəðəsneʔæ^nˆ	dəθineʔæ^nˆ	dəθneʔæ^nˆ
Tanacross	dihniⁿˑ	diⁿˑniⁿˑ	niⁿˑ	díhneⁿyˑˆ	díⁿˑneⁿyˑˆ	díˑneⁿyˑˆ
Alaskan Gwich'in	dihniaˑ	diⁿˑniaˑ	niaˑ	(lacking)	diðiⁿˑniaˑ	(lacking)
Canadian Gwich'in	dʒihnioˑ	dʒiˑnioˑ	nioˑ	diðihnioˑ	diðiˑnioˑ	dohnioˑ
Witsuwit'en	dəsni	dini	ni	we=dəzəsniʔ	we=dəziniʔ	we=dəsniʔ
Carrier	dəsni	dini	ni	ɬ=dəzəsnih	ɬ=dəzinih	ɬ=dəsnih
Chipewyan	desni	diⁿni	di, heni		(lacking)	
Navajo	dišní	díní	ní		(lacking)	
Hupa	diWneˑ	dinneˑ	neˑ		(lacking)	
Eyak 'to say'	dəxleh	diˑleh	dələh	dəxleˑɢ	diˑleˑɢ	dələˑɢ
Eyak 'to happen'	xleh	yileh	leh	xleˑɢ	yileˑɢ	leˑɢ
Tlingit 'to happen'	yuˑ=χad+ẏa	yuˑ=ʔiẏaniˑg	yuˑ=ẏaniˑg	yuˑ=χad+ʔuniˑg	yuˑ=ʔiˑniˑg	yuˑ=ʔuniˑg

TABLE 6.13. *Active Perfective 'To Say'*

	Afirmative/Realis			Negative/Irrealis		
	1.sg.	2.sg.	3.sg.	1.sg.	2.sg.	3.sg.
PA	*dəʁəyˤniʔ	*dəʁəɲʸəɲʸⁿniʔ	*dəʁəʁʸⁿniʔ	*dəˤʂniˑˑl-eˑ	*diˑˑŋʸⁿniˑˑl-eˑ	*diˑˑniˑˑl-eˑ
Ahtna	dʁasneʔ	dʁineʔ	dʁineʔ	desniˑle	diniˑle	diniˑle
Deg Hit'an	dəʁəsneʔ	dəʁenneʔ	dəʁeneʔ	dəsnel	denel	denel
Koyukon	dəʁəsniʔ	dəʁinniʔ	dəʁiniʔ	dəsnile	dinile	dinile
Lower Tanana	dəʁəsniʔ	dəʁinniʔ	dəʁiniʔ	dəsnilæⁿʌ	dinilæⁿʌ	dinilæⁿʌ
Tanacross	dihniⁿʔi	diⁿˑniⁿʔi	diⁿˑniⁿʔi	difhndiˑlʌ	diˤⁿndiˑlʌ	diˤⁿndiˑlʌ
Alaskan Gwich'in	diˑnìaⁿʔ	diⁿˑnìaⁿʔ	diⁿˑnìaⁿʔ		(lacking)	
Canadian Gwich'in	džìˑniʔ	džìˑniʔ	džiˑniʔ	džìhnìaˑ	džìˑnìaˑ	džìˑnìaˑ
Witsuwit'en	[disniʔ]	[diniʔ]	[diniʔ]	we=disnil	we=dinil	we=dinil
Carrier	disniʔ	daniʔ	daniʔ	ł=dəsnil	ł=dinil	ł=dinil
Chipewyan	deyiní	deyiⁿní	deyiⁿní		(lacking)	
Navajo	diˑniˑd	diˑníniˑd	diˑniˑd		(lacking)	
Hupa	diweˑneʔ	deˑnneʔ	deˑnneʔ		(lacking)	
Eyak 'to say'	disiłit	dəsełit	dəsełit	dəxsəłiɢ	dəsłiɢ	dəsłiɢ
Eyak 'to do'	siłit	sełit	sełit	ʔəxsəłiɢ	ʔəsłiɢ	ʔəsłiɢ
Tlingit	χad+wuˈniˈ	ʔiˈwaniˈ	wuˈniˈ	χad+wuniˈ	ʔiwuniˈ	wuniˈ

TABLE 6.14. Stative Imperfective 'To Be Lying (Down)'

	Affirmative/Realis			Negative/Irrealis		
	1.sg.	2.sg.	3.sg.	1.sg.	2.sg.	3.sg.
PA	*səyᵊte·ŋʸ	*səŋʸəŋʸᵊte·ŋʸ	*səte·ŋʸ	*hə`$te-he·	*hiʔ·ŋʸᵊte-he·	*hiʔ·te-he·
Ahtna	iste·n	zite·n	zte·n	ʔesteh	ʔiteh	ʔiteh
Deg Hit'an	ðəstaN	ðetaN	ðetaN	ʔəstaʔ	ʔentaʔ	ʔetaʔ
Koyukon	ɬəstæN	litæN	lətæN	ʔəstəʔæ	ʔintəʔæ	ʔitəʔæ
Lower Tanana	ðəstæN	ðitæN	ðətæN	ʔəstəʔænˆ	ʔintəʔænˆ	ʔitəʔænˆ
Tanacross	ðihte·ⁿ	ðinte·ⁿ	ʔe·te·ⁿ	ʔihte·y·ˆ	ʔínte·y·ˆ	ʔí·te·y·ˆ
Gwich'in	ði·tšiⁿ-	ðintšiⁿ-	ðitšiⁿ-	ʔihtšì·	ʔintšì·	ʔì·tšì·
Witsuwit'en	səstəy	sentəy	stəy	we=stɛh	we=ntɛh	we(y)tɛh
Carrier	səsti	sin ti	sti (Morice) (modern)	ɬ=əstoh	ɬ=intoh	ɬ=iteh
Chipewyan	θitiⁿ	θiʳtiⁿ	θɛtiⁿ		(lacking)	ɬ=itoh
Navajo	sétiⁿ	sínítiⁿ	sitiⁿ		(lacking)	
Hupa	se·tiŋ	sintiŋ	sitiŋ		(lacking)	
Eyak	siteɬ	səteɬ	səteɬ	ʔəxsteɬɢ	ʔəstehɬɢ	ʔəstehɬɢ
Tlingit: 'is sleeping'	χatá	ʔì`tá	tá	χʷatá	ʔì`tá	ʔutá
Tlingit 'is lying'	χasatá·n	ʔisatá·n	satá·n	χʷasata`n	ʔisata`n	ʔusta`n

TABLE 6.15. Stative Optative 'To Be Lying (Down)'

	Affirmative/Realis			Negative/Irrealis		
	1.sg.	2.sg.	3.sg.	1.sg.	2.sg.	3.sg.
PA	*ʁʊ$teʔ	*ʁʊɲjᵊteʔ	*ʁʊteʔ	*səʁʊ$teʔ-eˑ	*səʁʊɲjᵊteʔ-	*ʁʊsteʔ-heˑ
Ahtna	osteʔ	ʁuteʔ	oteʔ	zʁoteʔe	ʁusteʔe	osteʔe
Deg Hit'an	ʁostaʔ	ʁentaʔ	ʁetaʔ	ðeʁestaʔ	ðeʁentaʔ	ʁustaʔ
Koyukon	ʁostaʔ	ʁuntaʔ	ʁotaeʔ	leʁustaʔæ	leʁuntaʔæ	ʁotaʔæ
Lower Tanana	ɣostæʔ	ɣuntæʔ	ɣotæʔ	ðeɣustaʔænʌ	ðeɣuntaʔænʌ	ɣʊθtaʔænʌ
Tanacross	ɣuhteʔ	ɣunteʔ	ɣoteʔ	ɣúhtéʔᵛʌ	ɣúntéʔᵛʌ	ɣótéʔᵛʌ
Gwich'in	ʔoihtʃiʔ	ʔontʃiʔ	ʔoˑtʃiʔ	ðòihtʃiʔ	ðòntʃiʔ	ʔòhtʃiʔ
Witsuwit'en	ustɛʔ	untɛʔ	utɛʔ	we=sostɛʔ	we=sontɛʔ	we=stɛʔ
Carrier	husteʔ	honteʔ	huteʔ	łə=zusteʔ	łə=zonteʔ	ł=usteʔ
Chipewyan	ɣʷasté	ɣuⁿté	ɣʷaté		(lacking)	
			(Navajo and Hupa lacking)			
Eyak	yaʔ=ʔix	yaʔ=ʔiˑteʔ	yaʔ=ʔiˑteʔ		(lacking)	
Tlingit: hortative	naqata	naɢiˑta	naɢata or naɢʷata		naɢiˑta	ʔunɢata naɢʷata
Tlingit: potential or	ʔunqaˑt naqʷaˑt	naɢiyata	ʔunɢaˑta naɢʷaˑta	ʔunqata naqʷata	(same as affirmative)	

6.6 The Negative Imperfective Stem of Unsuffixed Open Roots

The reconstruction of the negative imperfective stem of unsuffixed open roots as *CV-he· in PA requires some comment. In some of the Alaskan Athabaskan languages (Deg Hit'an, Koyukon, Lower Tanana), the reflex of the negative imperfective stem plus enclitic is indistinguishable from the reflex of PA *CV ʔ-e·, as can be seen by comparing the reflex of the negative stative imperfective stems of 'to be lying' with the negative optative stems of the same verbs. In the other languages, however, the reflexes of these two stems are different. Glottal stop is crucially lacking in the negative stative imperfective stem in Tanacross and archaic Canadian Gwich'in, and both Ahtna and Carrier show clear evidence of PA *h rather than *ʔ. Note also that Ahtna and Carrier also have the reflex of reduced vowels before this *h. For this reason, I proposed in Leer 1979 that the negative suffix is to be reconstructed in PA as *-(h)e·, where the consonant *h appears only following an open stem. Furthermore, this consonant caused shortening of the stem vowel; that is, Pre-PA *CV·-he·> PA *CV-he·. This shortening is analogous to the shortening that occurs when *ʔ is suffixed to an open root: */CV· -ʔ/ > *CVʔ.

Why do Deg Hit'an, Koyukon, and Lower Tanana substitute glottal stop for *h? We should note that PA *h is a 'dummy' consonant that was probably added to vowel-initial stems where these were not preceded by a Cə- prefix, in which case Cə -V > CV. I also reconstruct the PA 'peg' prefix with this 'dummy' consonant *h. The reflexes of this 'dummy' consonant *h show a great degree of lexical variation. For example, the reflex of the *h of the 'peg' prefix is (nonphonemic) glottal stop in Alaskan and Pacific Coast Athabaskan languages, but in many Canadian languages it is h, and in Southern Athabaskan languages it is γ-. The reflex of the *h of a vowel-initial postposition such as PA *-(h)e·dən 'without', on the other hand, is glottal stop in virtually all languages that allow nouns to proceed postpositions without a resumptive pronoun. This is true in Koyukon and Gwich'in, languages where *h is preserved (and sometimes analogically extended) with vowel-initial nouns such as 'mother': PA *-(h)a·n, Koyukon -(h)ɔN, Gwich'in -han, and with vowel initial verb stems such as 'go [singular] {PROGRESSIVE}': PA *-(h)a·ɬ, Koyukon -(h)ɔɬ, Gwich'in -ha·. Thus Koyukon and Gwich'in have glottal stop for the reflex of *h in the 'peg' prefix and the postposition 'without', but preserve *h in the forms cited above. The negative suffix *-(h)e· (possibly historically related to PA *-(h)e·dən 'without') shows yet another pattern of reflexes for *h. Here the languages which have glottal stop as a reflex for *h, including Koyukon, also have the same reflex in the 'peg' prefix and the postposition 'without'. Only Ahtna and Carrier demonstrably have retained the *h of the negative suffix, this despite the fact that e.g. Ahtna has glottal stop as the reflex for the reflex of *h in the 'peg' prefix and the postposition 'without'.

6.7 Reconstruction of a PAET Negative Particle

The third-person negative stative imperfective form of the verb 'to be' can be reconstructed for PAET as *ʔɬeʔ 'it is not'. This is the source of the Pre-PA particle *(ʔ)ɬeʔ 'not'. It moreover seems probable that the Tlingit negative particle *l* is by origin a contraction of the prohibitive interjectional particle *(ʔi)ḵ* 'don't!', which is a phonologically perfect cognate with Pre-PA *(ʔi)łeʔ.²² See Table 6.16.

Although this particle is by origin the third person negative imperfective of 'to be', it appears to have been lexicalized as a particle meaning 'not' during the PAET stage. In none of the modern languages is it equivalent to a form meaning 'it is not'. The PA form with this meaning, for example, is reconstructable as *ʉi'·le-he·, hence Ahtna *ʉileh*, Koyukon *ʉiləʔœ*, Biblical Canadian Gwich'in *ʔi·li·*, Carrier (Morice) *ł=iləχ*, (Modern) *ł=iloh*.²³ The Eyak clause *dik' ʔaʔłe·ɢ* or *dik' ʔəłe·ɢ* 'it is not' /dik' ə-(ʔ-)łe·-ɢ 'not NEUTER.NEG-be-NEG'/ is likewise comparable with but not a direct cognate of this particle.²⁴

The longer form of Tlingit *ʔiḵ* 'don't!' is directly comparable with Central and Lower Ahtna *ʔeleʔ* 'not' and Canadian Gwich'in *ʔəlìt* (minus the final *-t*). The basic form underlying what is found in the Western and Mentasta dialects of Ahtna seems to be *liʔi*, which appears to have a suffix *-i*; this suffix could in turn have assimilated the stem vowel, i.e. *leʔ-i > liʔi. Both the contracted form of Tlingit *ḵ* 'don't!' and the Tlingit negative particle *l* are directly comparable with the Carrier negative preverbal proclitic *ł(ə)=*. The stem vowel correspondence PAE *e : T *i* is amply attested elsewhere, and that the final stigma correspondence PAE *ʔ: T Ø is amply attested with inalienably possessed nouns and with the negative/irrealis stigma Pre-PA *ʔ : T /ʔ/ (Ø ~ ' ~ ` ~ ·); see the chart in section 6.3 and the discussion of T /ʔ/ in the following paragraph. The phonological match between

TABLE 6.16. *AET Negative Particles and 'To Be' Forms*

		Prefix	Stem
		NEG	'to be'
Tlingit		(ʔi-)	łí
PAET		*(ʔi-)	łeʔ
Pre-PA		*(ʔi-)	łeʔ
Ahtna (Central, Lower)		ʔe-	leʔ
Ahtna (Western)			liʔ [-]i
Ahtna (Mentasta)		q'a	liʔ ([-]i)
	or	q'a	li·
Biblical Canadian Gwich'in		ʔə-	lì [-]t
Kaska		ʔe-	lá·
Carrier			ł(ə)=
Chilcotin			ła=
Galice			łah 'don't'
(Eyak		ʔə-(ʔ-)	łe·-ɢ)

TABLE 6.17. *V? Forms in Tlingit and Eyak*

Tlingit	Eyak	PA	
		Possessive form	Compounding form
+kú 'tail (of bird, fish)'	-ka? 'tail (of bird)'	*-kʸe? 'tail'	*-kʸe·-
+łú 'nose, point'	-ła? 'point, tip'	*-la? 'point, tip'	*-la·-
+tú 'inside (of deep container)'		*-ta? 'among'	*-ta·-
+tá 'head (of bay)' and +tá·(-g) 'bottom (of vessel, body of water)' cf. the preverbal proclitic	ta?= 'into water'	*ta'·= <*ta?= 'into water'	
+χ'é '(outer) mouth'	-q'a? 'edge'	*-q'a? 'edge'	
+šá 'head'	-tsiⁿ? 'neck'	*-tsi? 'head'	*-tsi'·- < *-tsi?-

the Athabaskan and Tlingit forms of this particle is thus perfect. However, note that Kaska *?elá·*, Chilcotin *ła=*, and Mattole *łah* 'don't' have the vowel *a*, which does not correspond to the vowel attested elsewhere. I have no explanation for the discrepancy in the vowels here. It is possible, however, that the vowel found in these forms is due to a suffix or enclitic added to the original particle—note also the as yet inexplicable suffixes in Ahtna *li ʔi* and Biblical Canadian Gwich'in *?əlìt*.

Another area of the lexicon where Tlingit stem-final V is found to correspond to PAE *V? is among possessed nouns (usually inalienable nouns) of the shape Tlingit +CV : PAE *-CV?. These are shown in Table 6.17. Here PAE(T) *-?is the postvocalic allomorph of the possessive suffix PAE(T) *-ə?. The stem form is usually underlyingly PAE(T) *CV·; this is attested as such in the Athabaskan compounding form of the noun.

6.8 The Perfective/Stative Suffix

The perfective/stative suffix, as mentioned previously, is reconstructible for Pre-PA and PAET as *-(ŋ)i. Only Athabaskan and Tlingit show overt reflexes of this suffix as seen in Table 6.18.

The Tlingit reflex of the PAET perfective/stative suffix is found in the realis telic perfective, in the telic perfective habitual, and in the realis stative imperfective. Its distribution may be more clearly seen in Table 6.19.

TABLE 6.18. *Perfective/Stative Suffix*

	Open stem	Closed stem
PAET	*-ŋi	-i
Pre-PA	*-ŋi	-i
PA	*-ŋ^{y25}	$\emptyset^{26}$
Tlingit	-·(ÿ)^{27}	$\emptyset^{28}$

TABLE 6.19. *Tlingit Suffixes*

Tlingit	Realis	Irrealis
Telic perfective 'it has gotten fat'	ʔuwatá· /ÿu-ÿa-ta-ÿ/	wutá /ÿu-ta-'/
Telic perfective habitual 'it (always) gets fat'	ʔutá·ÿdž /u-ta-ÿ-dž/^{29}	ʔutá·ÿdž /u-ta-ÿ-dž/
Stative imperfective 'it is good'	ÿak'é· /ÿa-k'e-ÿ/	ʔuk'é /u-k'e-ʔ/

From these examples, it can be seen that the stem variation in the telic perfective and stative imperfective of most Tlingit variable open verb stems is identical. I propose that this verb stem variation reflects rather closely that of the PAET stative. Compare, for example, the above Tlingit stative imperfective forms in Table 6.19 with the corresponding forms in PA, shown in Table 6.20.

What is remarkable about these Tlingit and PA stative imperfective forms is that they point toward a PAET reconstruction where both affirmative and negative stative imperfective forms had similar or identical prefixes and suffixes. The affirmative stative imperfective form had the stative/perfective prefix *(ŋ)i- and the stative/perfective suffix *-(ŋ)i. The negative stative imperfective form appears to have had the glottal-negative prefix * ñ- and to have lacked the stative/perfective suffix.

The correspondence would be even more perfect if the PA negative had the suffix *-ʔ, as does the Tlingit irrealis stative for many open stems. Although some Athabaskan languages do show a glottal stop in the negative stative imperfective stem of open verb roots, I argue in section 6.6 that this glottal stop comes from the negative suffix *-he· and is not historically part of the stem. Nor does Eyak show any sign of a suffix *-ʔ in the negative neuter imperfective. However, the reconstructed form PAET ñ-łeʔ 'not' < 'it is not' discussed in section 6.7 does have a glottalized stem. I therefore suspect that the Tlingit stem variation here

TABLE 6.20. *PA Stative Imperfective 'It is good'*

PA	Affirmative	Negative
Stative imperfective	*$*ŋ^y$əžu·ŋ^y$	*hi'·žu-he·
'it is good'	/ŋ^yə-žu·-ŋ^y/	/i'·-žu·-he·/

closely mirrors the PAET stem variation, and that the lack of *-$?$ in Athabaskan-Eyak here is innovative.

Further evidence in support of this hypothesis can be gotten by examining verbal nouns derived from stative verbs with open stems. Such verb stems are extremely rare; for PA we can cite only one example: PA *$*šu?$ 'goodness, beauty', also found as an adjectival enclitic =$žu?$ 'good, beautiful': Ahtna *su?-dze?* 'beautifully, nicely' and =$zu?$ 'good, pretty, handsome', Koyukon *su?* 'goodness' and =$zu?$ 'good', Gwich'in =$zu^n?$ 'good', Carrier *?əzu?, nzu?* 'goodness' and =$?əzu?$ 'good, fine', Chipewyan *sú-γá* 'good, all right, well' and *sú-dí* 'fun, laughable', Navajo *žò^n?* 'joy, fun thing'.[30] The semantically and morphologically corresponding (but not cognate) Tlingit form is *k'é* /k'e-?/ 'goodness', also found as an adjectival enclitic in the form *?a·-k'é* 'good one', where it is cliticized to the indefinite nominal *?a·* 'one'.

6.9 Tlingit Gerundives

The most productive class of Tlingit verbal nouns, called gerundives, resemble irrealis verb forms in all ways except that they lack the irrealis prefix /u-/. Specifically, like irrealis verb forms, they lack the I-element of the classifier, and where the irrealis verb stem differs from the realis stem, they take the irrealis stem. Two other verbal categories share these characteristics with the gerundive: the subordinative and the decessive. The subordinative is formed with the suffix /-(ÿ)i·/ (which is homomorphic with the possessed noun suffix); it is a quasi-nominal form that takes the free range of subject and object pronominals like a verb, and occurs with all the independent verb modes (tense-aspect categories of the verb), but functions syntactically as a complementized clause, forming PPs with certain postpositions and functioning as the possessor in constructions with certain relational nouns such as *?íd* 'place after/following'. The gerundive, in contrast, is not inflectable, and can occur in a possessive construction just like other common nouns. Compare, for example

Realis verb:
    yak'é· 'he/she/it is good'
Irrealis verb:
    g^wáł ?uk'é 'maybe he/she/it is good'
Gerundive:
    k'é 'goodness'
    du+k'e·-yí· (3.POSS+goodness-POSS) 'his/her goodness'

Subordinative:

    k'e·yí· 'the fact that he/she/it is good'

    k'e·yí·-dž 'because he/she/it is good'

    (*-dž* is the ergative postposition, also meaning 'because of' in some contexts)

Realis verb:

    ʔawsikú· 'he/she knows him/her/it'

    ʔad-wusikú· 'he/she knows things'

    (with the indefinite non-human object pronominal *ʔad+*)

Irrealis verb:

    gʷáł ʔawuskú 'maybe he/she knows him/her/it'

    gʷáł ʔad+wuskú 'maybe he/she knows things'

Gerundive:

    ʔad+wuskú 'knowledge'

    du+ ʔad+wusku·-wú· (3.POSS+knowledge-POSS) 'his/her knowledge'

Subordinative:

    (*yak'é·*) *ʔawusku·wú·* '(it is good) that he/she knows him/her/it'

    ʔawusku·wú·-dž 'because he/she knows him/her/it'

    ʔawusku·wú·-dáχ 'after he/she knows/knew him/her/it' (*-dáχ* 'from')

    ʔawusku·wú·-de· 'until he/she knows/knew him/her/it' (*-de·* 'to, toward')

    ʔawusku·wú+ ʔíd-náχ 'after he/she knows/knew him/her/it'

    (*ʔíd* 'place after/following, *-náχ* 'along')

The decessive is formed with the suffix *-(ÿ)i`n*. In general, the decessive denotes a situation that was true in the past (relative to the time denoted by the verb mode) but is no longer true. Like the subordinative, the decessive occurs with all the independent verb modes.

Imperfective:

    yak'é· 'he/she/it is good'

Decessive imperfective:

    k'é·yi·n 'he/she/it was good, used to be good (but is no longer good)'

Perfective:

    wu·k'e· 'he/she/it became good'

Decessive perfective:

    wuk'é·yi·n 'he/she/it had became good (but is no longer good)'

Future:

    ke·=gʷɢak'é· 'he/she/it will be/become good'

Decessive future:

    ke·=gʷɢak'é· yi·n 'he/she/it was going to be/become good (but no longer will)'

Perfective:

    ʔawsikú· 'he/she knows him/her/it'; 'he/she has come to know, has become acquainted with him/her/it'

Decessive perfective:

> *ʔawuskú·wu·n* 'he/she knew him/her/it, used to know him/her/it (but no longer does); he/she had come to know, had become acquainted with him/her/it (but no longer knows him/her/it)'

Future:

> *ʔaguχsakú·* 'he/she will know, become acquainted with him/her/it'

Decessive future:

> *ʔaguχsaku· wú· n* 'he/she was going to become acquainted with him/her/it (but no longer will)'

Habitual perfective:

> *ʔu·skú·wdž* 'he/she knows him/her/it (on every occasion)'

Decessive habitual perfective:

> *ʔu·skú·wdži·n* 'he/she used to know him/her/it (on every occasion, but no longer does)'

Potential:

> *ʔu·χsikú·* 'he/she might/could know him/her/it'

Decessive potential:

> *ʔu·χsakú· wu· n* 'he/she might/could have known him/her/it (but the possibility no longer exists)'

The attributive form of the decessive, i.e. the form added to the clause-final verb of a relative clause, usually immediately preceeding the head noun, lacks the final stigma plus n:

Attributive Perfective:

> *ʔawsikuwu qá·* 'a person that he/she/it knows'

Attributive Decessive Perfective:

> *ʔawuskú·wu qá·* 'a person that he/she used to know'

The subordinative and decessive are not mutually exclusive; their combination is expressed by adding the decessive enclitic =*yíyi·* /=ÿi·ÿi`/ to the subordinative form. This enclitic is also added to nouns, in this case meaning 'former, ex-':

du+šád 'his wife'
du+šád=yí·yi· 'his former wife, ex-wife'

ʔawusku·wú·-dž 'because he/she knows him/her/it' (subordinative)
ʔawusku·wú·=yí·yi·-dž 'because he/she used to know him/her/it' (subordinative decessive)

It seems probable that the decessive suffix /-(ÿ)i`n/ is by origin a shortened and morphologically reinterpreted version of the decessive enclitic =*ÿi·ÿi`*. The steps involved would be the shortening of /=ÿi·ÿi`/ to /=ÿi·ÿ/, the substitution of /n/ for the final /ÿ/,[31] and finally, the reinterpretation of this form as a suffix, so that it resembles other suffixes of the form /-(ÿ)i`(C)/.

A rather complex set of facts lends further support to this historical scenario. The possessed noun suffix /-(ÿ)i`/ appears to be cognate with the PA possessed noun suffix */-(ə)ʔ/. Here it would seem that the Tlingit stigma /ˈ/ corresponds to the PA stigma /ʔ/. I have already argued in section 6.6 that Tlingit stems of the shape /CV/ are historically derived from PAET stems of the shape /CVʔ/. When the possessive suffix is added to these stems, the result is /CV`-ÿi·/. The same is true of the subordinative suffix, which is phonologically identical with the possessed noun suffix.

However, when the decessive suffix is added to a verb stem of the shape /CV/, the result is /CVʔ-ÿi`n/ rather than /CV`-ÿi·n/. My hypothesis is at an early stage of Pre-Tlingit; both the stem and possessive suffix ended with glottal stop. There then arose in Pre-Tlingit a rule of glottal dissimilation, whereby the original */ʔ/ of *CVʔ stems was replaced by /ˈ/ before suffixes ending in a glottal stop, such as the possessive suffix. Subsequently, the glottal stop of the possessive suffix was also replaced by /ˈ/. This led to a further dissimilation rule, this time one operating rightward rather than leftward: the /ˈ/ of the possessive suffix, and in fact of all suffixes of the shape -(ÿ)i`(C), was replaced by /·/ after a stem with the stigma /ˈ/. Hence the modern Tlingit reflex /CV`ÿi·/ for this sequence. However, the original glottal stop of *CVʔ stems was not replaced by /ˈ/ before the decessive morpheme by the first glottal dissimilation rule, probably because it was at this time an enclitic rather than a suffix.[32] Therefore the original *ʔ of *CVʔ stems was preserved before the decessive morpheme. And in fact it was preserved only in this environment, since it was replaced by /ˈ/ before suffixes of the form /-(ÿ)i`(C)/ other than the decessive suffix, by /·/ before postpositions and suffixes of the form /-C/, and word-finally it zeroed out. Thus it is only in a decessive form such as (Northern Tlingit) *k'é· yi· n*, (Henya-Sanya Tlingit) *k'ê· yin*, (Tongass Tlingit) *k'eʔyin*, all from underlying /k'e-ʔ-(ÿ)i`n/ that the original glottal stop suffix of the irrealis verb stem is overtly realized as such, even if only in one now-extinct dialect of Tlingit.

There is strong external comparative evidence for this internal comparative hypotheses. The Tlingit decessive enclitic/suffix is undoubtedly cognate with the PA enclitic ≈ *=nəʔənə, whence Koyukon *=nəʔəN*, Sekani *-iⁿ*, Chipewyan *=niⁿ*, Navajo *-(y)éⁿeⁿʔ*, and Hupa *ne ʔin* //nəʔənə//. When added to nouns (most typically kin nouns) it usually means 'deceased'. In some languages it also occurs with a clausal verb. In Hupa, it forms a 'past tense' with a meaning similar to that of the Tlingit decessive. In Navajo, it functions as a relativizing enclitic denoting that the situation denoted by the verb in the relative clause is in the past relative to the time of the clause in which the relative clause is embedded; in other words, it has virtually the same function and meaning as the Tlingit decessive attributive. It seems likely, then, that the decessive construction was originally formed by adding the decessive enclitic to the nominalized form of the verb (that is, to a form identical to the subordinative but without the subordinative suffix /-(ÿ)i`/),[33] and that it evolved into its present form due to the remodeling of the decessive enclitic into a suffix when it immediately followed a verb stem.

6.10 The Gerundive and Subordinative

The gerundive and subordinative can thus be seen as more or less completely nominalized verb forms. The gerundive is clearly a category that can be identified as a verbal noun, whereas the subordinative functions as a dependent clause that is syntactically nominal in that it can function as the object of a postposition or the possessor of a possessed noun. Although the decessive synchronically functions as a dependent clause type, I argue in the preceding section that it evolved from the subordinative form of the verb (minus the suffix *-(ÿ)i`*) followed by the decessive enclitic. To capture the fact that these verb forms are all morphologically similar to the irrealis forms except that they lack the irrealis prefix /u-/, I found it useful to create the cover term "nonassertive" for these verbal categories. The term assertive therefore refers to the category of verbal forms that are not non-assertive, namely forms that are not gerundive, subordinative, or decessive. The irrealis/non-assertive category is definable by the lack of the I-element of the classifier, and the irrealis/non-assertive verb stem.[34] The irrealis category also requires the irrealis prefix. These characteristics are summed up in Table 6.21.

What do the non-assertive categories have in common with the irrealis category? I will propose as a working hypothesis that these categories, in general, share the semantic property that the embedded predication is in some way not asserted as being true. Thus, in the case of the irrealis, we find predications where the truth of a proposition is asserted, but the truth of the predication embedded within the proposition is not asserted as definitely true. The negative proposition 'it is not the case that P,' although making an assertion, does not assert that P is true. Likewise, dubitative propositions like 'maybe it is the case that P' or 'I guess it is the case that P' express reservations on the truth of P. The Tlingit optative construction, which requires the irrealis verb form, means 'I hope it is the case that P,' where again, the truth of P is not being asserted. The gerundive form is a verbal noun that might be paraphrased as 'the fact/quality of P,' where nothing is asserted. The subordinative form is always embedded in a higher predication whose truth is being asserted, but the truth of the proposition stated by the subordinative form is not explicitly being asserted. Finally, the decessive form can be paraphrased as 'it was but no longer is the case that P,' where the truth of P is not being asserted as true at the present time, or more precisely, at the time that the speaker has established as the effective now-point.

TABLE 6.21. *Tlingit Classifiers*

	Irrealis Prefix	Classifier	Stem
Realis assertive	—	±I	Realis assertive
Realis nonassertive	—	-I	Irrealis/nonassertive
Irrealis	u-	-I	Irrealis/nonassertive

6.11 Perfectivity and the Negative/Irrealis Morphology in AET

Although the formation of Athabaskan and Eyak verbal nouns is not as productive
and well-attested as that of Tlingit, the generalization holds that such verbal nouns
lack both the perfective/stative prefix and the perfective/stative suffix. One
example discussed in section 8 is PA *šuʔ* 'goodness'. Examples from Eyak are
easier to come by:

> Eyak *k'ahd* 'sickness, pain'; cf. *yi-k'ahd* 'he/she/it is sick, in pain'
> cf. Tlingit *ní·g*ʷ 'sickness, pain'; cf. *ÿa-ní·g*ʷ 'he/she/it is sick, in pain'
> and Navajo *di-ni·h* 'pain, ache'; cf. *di-ni·h* 'he/she/it is sore, aches, hurts'[35]

> Eyak *dǝ-tše·-l* 'hunger'; cf. *di-ši-tšeʔ-ł* 'I am hungry'
> cf. Navajo *di-tšin* 'hunger'

The Athabaskan-Eyak gerundive with prefix *s-* mentioned in section 4 allows
us a glimpse into the complex mystery of the Athabaskan-Eyak *sǝ-* perfective
prefix. We lack the space here to go into detail on this topic. However, it seems
quite likely that this prefix was originally composed of two elements: ≈ **s- and
**(ŋ)i-, the perfective/stative prefix. Where **(ŋ)i- was absent, the result was just
≈ **s-; but where both elements were present, the result was ≈ **si-, which shows
up in PA as *sǝ-/zǝ-* and in Eyak as *sǝ-*.[36] It would seem quite reasonable to infer
that the Athabaskan-Eyak gerundive with s- was originally the identical with the
s-component of the s-perfective, without the perfective/stative prefix **(ŋ)i-. Here
again, we see that the verbal noun lacks the perfective/stative prefix.

6.12 The Perfective/Stative Prefix and Suffix

More generally in AET, we have seen that the perfective/stative prefix (PAET
(ŋ)i-) and suffix (PAET *-(ŋ)i*) occur only in finite affirmative/realis verb forms.
They do not occur in negative/irrealis forms, nor do they occur in verbal nouns, nor
in forms that were presumably non-finite by origin. The correlation between degree
of perfectivity and degree of verbhood is hardly surprising. What is perhaps more
interesting is the correlation between the perfective and stative categories in AET.
In my dissertation (Leer 1991), I argue that two semantic operators are necessary
to account for the Tlingit perfective: PAST and RESULT. That is, the Tlingit realis
perfective asserts not only that a situation occurred in the past, but that the state
resulting from this occurrence persists into the present. In both Tlingit and Eyak,
the perfectives of event verbs (i.e., roughly, verbs containing the BECOME
operator) assert both the past event and the state resulting from the event, e.g. the
perfectives Tlingit *wudixʷédl*, Eyak *sǝgaʔł-iʾh* 'he/she became tired; he/she is
tired'. This was undoubtedly true also for PAE, as shown by comparisons such as
Eyak *sǝdahł-iʾh* 'he/she sat down; he/she is sitting' and the cognate PA *sǝda·*
'he/she is sitting'. The Eyak form is a perfective, and the PA form is morphologically identical with a perfective, but by PA times had been formally reinterpreted

as a stative imperfective—specifically, a subtype which we may call the s-stative imperfective so as to distinguish it from the Ø-stative imperfective to be discussed in the next paragraph.[37] We may thus conclude that for PAET event verbs, the perfective form had both past tense and resultative stative readings.

Athabaskan, Eyak, and Tlingit all have a class of state verbs (i.e., roughly, verbs containing the BE operator), whose imperfective asserts a state without reference to a past event. In Eyak and Tlingit, these verbs have stative imperfectives that differ formally from perfectives. Athabaskan state verbs have two major types of stative imperfective, the s-stative imperfective (historically derived from the s-perfective) discussed in the preceding paragraph, and the Ø-stative imperfective, which is not formally identical with any of the perfective types. The Eyak and Tlingit stative imperfectives and the Athabaskan Ø-stative imperfective all have similar morphological structures. First, they take the reflex of the the PAET stative/perfective prefix *(ŋ)i- but lack the prefixes that are specific to the perfective proper, namely Tlingit /ÿu-/, Eyak s(ə)-, and PA *zə/s(ə)-, *nə-, *ʁə-. In Athabaskan and sometimes in Tlingit they take the reflex of the PAET stative/perfective suffix *-(ŋ)i, but in Eyak they not only lack an overt reflex of this PAET suffix but also lack the Eyak perfective suffix -ł. Examples of this stative imperfective are Tlingit *ÿadáł* /ÿa-dał-ÿ/, Eyak *yida·s* /(y)i-da·s/, PA *ŋʸəda'·z /(ŋʸ)ə-da'·s-(ŋʸ)/ 'it is heavy'; Tlingit *ÿa-k'é·* /ÿa-k'e-ÿ/, PA *ŋʸəǰu·ŋʸ /(ŋʸ)ə-ǰu··(ŋʸ)/ 'it is good'; Eyak *yiłeh* /(y)i-łe/, PA *ŋʸəle·ŋʸ /(ŋʸ)ə-le··(ŋʸ)/ 'it is'. Such verbs thus exhibit the general morphological characteristics of the PAET perfective/stative but lack characteristics that are specifically perfective. Semantically, these verbs denote states that do not imply an event from which the state resulted, so that, for example, none of the forms cited above have the readings 'it became heavy', 'it became good', 'it became'. They are thus both morphologically and semantically distinct from the perfectives with resultative stative readings described in the last paragraph.

To sum up the discussion this far, then: the PAET perfective/stative affixes are found both in affirmative/realis perfectives and in affirmative/realis stative imperfectives. AET perfectives may both assert past action and present state resulting from past action (in the case of event verbs), whereas AET stative imperfectives assert present state, but not that the state results from past action (in the case of state verbs). It would thus be misleading to characterize both these categories either as simply "perfective"–thus implying that completed action is characteristic of both categories–or as simply "stative"–thus implying that present state is characteristic of both categories. This is why I have adhered to the cumbersome practice of referring to these affixes as "perfective/stative" in this chapter, rather than using the more common terms "perfective prefix" and "perfective suffix."

Nevertheless, the fact that these affixes are shared in common by perfective and stative imperfective verb forms leads us to wish to ascribe some common semantic feature to these categories. So does the fact that PA uses the glottal-negative prefix for the negatives of both these categories, whereas it uses the s-negative prefix for all other negatives.

If the perfective/stative affixes had an original common semantic factor which mirrored their formal characteristics, it must have been stativity rather than perfectivity. Stative imperfectives denoted states, and perfectives denoted past events and actions with persistent resultant state. The preceding formal analysis of the morphology of the AET perfective/stative affixes thus strongly suggests that PAET affirmative/realis perfectives necessarily implied resultant state, not just with event verbs, but with all active verbs, as is the case in Tlingit. For example, a PAET verb meaning 'I made it' would imply that the made object was still in existence and functioning, evaluated from the viewpoint of the speaker's now-window. If the made object were no longer in existence and functioning, then the corresponding PAET decessive form would be used, consisting of a nominalized form of this verb plus the decessive enclitic, just as its direct descendant is used in Tlingit. In other words, if form mirrored meaning in PAET, then Tlingit more or less faithfully reflects the correlation between stativity and verbhood inherited from AET, rather than the more well-known and universal correlation between perfectivity and verbhood.

And ultimately, at a time too far in the past to see clearly from our viewpoint, the PAET perfective/stative prefixes and suffixes we have studied here probably originated as auxiliary verbs:

Pre-PAET $\approx$ **ŋi 'is'
Pre-PAET $\approx$ **ʔi 'is not'

But that is another story.

Notes

Throughout this essay, I use the notation (C) to designate a consonant that occurs in the postvocalic allomorph of a prefix, suffix, or clitic; the postconsonantal allomorph lacks this consonant. A few other notational and terminological innovations used here depart from those usually found in writings about the Athabaskan languages. The symbol = represents clitic boundary and # represents word boundary; in Tlingit, + represents an incorporate/compound boundary. The symbol ~ after a Tlingit or Eyak verb root means that the root has variable stigma (glottal marking); ~ followed by a stigma indicates the type of stigmatic marking that characterizes the variation. For more on Tlingit, see Leer 1991, chapter 5. The symbol $\approx$*(*) denotes an approximate reconstruction, one that is indeterminate to some degree. AET classifiers are notated by indicating the classifier components, so that in Athabaskan, for example, D- represents the "d- classifier" and l-D-represents the "l-classifier." And finally, the term *stative* here has its universally understood sense. Athabaskanists have long used the more obscure term *neuter* to refer to a stative verb form; I depart from Athabaskanist tradition on this point.

1. The Athabaskan negative suffix PA *-*(h)e·* appears to be related to the postposition PA *-*(h)e·-dən* 'without'. The form PA **k'ʸ-e·-dən* 'without something/anything' is comparable with the Eyak adverb *k'a·dih* 'absent'.

2. The initial consonant of the 'peg' prefix is omitted from these paradigms, namely in all the negative perfective/stative forms and in the third person negative active imperfective, since it is more of a hindrance than a help to visualizing the data. The Alaskan Athabaskan forms were provided by Jim Kari and Michael Krauss (p.c.), supplemented by Jetté's

grammar in the case of Koyukon and Kari's Ahtna Dictionary in the case of Ahtna (Kari 1990). The Gwich'in forms have not yet been thoroughly documented, but are still found in certain lexicalized verb forms. The Witsuwit'en forms were provided by Sharon Hargus (p.c.). The Carrier forms are cited from Morice's grammar (Morice 1932). The Chilcotin forms cited here were abstracted from Cook 1989. And finally, the Chipewyan prefixes were inferred from paradigms of fossilized negative stative imperfectives found in Li's data.

3. Here H represents a zero onset, historically from a voiced fricative, in this case *y < *z̧.

4. Here H < *ʁ.

5. For phonological reasons, the 'peg' prefix (PA *hə -) is required before a prefix consisting of a single consonant (e.g. *s-, *ɬ-) without a preceding conjunct prefix. Since such prefixes can occur only in coda position, the addition of the 'peg' prefix *hə- provides an onset and nucleus, thus resulting in a canonical syllable.

6. In Koyukon, however, the vowel ə of an object prefix lengthens to i (ordinarily < PA *i·-) after object prefixes; with prefixes which occur to the right of the 'deictic subject' prefixes, on the other hand, the vowel ə lengthens to æ (ordinarily < PA *e·-).

7. Krauss evidently assigned the glottal-negative prefix and the neuter prefix to the same prefix position because they are in complementary distribution, attributing the fact that the glottal-negative prefix precedes the subject pronoun to metathesis.

8. In this chart (ʔV) denotes ʔV- in absolute initial position and elsewhere. In all cases this (ʔV) is underlyingly /(ə-)/. Forms with the vowel i in the paradigmatic prefix string (including those with i in the classifier, and the 1.sg. affirmative perfective prefix si-) undergo a vowel harmony rule such that, in a Cə- prefix immediately preceding the paradigmatic prefix string, ə > i; furthermore, Ci-yi- > Ci·- and Cu-yi- > Cu·-. Also, in the negative neuter paradigm, ə > a / ʔ.

A subset of neuter imperfective verbs lack the prefix /(ə-)/—in this case surfacing as (ʔi)—in their affirmative paradigm; compare for example the copular verb requiring a predicate complement, e.g. 3. & 2.sg. yiɬeh 'he/she/it is; you are', 1.sg. xiɬeh 'I am', with that requiring a complement of manner, e.g. 3. & 2.sg. (wəχ) ʔit'eh 'he/she/it is (so); you are (so); 1.sg. (wəχ) ʔixiɬeh 'I am (so)'. Neuter perfective verbs always take the prefix /(ə-)/.

9. The core clause is the main part of the clause, excluding focused phrases which precede the core clause and 'afterthought' phrases which follow the core clause.

10. Furthermore, the irrealis prefix, or a prefix homomorphic with it, can occur as a thematic prefix. This thematic /u-/ is in complementary distribution with a nearly homomorphic thematic prefix /u(·)-/; these thus appear to be alloforms of a single prefix. Thematic /u-/~ /u(·)-/ has all the same cooccurrence restrictions as irrealis /u-/. When these two prefixes are in competition, irrealis /u-/ prevails: thematic /u(·)-/ zeroes out in the presence of the irrealis prefix.

11. The AET source of Tlingit tɬé·k' 'no' will not be fully explored in this paper. My present hypothesis is that it is a doublet with Tlingit tɬé·x' 'one' < PAET *də =N̑-q' 'one; together, all'. Tlingit tɬé·x' 'one' can occasionally be translated as '(all) together (i.e. as a group)'. Assuming that this meaning was inherited from PAET, Tlingit tɬé·ɬ < tɬék'=ɬ 'not' may once have been structurally analogous to French 'pas (=ɬ) du tout (tɬék')'.

12. The three verb themes meaning 'to be' or 'to exist', all with the stem -ti~, have a unique realis/irrealis pair of stem markings: the realis stem has stigma Γ/, and the irrealis stem has stigma /ʔ/. The theme in this case is MANNER Ø-ti~ 'to be (so)', where the default manner adverbial is yé· 'thus'.

13. The irrealis prefix is deleted in the presence of the perfective prefix wu- /ÿu-/ as well as subject prefixes containing high vowels (i, u).

14. This particle can perhaps be glossed as '(how) could it be?'. Compare the related particle cited under (b) above and the particle/enclitic gʷá· 'wow!; is that so?!', as an enclitic

$=g^w\acute{a}\cdot$ also meaning 'could it be...?', 'or (rather)...?', as in *hí· n=g^wá· ñ-tuwá' sigú,̓ tšá yu`=g^wá·* 'do you want water or tea?'

15. See Krauss' *Eyak Dictionary*, p. 91, for both these constructions. There is also a related interrogative *tła·-χ* 'where?' (usually, but not always, implying strong skepticism, disbelief, or denial that S does indeed exist anywhere), which does not, however, select the optative mode.

16. If I were to hazard a guess at the moment, it would be that Eyak *tła·ʰ* and *tła·*, perhaps to be glossed something like 'where could it be?', correspond functionally and semantically with Tlingit *gu ʔa'* '(how) could it be?', not with Tlingit *ł=*.

17. The prefix /u-/ also occurs in the telic perfective habitual mode. This prefix is formally virtually identical with the irrealis prefix, but I now believe it has a different origin and should be considered a different morpheme from irrealis /u-/.

18. I refer here to Krauss' 'y-component' and 'd-component' of the classifiers, respectively, as the 'I-element' and 'D-element'. In Athabaskan-Eyak, the classifiers with D-element are reconstructible as PAE *dǝ*- and *łǝ*-. With the addition of the I-element, these become PAE *di-* and *łi-*. In Athabaskan, however, the contrast between PAE *ǝ* and PAE (short) *i* is lost, so that PAE *dǝ*- and *di-* merge as PA *dǝ*-, and PAE *łǝ*- and *łi-* merge as PA *łǝ* - ~ *l(ǝ)*-. The former existence of the I-element of these classifiers, however, is reflected by the addition of **y* to originally vowel-initial verb stems.

19. In Tlingit, this 'peg' prefix *ñ-* is inserted only before consonantal classifiers (*ł-, s-, š-*) in word-initial position.

20. Krauss 1969 offers an interesting alternative to the comparisons given here, linking the Tlingit s-classifier in the theme *s-ta~`* with the AE s-perfective prefix. I believe, however, that Krauss' hypothesis does not bear up under careful scrutiny.

21. The deletion of short high vowels in clitic particles is attested elsewhere, e.g. in the contraction of the yes/no interrogative particle *=gí > g=* / after *ʔá* and before a demonstrative clitic, e.g. *ʔá=g=wé* 'is that . . .?', and in the clitic particle *(=)gu- > (=)g^w* discussed in 3.1.

22. The morphologically conservative Alaskan Athabaskan languages (Ahtna, Deg Hit'an, Koyukon, and Lower Tanana, among others) exhibit a unique irregularity in the negative stative imperfective: the glottal-negative prefix is preceded by PA *ʁǝ*- < Pre-PA *Gǝ*-. In Carrier, however, the ordinary paradigm is found.

23. The form *ʔǝłe·G* is attested in the Eyak Dictionary as a variant of *ʔa ʔłe·G*. This form is irregular in that it lacks the glottal-negative prefix, but interestingly enough, it corresponds more closely to the posited reconstruction PAET *ñłe ʔ* than does the regular form.

24. This suffix does not appear with stems that originally ended with a sonorant (generally **y* or **w*) in Pre-PA. These sonorants disappeared in the transition from Pre-PA to PA, so that the PA stem constitutes an open syllable without the suffix *-ŋ^y*.

25. With closed stems ending in an obstruent, the obstruent fails to undergo spirantization in PA. As explained in Leer 1979, this fact can be explained by assuming that Pre-PA had a vocalic allomorph of the perfective/stative suffix after closed stems.

26. The allomorph *-·ÿ* occurs only in the telic habitual perfective, where it is followed by the habitual perfective suffix *-dž*. My hypothesis here is that the habitual perfective suffix *-dž* provided an environment where the suffixal *ÿ* was preserved overtly; elsewhere, *ÿ* was dropped.

27. Although Tlingit has no overt reflex of *ÿ* here, stem vowel reduction occurs. Stem vowel reduction occurs elsewhere only when a consonantal suffix follows the stem. My hypothesis here is that stem vowel reduction is conditioned by the former occurrence of suffixal *ÿ*.

28. Note that the Tlingit telic perfective habitual takes the prefix /u-/. Although in my dissertation (Leer 1991) I identify this prefix with the irrealis prefix, I now believe that this prefix is an allomorph of the perfective prefix /ÿu-/, one that is also found in the telic perfective, e.g. in *ʔuwatá· /ÿu-ya-t'a-ÿ/* 'it got fat', cited above. Even synchronically, there

is a minor but telling difference between the irrealis prefix /u-/ and the telic perfective habitual prefix /u-/: with indefinite human subject, /u-/ is (optionally for many speakers) found before the indefinite human sub ject prefix /du-/ in the telic perfective habitual, but never in irrealis forms.

29. The nasalization in the Gwich'in and Navajo forms is apparently analogical; the corresponding stative verbs have nasalized stems.

30. In Krauss and Leer (1981, pp. 146-160) I present evidence that Tlingit /ỹ/ < Pre-Tlingit */ŋ/, i.e. that /ỹ/ was originally a nasal sonorant. Furthermore, Tlingit has two other suffixes, both of the form /-in/, that end with /n/, whereas no suffix ends with /ỹ/. It is thus easy to see how /n/ would have been substituted for /ỹ/ when the decessive enclitic was reinterpreted as a suffix.

31. Even if it had already been reinterpreted a suffix at this point, its stigma was /·/ rather than glottal stop, and would therefore not have triggered the first glottal dissimilation rule.

32. In a few constructions we find subordinative verb forms that lack the suffix /-(ỹ)i`/; see Leer 1991, pp. 487-88.

33. Note that the corresponding assertive form may or may not take the I-element in the classifier, and that the non-assertive verb stem may or may not be different from the non-assertive verb stem. Furthermore, the irrealis prefix (or if you will, a prefix homomorphic with the irrealis prefix) may occur as a thematic prefix, in which case it is present in both realis and irrealis forms of the verb.

34. The verbal noun *di-ni·h* < PA **də-nə'xʸ-X'* < Pre-PA **də-nig-X'* (where -X' is unidentified glottal obstruent), whereas the verb *di-ni·h* < PA **də-nə'xʸ-X'* < Pre-PA **di-nig-X'*, where Pre-PA **di-*, identical with Eyak and Tlingit *di-*, contains the I-element of the classifier ultimately from the PAET perfective/stative prefix **(ŋ)i-*. Because of the merger of short **i* with **ə*, however, the classifiers **də* - and **di-* have fallen together in Athabaskan.

35. I must stress that this is an extremely idealized statement. For example, the Eyak 1.sg. perfective prefix string is quite irregularly *si-*. Moreover, Athabaskan **sə-/zə-* appears to have been generalized to all forms where a non-zero subject prefix occurs.

36. Sapir and his students refer to such forms as 'neuter perfective' forms; this terminology is still used, particularly by students of languages such as Navajo and Hupa, where there is no formal evidence that forces the interpretation of such forms as imperfectives. Such evidence comes primarily from Northern Athabaskan languages, on the basis of which we can reconstruct a complete set of modes corresponding to stative imperfectives such as **səda·*, e.g the stative perfective form **вəŋʸədaʔ* 'he/she was sitting'. Furthermore, in languages that retain the negative paradigms, the negative form corresponding to **səda·* takes the negative stative imperfective stem (**-da-he·*) rather than the negative perfective stem (**-da·ł-e·*). . Finally, we note that unlike Eyak *sədaɫ-i·h*, PA **səda·* means only 'he/she is sitting', not 'he/she sat down'; the latter meaning is supplied by the active perfective PA **ne'zᵉda·*.

References

Boas, Franz. 1917. *Grammatical Notes on theLanguage of the Tlingit Indians.* University of Pennsylvania Museum, Anthropological Publications 7 (Philadelphia).

Cook, Eung-Do. 1989. Chilcotin Tone and Verb Paradigms. In *Athabaskan Linguistics: CurrentPerspectives on a Language Family*, eds. Eung-Do Cook and Keren Rice, Trends in Linguistics State-of-the-Art Reports 15, Mouton de Gruyter (Berlin, New York), pp. 145-198

Hargus, Sharon. 1989. Sekani Ghə: Conjugation or Mode Prefix? In *Athabaskan Linguistics: Current Perspectives on a Language Family*, eds. Eung-Do Cook and Keren Rice, Trends in Linguistics State-of-the-Art Reports 15, Mouton de Gruyter (Berlin, New York), pp. 199-227.

Hargus, Sharon. 1991. The Disjunct Boundary in Babine-Witsuwit'en. *IJAL* 57: 487-513

Hargus, Sharon. 1996. Conjugation, Negativity, and Mode in Babine-Witsuwit'en. Paper presented at the 23rd meeting of the Alaskan Anthropological Association, Fairbanks, Alaska.

Jetté, Jules. 1940. *Ten'a Grammar*. ms.

Kari, James. 1990. *Ahtna Athabaskan Dictionary*. Alaska Native Language Center (Fairbanks).

Krauss, Michael E. 1965. Eyak: a Preliminary Report. *Canadian Journal of Linguistics* 10(2,3): 167-18

Krauss, Michael E. 1969. On the Classifiers in the Athapaskan, Eyak and Tlingit Verb, Indiana University Publications in Anthropology and Linguistics, Memoir 24 of *IJAL*, supplement to 35(4).

Krauss, Michael E. 1970. *Eyak Dictionary*. ms. Alaska Native Language Center.

Krauss, Michael E. and Jeff Leer. 1981. *Athabaskan, Eyak, and Tlingit Sonorants*. Alaska Native Language Center Research Papers 5 (Fairbanks).

Leer, Jeff. 1979. *Proto-Athabaskan Verb Stem Variation, Part One: Phonology*. Alaska Native Language Center Research Papers 1 (Fairbanks).

Leer, Jeff. 1991. *The Schetic Categories of the Tlingit Verb*. Ph. D. dissertation, Department of Linguistics, University of Chicago.

Morice, A. G. 1932. *The Carrier Language*. Anthropos (St.-Gabriel-Mödling, Winnipeg).

Rice, Keren. 1989. *A Grammar of Slave*. Mouton de Gruyter (Berlin, New York).

Rice, Keren. 1985. The Optative and *s and *n Conjugation Marking in Slave. International *Journal of American Linguistics* 51: 282-301.

Rice, Keren and Sharon Hargus. 1989. Conjugation and Mode in Athapaskan Languages: Evidence for Two Positions. In *Athabaskan linguistics: Current Perspectives on a Language Family*, eds. Eung-Do Cook and Keren Rice, Trends in Linguistics State-of-the-Art Reports 15, Mouton de Gruyter (Berlin, New York), pp. 265-315.

Story, Gillian L. 1996. *A Morphological Study of Tlingit*. M.A. thesis, School of Oriental and African Languages, University of London.

Young, Robert and William Morgan. 1992. *Analytical Lexicon of Navajo*. University of New Mexico Press (Albuquerque).

7

ON A BIPARTITE MODEL OF
THE ATHABASKAN VERB

Joyce McDonough

*All the Carrier verbs are made up of at least two parts, the first of which
denotes the tense and person, while the second, namely the ending or stem,
contains the main signification of the word.*

A.G. Morice (1932), The Carrier Language

*The Na-Dene languages are not one-third as synthetic as they look. . . .
Haida in particular, I find, is extremely analytic. . . . What Swanton calls
affixes are all independent stems entering into composition, or even little
verbs. . . . It all crumbles into pieces at the least touch. I think the same will
prove to be true of Athabaskan-Tlingit.*

Edward Sapir (1921),
excerpt from a letter to A. L. Kroeber

A concise and motivated model of verbal morphology is essential to any investigation of the Athabaskan sound and morphosyntactic systems because assumptions about the morphophonemic structure necessarily underlie these analyses.
There are several often conflicting models of the morphological structure of the
Athabaskan verbal complex (Morice 1932, Sapir and Hoijer 1967, Kari 1976,
1990, McDonough 1990, Halpern 1992, Hargus 1994), although, for most

purposes, a version of the abstract slot-and-filler or position class template used in Young and Morgan (1987, 1992) is assumed.

There are several reasons for disputing this template as a basis of a speaker's working knowledge of the language. First, it was never intended to represent this knowledge; it was invented as a diachronic device for cross-linguistic comparison Li (1946). It is an excellent and valuable tool for this purpose. McDonough (1990) and Kari (1989) have pointed out that the positions in the template do not represent morphological structure, only linear relationships between proposed morphemes.[1] It is only assumed that the linear relationships represented by the positions in the template reflect morphological structure of the verb.

Second, as a morphological type, position classes have an odd status. The position classes exist because of ordering considerations among morphemes: they arise crucially when concatenation cannot be accounted for either by prosodic morphology or affixation to stem without the prosthesis of the template.[2] Position classes are unlike base-and-affix morphology because position classes have no formal status in the morphology outside of their role as placeholders. In addition, or perhaps because of this, in Athabaskan particularly, the position classes are ill defined with respect to each other, even within the same template. In Athabaskan, some position classes are marked by clear semantic or functional properties, such as the subject agreement position class (position "ix" in Young and Morgan 1987). But other positions have little or no internal consistency, such as the morphemes of position "vi a, b, and c," which are basically a set of ill-defined position classes that are grouped together mainly by their falling between two more well-defined classes, and they also apparently observe some phonologically determined ordering (Wright 1983), which, if defendable, obviates a need for position classes here. Sometimes a position is invented for a single morpheme.[3] Sometimes morphemes from two position classes never co-occur, such as morphemes from positions "iv" and "v" in the template, making the relationship between the two positions nonlinear. It is this sort of grab-bag property that Simpson and Withgott (1986) argued was the outstanding characteristic of position class morphologies; they were defined exactly by being unlike other morphologies, a last-resort morphology. The opacity of the structure of position classes is further reflected in the lack of agreement in Athabaskan on the actual number and kind of positions for a language. And finally, the affix-to-base concatenation type for position classes is weakened because it requires the additional prosthesis of extensive morphosyntactic constraints to account for the co-occurrence restrictions that are often a direct effect of ordering the morphemes via the position classes.

Position class morphologies are also unlike prosodic or nonconcatenative morphologies. In these morphologies, the morphological primes are phonologically defined and word formation processes are motivated by phonological principles. Thus it remains unclear what formal devices underlie the position classes and concatenation of position class morphemes. If position classes are a kind of morphology, we expect to be able to motivate them. In effect, position classes have little or no predictive power and exist as a descriptive device, albeit powerful and useful, but questionable as a morphological type comparable to stem-and-affix or prosodic morphologies.

A third reason for questioning the position class template as a morphological device is an interaction between the phonology and morphology. Phonological analyses based on the position class template result in Athabaskan in a considerable mismatch between the phonology and morphology, to the extent that it has been claimed that this mismatch is a component of Athabaskan phonology and represents the possible existence of such mismatches (Hargus 1995). A mismatch of this type is extremely expensive to maintain because it makes morphophonemic structure very abstract. If knowledge of form, or morphophonemics, is prior to a speaker's knowledge of morphosyntax and phonemic structure, as it is generally assumed, then it is an inopportune area to be highly marked. This is one of the strongest arguments against assuming a position class template in Athabaskan. A language with both a rich inflectional morphology and a highly marked structure is at a distinct disadvantage, and probably at least unstable. Rather than presupposing this structure, arguments for the marked structure need to be developed independent of that structure, in the same way that arguments for a marked phonological structure are developed. Fourth, several early investigators, including Morice and Sapir, have proposed that a much simpler structure underlies the composition of the verb. And finally, but not least, speakers and teachers of Navajo themselves find the template counterintuitive and opaque as a learning device.

In this chapter I will lay out a different, simpler model of the morphological structure of the Athabaskan verb, called the bipartite constituent model. This model does not use position classes as a structural base for word formation. In this model, the basic verb is a compound of two constituents, a verb and an auxiliary or "infl" constituent. Each constituent has a base, called a "stem" in this chapter, and a single set of prefixes. A third set of prefixes is the agreement markers attached either to the left edge of the infl constituent or to the compounded constituents. This bipartite compound takes a rich set of proclitics and proclitic "postpositions" which leave the left edge of the verb word often weakly defined. The arguments developed for this model represent a conspiracy of evidence for this "bipartite" structure. In this chapter, we will mostly be concerned with evidence from the phonological patterns in Navajo. This model draws on several sources, both early work on the Athabaskan verb and the work of Kari and others who have attempted to come to terms with the position classes as a morphological model. The bipartite model is intended to represent a native speaker's working knowledge of the structure of the verbal complex. As such it is designed to serve both the morphophonemics and morphosyntax in a maximally transparent way.

7.1 The Verbal Domains

The minimal verb in Navajo (and in Athabaskan in general) is marked for tense/mode,[4] subject, person and number (Sapir and Hoijer 1967, Jelinek 1984,

Young and Morgan 1987) and can stand alone as a proposition. The following is an example of a basic Navajo verbal form, the verb stem is <bą́ą́s>.[5]

(1)   *hasébą́ą́s* 'I drove it up.'
       ha   #   *sé-*   /   *bą́ą́s*
       'up'   #   s-perf/1s - classifier   /   'handle globular object':perf
       1   2   3

The basic verb divides into three well-established domains: the proclitic "disjunct" (1) and inflectional "conjunct" (2) domains and the verb stem (3) (Sapir and Hoijer 1967, Kari 1989, 1976):

(2)   A schema of the morphological domains in the Athabaskan verb:

       [disjunct   #   conjunct   /   verb stem]$_{Wdverb}$
       1   2   3

The disjunct domain (1) contains a group of morphemes with clitic-like properties. The domain is optional in the sense that the morphemes in this domain are optional, though there are subcategorization constraints that may require some proclitics (such as the dual marker <na->). The boundary between the disjunct and conjunct domains, marked with a #, is well established in the literature. It is marked as a domain edge in the phonology and as a boundary marker for morphophonemic rules (Sapir and Hoijer 1967, Kari 1976, Young and Morgan 1980, 1987). I refer the reader to the literature on the subject. We will adopt this # notation as marking the boundary between disjunct and conjunct domains, domains (1) and (2) respectively, in the chapter. The conjunct domain (2) contains a set of morphemes, some of which are obligatory in the verb. This domain is from one to several syllables long, marked as containing five position classes in Young and Morgan's template. Two of these positions are obligatory: the tense/mode and subject morphemes. I will argue that the tense/mode and subject morphemes often appear as a single portmanteau or synthetic morpheme (<sé> in (1) is the s-perfective / first-person singular form of the subject and tense morphemes). They combine to form an independent morphological category, a "stem"—that is, these morphemes are not prefixes. This polysynthetic stem is the base of this domain. In the classic view, the third domain (3) is the verb stem domain. In Navajo, this is the final syllable in the verb word. I will argue that the "classifier" prefix is part of this domain and not the conjunct (2) domain (as it is in Young and Morgan).

Thus every verb in Athabaskan has morphemes from at least two domains: conjunct (tense/subject) and the verb stem. These two domains, (2) and (3), are the two basic units of the verb and provide a simple account for the fact that the verb is always at least bisyllabic. We will take this up again later. Some examples and glosses of verbal constructions are provided below. The two obligatory morphemes (tense/subject and verb stem) are underlined. The disjunct (3), conjunct (2), and verb stem (1) domains are marked:

(3) a. *hasébą́ą́s* 'I drove it up.' (Young and Morgan 1987:48)

   ha # *sé-*   / *bą́ą́s*
   'up' # sperf/1s - cl / 'move hooplike object': perf
   1   2   3

   b. *honílįid* 'I/he appeared/came.' (YM1987:76)

   h + *ní*   / *lįid*
   3s + nper/1/3/s / 'appeared, came':perf
        2   3

   c. *yishcha* 'I cry.' (YM1987:779)

   (*y*)*ish* / *cha*
   øimp/1s / cry:imp
   2   3

The form in (3a) has morphemes from all three domains, (3b) contains two conjunct morphemes and the verb stem; no disjunct morphemes. In (3c) is the minimal verb, with the two obligatory morphemes, the tense/subject portmanteau <ish> (first-person singular imperfective) and the verb stem <cha>, both underlined.

In the next section I will take up issues concerning the boundary between the conjunct or inflectional domain (2) and the verb stem (3).

7.1.1 The Conjunct-Stem Boundary

The first evidence that the conjunct and stem form separate domains is the consistent existence of a consonant cluster between the ultimate and penult syllables (McDonough 1990, Halpern 1992). Codas appear in restricted places; in word final position and in postpositions, and in the penult syllable in the word.[6] Note the following Navajo forms. The syllables, separated by a period, are constructed by a conventional syllabic algorithm that maximizes onsets (Kahn 1976).

(4) a. *ni.hozh*   'You tickle it.'
    yis.gan   'He dried it.'
    nil.gha: 'You eat meat.'   K:50
    wo:.gha: 'You (pl) eat meat.'
    dish.lid   'I am burning.'   K:51
    nish.chééh 'I flee.'   YM 1992:77

   b. *haash.zhee'* 'He hunted.'   K:50
    yiil.gozh   'We tickle it.'
    yiil.ziih   'We miss it.'   K:53

    c.   *sí.nił.gan*   'You dried it.'
         ha.shí.níl.zhee' 'You hunted.'   K:50
         ha.iil.zheeh   'We hunt.'   K:53
         yi.di.yooł.hééł 'He'll kill it.'   K:55

The appearance of the cluster between the ultimate and penult syllable is problematic because it is a distribution restriction on codas, apparently *inside* the word. Syllabic constraints codify the syllable types found in a given language, and, crucially, they cannot govern the distribution of syllable types in the word. Navajo either allows codas or it doesn't. If it allows them, then syllables with codas will occur; if they do not, or if they put constraints on codas, then syllable types that violate these constraints will simply not occur, except as a possible edge effect. In English, for instance, consonant clusters found at the edge of words are not allowed within them, as in <strengths> ([strɛnθs]) or <sixths> ([sɪksθs]). This type of edge phenomena is called extraprosodicity or extrametricality. Extraprosodicity has been shown to account for the odd or illegal syllable type at the edge of a domain, and the existence of illegal syllable types indicates domain edges.

    It has been claimed that Navajo syllable structure is CV(V)(C), because of forms like those in (4). However, there are two problems with analysis of Navajo syllable structure. One is the distribution problem just mentioned. If there were codas, we would not expect to see distribution restrictions like we see in Navajo. The second problem concerns epenthesis. McDonough (1995) has presented evidence for epenthetic alternations in the vowels of the conjunct prefixes.[7] If a morpheme is prefixed to a vowel initial base (C+V) (5a) it appears in the onset of the syllable; if it is prefixed to a consonant initial base (C+CV) (5b), an epenthetic vowel appears (CiCV). If there are two prefixes, epenthesis produces CVCVCV (5c).

(5)   a.   *yismáás* 'I rolled.' (YM1987:776)
         [*ish*]   [*máás*]
         [óimp/1s] [impf 'roll']

     b.   *dismáás* 'I started to roll.' (YM1987:331)
         [*d - ish*]   [*ł - máás*]
         [incpt - óimp/1s] [cl - impf 'roll']

         dishchííd 'I extend my arm.' (YM 1987:325)
         [*d - ish*]   [*l - chííd*]
         [QU - óimp/1s] [CL - imp 'act with arms']

     c.   *bijáátah*[8] *dinishchííd* 'I trip him.'[9] (YM 1987:325)
         [*d - nish*]   [*l - chííd*]
         [QU - nimpf/1s] [CL - imp 'act with arms']

In this case, the epenthetic alternations are using a CV template, not CVC. If it were using a CVC algorithm, we would find epenthesis building CVCCV and not CVCVCV sequences.

If the syllable structure is CV(V), and codas fall at domain boundaries and in the penult syllable, the existence of a coda in the penult syllable indicates a juncture between the last two syllables. In (6), this domain boundary is marked by x, the final boundary by y:

(6) *dish.lid* 'I am burning.'

  $d\ i\ sh]\ _x\ l\ i\ d]\ _y$

Since we have no evidence to the contrary, we will assume that the boundary at x is equal in strength to the word final boundary at y. We will call this the Navajo internal boundary hypothesis:

(7) *Navajo internal boundary hypothesis:* In (6), x and y are the edges of domains, and the domain boundaries x and y are equivalent.

The existence of a juncture here is a serious problem for the assumption of the position class template that the verb stem is the base of prefixation in the verb.

I take no stand here on what kind of morphological category this boundary defines (root, stem, word, or Wd[-1]), only that the two categories are, for present purposes, equivalent. Since the two obligatory parts of the verb (tense/subject and verb stem) are in the penult and ultimate syllables, they fall into two separate domains, and the Navajo verb is a compound of two domains. This is the basis of the bipartite structure.

The right domain, y, is the verb stem, and we will call this the verb constituent. There are several questions. One, if x represents a domain edge, what domain is it the right edge of and what is the structure of that domain? A second question, which we will take up next, relates to the phonology and domain affiliation of the "classifier" prefix class, the position class adjacent to the verb stem in the template.

7.1.2 The Classifier Prefixes

The rightmost domain is the verb domain; it comprises the final syllable of the word and contains at least the verb stem morpheme, as stated. The position classes that precede the verb stem are listed here, with the number of their position class[10] (from Young and Morgan 1987) beneath them:

(8) tense/mode Subject classifiers verb stem
  vii   viii   ix   verb stem

The misnamed *classifier* (cl) prefixes (<l, ł, d, ø>) of position 9 are generally considered to mark valence on the verb (Thompson 1993). As such, this prefix is an operator on the argument structure of the verb. For this reason, we will adopt the hypothesis that the classifier morpheme is a prefix on the verb in the verb domain (McDonough 1990). In this view, the verb domain consists of two morphemes, the classifier and verb stem:

(9) $]_x$ [cl - verb]$_y$ = Verb

If the verb stem has a prefix, the prefix is in this domain, and the verb stem is always the final syllable, why is the domain boundary between the last two syllables? The answer to this question concerns the unique prosodic distribution properties of the classifier prefixes. The following observations about the classifier patterns follow the extensive literature on the classifier phonology in the Athabaskan family (Sapir and Hoijer 1967, Hale 1972, Hale and Honie 1972, Howren 1971, Kari 1976, Hargus 1985, Young and Morgan 1987, Randoja 1989).

   Because the classifiers are consonantal prefixes, prefixation of a classifier to the consonantal initial verb stem results in an illegal sequence, CC. Because of the epenthesis process available in Navajo, we would expect one of the following forms to occur with the prefixation of one of the classifier morphemes to a consonant initial stem, depending on the syllable algorithm and the boundary effects (presented in b, c and f of (10)):

(10)   If the classifier is preceded by a closed syllable:

          C + C + C   (a)   → CiCiC
                       (b)   → CCiC
                       (c)   → CiCC

       If the classifier is preceded by an open syllable:

          CV + C + C   (e)   → CVCiC
                       (f)   → CVCC

Given a CV syllable algorithm (with simple onsets) and a domain boundary as outlined above, we predict b, e, or f to occur. In fact, the only one of the forms that occurs in Navajo is the one in f; that is, these classifier prefixes do not use epenthesis to fix up the illegal sequences produced when they are attached to the verb stem. Instead, in Navajo the classifiers delete. (Forms in e and f occur in languages where the classifiers epenthesize (see Golla 1970 on Hupa and the coastal Athabaskan languages and Hargus and Tuttle 1995).

(11)   The classifier prefix algorithm:

classifier
C] [C + C → CC
     ↓
     ø

If the coda of the preceding syllable (which is in the left domain by (9)) is open, they will incorporate into that syllable. Examples follow of the first-person perfective (a) and imperfective (b) forms of the verb <ch'al>. The domains are bracketed. In the first example the classifier surfaces in the coda of the preceding syllable, <yí> the morpheme for the first-person perfective. In the second example, the classifier <ł> is deleted after the imperfective <yish> form:

(12)   a.   *yíŁchæal*   'I lapped it up.'   (YM1987:779)

   [*í*]₁   [Ł - *chæal*]ᵥ
   [óperfective/1s]₁   [cl - perf]ᵥ

   b.   *yishch'al*   'I lap it up.'   (YM1987:779)

   [*ish*]₁   [*ł ch'al*]ᵥ
                        ↓
                        ø

The <d> classifier is even more constrained. It is apparently also barred from the coda position; the <d> will surface only in the rare case of a vowel initial stem, otherwise it deletes and causes a series of phonological mutations on the verb stem called the "d-effects" (Sapir and Hoijer 1967, Howren 1971, Bennet 1987, McDonough 1999b). In the d-effects, the fricatives <z, zh, l> mutate to the affricates <dz, j, dl> after the <d>.

(13)   The d-effects (fricative to affricate alternation):

séloh 'I lassoed it.'	*yisdloh* 'It was lassoed.'
[*sé*] [*loh*]	[*yis*] [*d- loh*]
[sperf/1Su] [perf 'lasso']	[yperf/3Su] [cl - perf 'lasso']

yiih yiyííziid 'He poured it into it.'	*biih yidziid* 'It was poured into it.'
[(*y*)*i* - [*yíí*] [*ziid*]]	[*yi*] [*d- ziid*]
'it' [3Oj [yperf/3Su] [perf 'pour']]	'it' [øperf/3Su] [cl - perf 'pour']

The lateral classifiers also have a phonological effect on the stem: they determine the voicing of the stem initial fricatives (Hale and Honie 1972, Kari 1976, Young and Morgan 1987). The general distribution pattern is this: the classifiers will incorporate into the onset of a (rare) vowel initial stem or incorporate into the preceding open syllable. And, if neither of these positions is available, they delete. In effect, the stem maintains an identity between its edge and the edges of the verb domain. There is supporting synchronic and diachronic evidence that the stem resists affixation altogether; the stem absorbs both prefixes and suffixes (from the d-effects, and tonogenesis and the origins of the vocalic nasality contrasts respectively; see discussion of these topics in Leer 1979, 1982, Krauss 1964, 1986, Hombert 1975, Kingston 1990, Hargus 1985, Randoja 1989, and McDonough 1999a).

The two morpheme classes to the immediate left of the classifier position are the subject marker and tense markers, in positions viii and vii respectively:

(14) tense/mode   Subject classifiers   stem
      vii   viii   ix   verb stem

In the view proposed here, the classifiers are in the verb domain, and the domain boundary falls between the subject and classifier morphemes:

(15) tense/mode   Subject]   [classifiers   stem]
      vii   viii   ]   [ix   stem]

The classifiers (which spread features to the stem initial fricatives independent of whether they surface or not) will delete unless they can incorporate into the preceding syllable. The incorporation of the classifier prefix into the preceding syllable is across the domain boundary. This will allow us to affiliate the classifier prefixes with the verb domain, as valance markers and operators on the arguments of the verb stem.

In the next section we turn to the question of the left domain: what its structure is and what kind of domain it is. I will argue that the left domain is best characterized as an infl domain consisting of a base with the morphological status of a stem and a set of prefixes, mirroring the verb domain in structure. We'll call this the infl domain (ID) hypothesis.

7.2   The Infl Domain (ID)

7.2.1   The Infl Stem

Along with the verb stem, the minimal morphemes needed to produce a verb word are the tense/mode and the subject prefixes.[11] In the infl domain hypothesis, the tense/mode and subject morphemes come from two positions in the template that are adjacent to the right edge of the infl domain (in (15)).

These two morphemes often combine into a single opaque or polysynthetic morpheme of tense/mode marked for person and number. Young and Morgan call these morphemes "essentially paradigmatic elements" (Young and Morgan 1987:39). The synthetic nature of many of these morpheme concatenations is easiest to see when we consider that the surface realizations far outnumber the combinatory possibilities of the morphemes of these two position classes in number and kind. In the first two columns in (16) are the proposed (position class) morphemes for position (7) and the morpheme for the first-person subject in (8), <(y)ish>.[12] In the last two columns are the surface (occurring) synthetic forms of the imperfective and perfective tense/mode and first-person subject morphemes.

(16)   From Young and Morgan (1987:200)

| Proposed for First Person | | Occurring in First Person | |
Tense/mode (vii)	Subject (viii)	Imperfective	Perfective
í	(y)ish	(y)ish	yí
i		nish	ní
ni		shish	sé
si		yiish	sis
yi			yii
ó			deesh
null			(w)ósh

Extensive and often highly abstract morphophonemic rules are needed to adjust the underlying morpheme concatenations to the existing surface forms, especially in the perfective paradigms[13] (Hale and Honie 1971, Kari 1976). Such extensive morphophonemic constraints on morpheme concatenations are the hallmark of polysynthesis. The insight of the bipartite view is that these morpheme "positions" represent a single morphological entity, a portmanteau of tense, person, and number. This entity is the base of affixation in the infl domain. We will call this entity by the morphological category "stem." The reason for doing so is that this morpheme mirrors the verb stem in sitting at the right edge of the domain, in having long vowels and codas, in being derived (the roots are marked for aspect). It is when this morpheme has a coda that the classifiers will delete.

In this view, the form <yischa> ('I cry') is comprised of two morphemes: a verb stem <cha> and an infl stem <(y)ish>. The <(y)ish> is the first-person form of the imperfective conjugation. The <cha> is the imperfective form of the verb root <CHA>. These two morphemes always agree in tense/mode.

If the tense/mode entity is the base of affixation, what are the affixes? In the view proposed here the tense/mode and subject are a single entity, a stem. We'll refer to this as the infl stem (Istem) or "tns/Su":

(17)   tns/Su]   [classifiers   stem]
       Istem]   [ix   Vstem]
       (vii/viii)

In this view the morpheme gloss of a minimal verb form like <yíłch 'al>, is as in (12) repeated here as (18). There are two constituents, infl and verb, and each constituent has a base, the Istem and Vstem, respectively. The verb constituent in <yiłch 'al> has a prefix, the classifier <ł>:

(18) *yiłch'al* 'I lapped it up.'   (YM1987:779)
      [*í*]$_{infl}$ [*ł - chæal*]$_{verb}$
      [óperf/1s]$_{I}$ [cl - perf]$_{v}$

In the Young and Morgan 1987 position class template, there are three position classes (iv, v, vi) and three subposition classes (vi a, b, and c) to the left of the Istem.

(19) #   obj deictic sub   qualifiers   tns/Su] [cl   stem   ]
           iv   v   vi   Istem] [ix   Vstem]
                        a   b   c

The position class iv sits at the left edge of the conjunct domain at the boundary between domain (1) and (2) in (2), the disjunct-conjunct boundary (#). In the model, these position classes to the left of the tns/Su morpheme fall into two groups, the qualifiers (qu) and the agreement markers (agr).

    In the version of the bipartite model that is being presented here, the qualifiers are prefixes attaching to the Istem base; the Istem and the qualifiers are the two morphemes of the Infl domain.

(20) [Qu   tns/Su]$_{infl}$ [cl   stem   ]$_{verb}$
      [vi   Istem   ]   [ix Vstem]
             (vii/viii)

The agreement markers are attached to the Istem but are outside that constituent.

(21) #   Agr [Qu   tns/Su]$_{infl}$ [cl   stem   ]$_{verb}$
           iv/v [vi   Istem   ]   [ix Vstem]
                      (vii/viii)

I will lay out the arguments for this structure in the two following sections.

7.2.2 The Qualifiers

In the position class template, the positions adjacent to the tense/mode and subject morpheme classes are the position vi morphemes. This class of morphemes has three subdivisions, vi a, vi b, and vi c.

(22)   Qu -   tns/Su]   [cl -   stem   ]
       vi a,b,c Istem   ]   [ix   Vstem   ]

The morphemes from position vi represent a group of "aspectual" prefixes that Young and Morgan call "representing an ancient stratum in the language" (1987:80). They represent a difficult class of morphemes. Some have termed some qualifier prefixes as "derivative" or "adverbial," but this classification is not based on a formal definition. In fact, the function and meaning of many of these prefixes has become opaque and nonproductive (see the extensive discussion of these prefixes, with examples, in Young and Morgan 1987:81ff). In his 1989 article on zones in the verbal complex, Kari calls this group of morphemes the "Qualifiers" (qu). I use this name in this chapter to avoid confusion with the technical term "aspect"; these are not rightly aspectual prefixes per se, and understanding their origin, meaning, and function in the word is often difficult. We assume Young and Morgan's prescription that many of these morphemes have lost their semantic transparency and functional productivity. These qualifier morphemes play an important role in the meaning bases of the verb and in the definition of traditional Athabaskan terminology like "verb theme" and "verb base."[14]

From the point of view of the phonology, this morpheme group has two salient properties. First, there is a great deal of homophony among these prefixes. For instance, Young and Morgan (1980:100) list 14 different <di> prefixes. We assume this homophony has arisen through or in conjunction with the collapse of semantic and functional transparency. For our purposes we note that there are only a handful of phonologically distinct prefixes; some of them, such as <łi>, have very limited distribution:

(23)   Phonological shapes of the morphemes in position class vi

vi a	vi b	vi c
di/dí	ni/ní	yi
dzi/ji		
hi/hí		
si/shi		
yi/yí		
łi		

Second, this is the one morpheme group outside the clitic group in domain (1) in which more than one morpheme from the group may appear. When these concatenate, their concatenation appears determined by some kind of sonority algorithm (reflected in the template subpositions vi a, b, and c—that is, their position is phonologically governed. This kind of ordering is different in nature from the ordering of the morphemes of the other position classes and could be formally handled by phonological principles (Wright 1984, Kari 1989). The principles behind this sonority ordering have yet to be worked through and are dependent on an analysis of the glide-fricative alternations in Navajo and the semantics of aspectual markers. The most complete description of these position vi qualifier prefixes and their distributional and semantic properties and co-occurrence restriction morphemes is in Young and Morgan 1987; I refer the reader to the grammars. The point here is that the subpositions do not determine ordering, they reflect it.

In (24a) are forms without qualifier prefixes; in (24b) the qu prefix <h> seriative is attached to the Istems <(y)ish> and <sé>,[15] the first-person ø-imperfective (column a) and s-perfective (column b) tns/Su forms. The verb stem is <ne'> 'chop (SRO)' in the imperfective and perfective forms.

(24)   Repetitive form of <ne'> 'move swiftly through the air (SRO)'

    a.   *yishne'*   *yítne'* '(I) chop (SRO).'

       [*yish*]$_{infl}$ [*ɬ- ne'*]$_{verb}$ [*yí*]$_{infl}$ [*ɬ-ne'*]$_{verb}$
       øimp/1Su cl- imp   yiperf/1Su cl- imp

    b.   with seriative <h->:
       hishne'   *héɬne'*   '(I) chop a series (of SRO).'

       [*h- ish*]$_{infl}$ [*ɬ ne'*]$_{verb}$ [*h - sé*]$_{infl}$ [*ɬ ne'*]$_{verb}$
       [ser - øimp/1Su] [cl- imp]   [ser - sperf/1Su] [cl- imp]

It is possible to have more than one qualifier prefix from this group, the insight behind the subpositions a, b, and c in the template. In the following, the first-person Istems <(y)ish> and <sé> are prefixed by two qualifiers, <h> "seriative" and the <d> "terminative." There is no classifier (zero morpheme) in the verb domain:

(25)   '(1s SU) start to live' in the ø-imperfective and s-perfective, intransitive
    (root <nááh> 'move', YM 1987:338)

    hidishnááh | *hidéna'*

    [h-d- ish]   [nááh] | [h- d- sé]   [na']
    [ser- term- 1s/øimp] [imperf 'move'] | [ser- term- 1s/sperf] [perf 'move']

An epenthetic vowel <i> appears to fix up the illegal clusters.

    The qualifier and agreement morphemes exhibit one of the principal formal problems of the position class template; the notion of what constitutes a position in the template is ill defined.

7.2.3 Agreement Prefixes

The agreement prefixes fall to the left of the qualifiers. These are assigned two position classes in the template, iv and v. However, as Young and Morgan (1987:74) note, morphemes from positions iv and v do not co-occur.[16] Therefore these two positions do not represent linear ordering. Position iv is the direct object of transitive constructions, position v (the "deictic" subject markers) the impersonal third-person subject of intransitives. An example of this follows; the agreement prefixes are <n> second-person object, <sh> first-person object, and < '(a)> (an existential qualifier). They are adjoined to the infl constituent which contains the n-imperfective first-person singular stem <nish>:

(26) *baa ninishteeh* 'I give you to him.' (YM 1987:217)
      n - [*nish*]   [*ł - teeh*]
      2s -[nimp/1s] [CL - imp 'handle animate object']

      baa shinił!teeh 'You give me to him.' (YM 1987:217)
      sh -[*ní*]   [*ł - teeh*]
      1s - [nimp/2s] [CL - imp 'handle animate object']

      'anisbaas 'I arrive driving (something)' (YM 1987:217)
      ' - [*nish*]   [*ł - ba7a7s*]
      3o - [nimp/1s] [CL - imp 'roll globular object']

Important to the point is the fact that these prefixes appear outside the qualifier prefixes, as we can see below. The existential quantifier <'(a)> is an agreement marker and means 'something':

(27) *'anidló* 'killed by frost' (YM 1987:115)
      ' - [*n- i*]$_{infl}$ [*d dlí*]$_{verb}$
      3iobj/su - [term - impf/3Su]$_{infl}$ [cl - imperf 'freeze to death']

The phonological arguments for putting the agreement markers outside the whole infl constituent are less strong. One of them comes from consonant harmony. Navajo is a consonant harmony language. Harmony is the reason for <s> / <sh> alternations in the first person marker <(y)ish> below.

(28) *yishteeh* 'I handle it (animate object).'
      [(*y)ish*]$_{infl}$ [*ł - teeh*]$_{verb}$
      [1s/øimp] [cl - imperf 'handle IO']

      yists'ééh 'I chew it (something mushy).' (YM 1987:778)
      [(*y)ish*]$_{infl}$ [*ł ts'ą́ąh*]$_{verb}$
      [1s/øimp] [cl - imperf 'chew something mushy']

While harmony is imposed within roots and stems (both Istems and Vstems; see root and stem dictionary in Young and Morgan 1987:302ff) and across the infl and verb domains (see the preceding), there is dialect difference in whether the agreement markers harmonize or not. In some dialects, the agreement prefixes are harmonized, in others they are not; speakers have strong reactions to the dialect differences (C. Christ and M. Willie, personal communication).[17] The agreement marker on the noun is harmonized in (29a) and not harmonized in (29b). In neither case is the rule optional. The underlying form for both is

<shi - k'is>: <shi> first-person agreement marker, <k'is> is a kinship term. The forms mean 'my friend' (<hak'is> 'same sex sibling').

(29) (Dialect a)   <sik'is>   (Dialect b)   <shik'is>

The agreement markers are attached to the noun base.

The dialect difference in the harmony constraint seen here does not affect the relationship between the two stems. The <-sh> in the øimp/1SU <(y)ish> must harmonize to the stem's anterior coronal fricative [s] in <-mas>. The form *<yishmas> is ungrammatical in Navajo:

(30) *yismas* 'I rolled it along.' (YM 1987:776)
      [(*y*)*ish*]ᵢₙₙ [*ł* - *mas*]ᵥₑᵣᵦ
      [øimp/1SU]   [cl - impf: 'roll globular O']

The generalization is that the two domains, verb and infl, cannot have opposing values for coronality. In forms like <yishcha> they share [–ant], in <yismas>, [+ant]. As we can see in (30) (and throughout the Young and Morgan dictionaries), the infl stem exhibits the alternation, which means that it harmonizes to the verb domain (McDonough 1991). There are no dialect differences in this harmony rule.

However, as with the agreement marking on the noun, dialects differ in whether or not they require the agreement markers on the verb to harmonize. Both forms appear in (31):[18]

(31) *dzizdiz* / *jizdiz* 'She spun it.' (YM 1987:77)
      j - [*iz*]   [*diz*]
      'fourth per' [sperf/3Su]   [perf:twist[19]]

These facts indicate that the difference between the harmony between the two stems and the harmony here is best understood as a structural difference. The argument is that the difference may be viewed as a constraint which either includes the agreement markers or does not. Dialect (a) in (29) includes the entire conjunct domain (2) in the domain for harmony, up to the # boundary in (2); the agreement markers are within the conjunct domain, to the right of the domain boundary (#), and they are under the constraint to harmonize. In dialect (b), where the agreement markers do not harmonize, the harmony domain excludes the agreement markers. In the version of the bipartite model presented in this chapter, the agreement markers are represented outside the infl constituent as in (21) and outside the harmony domain of the two constituents, infl and verb. In a third view, where the arg markers are inside the infl constituent, we would expect more intra- and/or interspeaker variation. It remains to be seen whether there is supporting evidence from the morphosyntax and semantics for this structure (see Willie and Jelinek, Chapter 11, this volume).

7.2.4 Disjunct Morphemes

The disjunct morphemes are a group of morphemes with clitic-like properties that attach to the left edge of the conjunct domain:

(32) A schema of the morphological domains in the Athabaskan verb:

[disjunct   #   conjunct / verb stem]$_{Wdverb}$
1   2   3

The following are examples of verbal forms with disjunct morphemes, examples (b) in (33) and (34):

(33) a.   (*taah*) *yishkaad* 'I toss it (into the water).'   (YM 1987:784)
            [*ish*] [*ł - kaad*]

       b.   *naashkaad* 'I drop it (downward).'
            na # [*ish*] [*ł - kaad*]   (YM 1987:597)

(34) *nóshkaad* 'Drive them into it, herd them.'   (YM 1987:659/56)
      [*n - ósh*]   [*ł - kaad*]
      [term - opt/1s] [CL - opt 'move in a spreading manner']

      ninóshkaad 'Stop herding them.'   (YM 1987:650/648)

      ni   # [*n - ósh*]   [*ł - kaad*]
      term # [theme - opt/1s] [CL - opt 'move in a spreading manner']

Included in the disjunct domain are morphemes Young and Morgan 1987:38 call "postpositional stems," as well as indirect objects, including reflexives and reciprocals. See the discussion in Young and Morgan. The point here is that the left edge of this domain is less well defined than the right edge, meaning that the left edge of the word is less well defined. This is reflected in speakers' intuitions about whether certain disjunct prefixes 'belong' in a word or not. Note that the right edge of the word is the verb domain and the rightmost morpheme is the verb stem. The verb stem has many distinct properties that make this morpheme prominent in the word (McDonough 1995, 1999c). The consonants and vowels in the stem are longer than consonants and vowels in other places in the word. The full set of both consonantal and vocalic contrast only occur in the stem. The pitch range in stems is expanded. Longer duration and expanded pitch range are classic properties associated with auditory prominence and stress. Thus the right edge of the verb word is clearly identifiable. In the bipartite model we will simply assume that this is the case; the left edge of the word is less well defined than the right edge. We predict that word processing studies will show that this is the case.

7.3   Minimal Verbword

Important evidence for the bipartite structure comes from the so-called minimal word constraints across Athabaskan. In the final section of this chapter, I will discuss this.

In Navajo, nouns and verbs have different constraints: while nouns can be monosyllabic, verbs are minimally bisyllabic.

(35)   nouns: monomoraic   [t^{w}o]   'water'
       verbs: bisyllabic   [yicha]   'I cry'

In the template view, this difference falls out from nothing, it must be stipulated. In the bipartite view, this is an effect of the morphological structure of verbs versus nouns: verbs are made up of two constituents, infl and verb, each constituent is realized, verbs are two syllables.[20]

7.3.1   Position Class Minimality

In the position class template view, several positions have zero morphs (Young and Morgan's "Primary Inflectional Determinants," 1987:200); not coincidentally, these positions represent the obligatory inflection in a word. The positions with zero morphs are the mode, subject, and classifier prefixes.[21]

To the present issue: the morphemes from this "primary" or obligatory group have default values, in which case they are represented by a null or zero morph. It is possible to have all the obligatory morphs null, the null imperfective, the null third-person subject and null classifier. In this case, the verb is comprised of a single stem, in the template view:

(36)   *yicha*   'He cries.'   (YM 1987:779)

    ø   ø   ø   -cha
    impf - 3s - cl   -stem$_v$

The presence of the surface <yi> in <yicha> is the result of a strategy by which the grammar has to expand the verb to its bisyllabic size. An extra syllable is added to meet stipulated syllabic requirements; verbs are at least two syllables long. The syllable receives default values according to the grammar:

(37)   Wd$_v$ = 2 σ
    σ   σ
    [*i*]   *ch a* → *yicha*

Navajo has an onset condition and its default vowel is <i>; thus <yi> is the shape of the default syllable.

7.3.2 Bipartite Minimality

In the bipartite view, the verb is minimally two syllables because there are two stems in a word. In the following example, the infl constituent is arguably an empty morpheme, the third singular of the ó imperfective conjugation, as in the preceding.

(38) *yicha* 'He cries.'

　　[ ]ᵢ　　　　　[*cha*]ᵥ
　　[ø imp/3]ᵢ　　[imperf]ᵥ

Each constituent must have a phonological realization. The prosodic imperative is only that stems have content. It is not based on metrical constraints. Content is provided by the epenthetic vowel ([i]) for which there is independent evidence as we have seen:

(39) [*i*]stemᵢ]ᵢ [[*cha*] stemᵥ]ᵥ

The minimality effects are the result of the morphological structure of the verb; they have two stems. In the version of the bipartite structure offered in this chapter, we will assume that there are two instances when the Istem is empty: when the third-person imperfective is a null morpheme and when the subject argument is bound outside the Infl constituent in certain morphosyntactic construction such as the mediopassives. In the following forms, the third indefinite marker <'(a)> is used to bind the subject argument to the existential quantifier. The differences in tense/mode conjugations show up in the Istem (<i> øimperfective versus <iz> yperfective versus <doo> future) . This is evidence that the <i> carries morphosyntactic features (third singular øimperfective):

(40) From Young and Morgan 1987:75

a. *'átah 'aleeh* 'A meeting convenes.'
　　meeting ' + [[*i*]ᵢₙₙ　　+ [*l leeh*]ᵥₑᵣᵦ]ᵢ/ᵥ
　　3i　　　+ [[imperf3s] + [cl + 'come'ᵢₘₚf]]

b. *'átah 'azlį́į́'* 'A meeting convened.'
　　meeting ' + [[*iz*]ᵢₙₙ　　+ [*l leeh*]ᵥₑᵣᵦ]ᵢ/ᵥ
　　3i　　　+ [[yperf/3s] + [cl + 'come'ₚₑᵣf]]

c. *'átah 'adooleeł* 'A meeting will convene.'
　　meeting ' + [[*doo*]ᵢₙₙ + [*l leeh*]ᵥₑᵣᵦ]ᵢ/ᵥ
　　3i　　　+ [[fut/3s] + [cl + 'come'fᵤₜ]]

In either case, the constraint that the stem have phonological content will insure that the epenthetic vowel <i> is inserted as in (39). The Navajo minimality is not a prosodically motivated word minimality constraint. It is due to its morphological structure; minimally two constituents, minimally two syllables.

7.3.3 Other Athabaskan Languages

Examples in (41) show that the tense/subject morpheme is always phonologically realized in other Athabaskan languages, even when the default vowel is a schwa.

In these cases the tense/subject morpheme is arguably the null morpheme, the 3s/imperf form of the verb. These are similar to the Navajo <yi> cases discussed here. These languages vary according to the features of the default vowel (/i/ versus /ə/ versus /ɛ/) and to whether or not there is an onset condition in the language (i.e., Navajo has an onset condition; Salcha and Sekani do not). The examples in (42) are glosses of the forms [əɬtsəəyh] (Salcha) and [əbil] (Sekani) in the bipartite model.

(41) Minimality effects in other Athabaskan languages (adapted from Hargus and Tuttle 1995:1)[22]

Language	3S/Imperf		Source[23]
Babine	*həwes*	'S/he's ticklish.'	Hargus and Kari
	həɬɣis	'S/he itches.'	Hargus and Kari
Deg Xinag	*ələχ*	'It (fish) swims.'	Kari and Hargus
	oyh əɬtse	'S/he makes snowshoes.'	Kari and Hargus
Koyukon	*o ahonh*	'He is eating o.'	Jones, Thompson and Axelrod 1982
Navajo	*yile:h*	'S/he becomes.'	Young and Morgan 1987
Salcha	*əɬtsəəyh*	'It's windy.'	Tuttle
Sekani	*əbil*	'S/he swings.'	Hargus
	o ahgək	'S/he rubs, massages o.'	Hargus
Slave	*o ɛhtʃɛh*	'S/he boils o.'	Rice 1989:488
S. Slavey	*ɛzi*	'It's roasting.'	Howard 1990:800

(42) *əɬtsəəyh* 'It's windy.'

 [ə]ᵢₙfl   [ɬ ɬ- tsəəyh]ᵥₑᵣb
 [imprf:3s] [cl-stem]

 əbil 'S/he swings.'

 [ə]ᵢₙfl   [*bil*]ᵥₑᵣb
 [imprf:3s] [stem]

As in Navajo, the tns/Su stem is always realized, and this is the minimal morpheme in the infl constituent:

(43) [tns/Su]   [verb]
      [stem₁]   +   [stemᵥ]]
      Infl   +   **Verb**

There are two cases where the bipartite model makes interesting predictions about what is possible in Athabaskan. Recall that Navajo 'classifiers' do not epenthesize and the verb stem is a single syllable long. In a given Athabaskan language, if the classifier epenthesizes, and/or if the verb stem itself is bisyllabic, the bipartite model stipulates that the verb compound will be minimally three syllables long. The verb will always have a tense/subject morpheme as the base of the infl constituent.

In the following forms are verbs where the verb constituent is bisyllabic. In these forms the verbs are three syllables long.

(44) Bisyllabic verb constituents (from Hargus and Tuttle 1995)

Language	3S/Imperf		Source
Deg Xinag	*ədəjał*	'S/he is busy.'	Kari and Hargus
	ədəɢəsr	'S/he arrived (crawling).'	"
	ɣəqən xətux ələvənh	'Yukon is filling up.'	"
	ələɢok	'S/he arrived (running).'	"
	ələɣanh, ləɣanh	'S/he is fat.'	"

A gloss of [ələɢok], 'she arrived running,' follows; the verb stem is /ɢok/, the classifier is the /l/ classifier. A (possible) epenthetic [ə] appears between the two consonants, the verb constituent is bisyllabic, and the word is three syllables long:

(45) *ələɢok*
      [ə]ᵢₙfl   [lə - ɢok]ᵥₑᵣb
      [impf/3s]   [cl - impf]

Hargus and Tuttle point out, correctly, that the existence of these forms in Athabaskan weakens considerably the argument that the prosody is the regulator of verbal minimality because word size is accounted for by the number of morphemes and by the number of constituents alone, without the addition of prosodic or metrical constraints. The bipartite structure offers a straightforward explanation of these effects: the verb is a compound, the noun is not. The difference between verbs and nouns is due to the differences in their morphological structure.

7.4 What Is Acquired?

Is the difference between English morphology and Navajo morphology a difference in type? If Navajo represents a position class morphology, this can only be true if the prosthetic template is a morphological type. While independent evidence for the existence of stem and affix and prosodic morphology is abundant, the opposite is true of position classes which have proved notoriously difficult to characterize. One way of establishing evidence is to uncover the formal properties of position classes. Stump (1991) has attempted to do so by building an algorithm for position class concatenation. However, his models work equally well in Navajo for both the position class and the bipartite models (McDonough 1999c)—that is, they are too powerful. Part of the reason for their power is that the model is not constrained by morphophonemic structure. Morphosyntactic and morphophonological models that assume position classes are not evidence for the existence of position classes.

In English, the affixation is to a word level entity. Is there a principle that ensures this as a fact about English morphology? In one strong sense the answer is no. It is simply, as Williams (1996) has noted, a pattern in the lexicon. In fact, English does have (limited) stem level affixation (as in '-mit' constructions of 'remit', 'permit', 'submit') and prosodically governed affixation ("expletive" insertion). Does English have position classes? If it doesn't, why not? The answer cannot be that English does not have as complex a set of morphemes as Navajo, because that begs the very question it seeks to answer: what's the status of the morphemes in the grammar? In English they are "words" and affixes. The question best asked then is, what are the patterns in the Navajo lexicon?

The template claims that most verbal morphemes are "prefixes," although some are "stems." This is an empirical issue. We have argued that the status of many morphemes classified as "prefix" is maintained only at the cost of the loss of important generalizations. Use of the template obscures the structure that is there. The answer I have offered is that speakers do not find the template in lexical patterns. The claim of the bipartite model is that it represents these patterns better than the position classes.

The "bipartite model" is a proposal that begins with the assumption that the structure of the verb in Athabaskan is transparent to learners. Particular information about morphological structure must be partially or even fully recoverable from the phonetics and phonology of the language. In this sense morphology is different from what happens above the level "word"; sound, structure, and meaning are more finely enmeshed below the level "word." It may be in fact that this is what "word" level is, the point above which structure achieves some autonomy from sound.

Thus it is in the phonetics and phonology that we can turn for evidence of morphological structure. That the sound system is sustained or supported by more abstract notions like inflectional or syntactic categories is not at issue. But formal or abstract devices supporting the sound system that are themselves unique or odd must be either recoverable or inferred, and exist only at some cost to the system. Many have noted that the structure of the Athabaskan verb is bipartite. I suggest that we need to return to this view.

Finally I repeat the main claims of the bipartite model: the verb is divided into three domains, disjunct clitics, an inflectional or "conjunct" domain, and a verb domain. The verb domain is the last syllable in the verb word. The verb domain consists of two morphemes, a verb stem which is the base of affixation of its domain and a set of valence markers or classifiers. The second domain is the infl domain. This is adjacent to the verb domain. It mirrors the verb domain in structure: it consists of a stem as a base of affixation and a set of prefixes. The stem is a portmanteau of tense (or mode) and subject marking. The variations among these morphemes can be construed as conjugational paradigms, such as the imperfective paradigm. This is the way, in fact, that these are listed in Young and Morgan. The set of prefixes are the qualifiers (QU) ("aspectual" in Young and Morgan's template). To the left of this domain, outside the domain are the agreement markers (AGR). The agreement markers are the leftmost morphemes in the inflectional or conjunct domain. To the left of the conjunct is the disjunct or clitic domain. The schema of this model follows:

(46)   The bipartite model of the morphological structure of the Navajo verb:

   disjunct clitics   # (AGR)   [(QU) Istem]$_{infl}$ [(CL) Vstem]$_{verb}$]$_{wd}$

Finally I give glosses of several verbs in the bipartite model:

(47)   a.   *jiyą́*   'He's eating it.'

   j + [*i*]$_{infl}$ [*yą́*]$_{verb}$]$_{wd}$
   3a [øimper/3s] [imp:'eat']

   b.   *'ajiyą́*   'He's eating.'

   '+ j [[*i*]$_{infl}$ [*yą́*]$_{verb}$]$_{wd}$
   3s - 3a [[ø imper/3s] [imp:'eat']]

   c.   *jileeh*   'He becomes.'

   j +   [[*i*]$_{infl}$ [*leeh*]$_{verb}$]$_{i/v}$
   3a   [[ø imper/3s] [imp:'becomes']]]

   d.   *njighá*   'He's going about.'

   n # j [*i*]$_{infl}$ [*ghá*]$_{verb}$]$_{wd}$
   'around' # 3a [øimper/3s] [imp: 'go']]

   e.   *dah díníishkaad*   'I started off with the herd.'   (YM 1987:330)

   dah [*dí ní yi ish*]$_{infl}$ [*ł - kaad*]$_{verb}$
       [incep - thematic - transitional øimpf/1Su] [cl - imper: '[herd]'[24]]

f.   *ch'éhésht'e'*   'I tossed them out (one after another).' (YM 1987:277)

   ch'í # [*h- ish*]   [*ł- t'e'*]
   'out'   [ser - øimp/1Su] [cl - impf: cause to move (SSO/AnO)']

Notes

I thank the teachers, staff, and students at Navajo Community College in Shiprock, New Mexico, and the members of the Summer 1993 Navajo Language Endorsement Program in Monument Valley, Arizona, as well as the community of speakers on Navajo Mountain who so kindly worked with us. Particular mention goes to Mary Willie of the University of Arizona, Helen George of the University of California, Los Angeles, and Martha Austin of NCC. Also I thank Ken Hale, Emmon Bach, and Eloise Jelinek for reading many versions of this essay and discussing these ideas with me. Although they are not responsible for the mistakes here, they surely are responsible for the good in this essay. Besides funding by the NSF, this work was supported by the National Institute on Deafness and Other Communication Disorders, and a grant from the Phillips Fund of the American Philosophical Society.

1.   Young and Morgan in fact appear to hold a less rigid view of the template than is often assumed; they refer to the prefixes as 'normally' appearing in a 'fixed relative order as components of the verb' (Young and Morgan 1987:39). They make no assumptions or claims about the template's role as a representation of a speaker's working knowledge of their language.

2.   The essentially prosthetic nature of the position classes is one of the stronger reasons for seeking independent evidence for this type of morphology.

3.   See the position 6b in Young and Morgan 1980, dropped in the 1987 version.

4.   There is no tense marking per se in Navajo. Mode refers to the conjugations, perfective, imperfective optative, future, etc., in Young and Morgan 1986:200ff. I use the term 'tense/mode' here to distinguish this morpheme from another class of morphemes in the conjunct domain that are referred to as 'aspectual' in Young and Morgan (position 6) and other works. In this chapter, I have referred to these aspectual morphemes as 'qualifiers' after Kari 1989, to further disambiguate the terminology. See discussion in section 7.1.2.

5.   I assume the orthography used in Young and Morgan 1987, the standard Navajo orthography. Words written in the Navajo orthography are in angle brakets (<hasébą́ą́s>) in the text. The terms for the mode conjugations (s-perfective, n-perfective, ø-imperfective, yi-perfective) are taken from Young and Morgan and Kari (1976). Terms for the aspect (inceptive, terminative, seriative) are taken from Young and Morgan 1987. Subject agreement is 'Su', object is 'Ob'. All morpheme glosses unless otherwise noted are derived from the morpheme glosses given in Young and Morgan 1987; page numbers are noted for the forms. The main difference between the glosses used in this paper and the glosses of Young and Morgan are in the tense/mode and Subject agreement. Young and Morgan report these as two separate morphemes; I report them as a single synthetic stem morpheme, (øimper/1Su) reads the ø-imperfective, first-person subject agreement. The names for the classes of

morphemes are 'cl' classifiers, 'qu' qualifiers, 'Istem' and 'Vstem' the bases of the infl and verb domains respectively, 'agr' agreement markers (position 'vi' and 'v' in Young and Morgan), 'tns/Su' the tense/mode and subject portmanteau (Istem) that is the base of the infl constituent.

6. The fourth-person marker <ji> can metathesize into a coda in the conjunct domain. See Kari (1976) and Young and Morgan (1987).

7. Young and Morgan note: "The prefixes of positions IV–VI, inclusive, are all composed of a consonant (C) + the vowel /i/ . . . for the most part the slots do not have inherent . . . tone" (1987:39).

8. The <-jáá> relates to the gap between the legs, <-tah> 'mixed in with'; thus [bijáátah] 'between his legs' (Young and Morgan 1987:368). The l-classifier-Vstem [l-chííd] means 'act with the hands, reach' (325).

9. (By sticking my hand between his legs), see note 8.

10. Young and Morgan use uppercase roman numerals for their position classes; I use lowercase.

11. The classifier morphemes, as valence markers, are also considered obligatory. However, one of the classifiers is the null morpheme <ø>, a zero morpheme which marks intransitivity. In the view put forth in this bipartite proposal, this morpheme represents the default specification, intransitive. For the purpose of this essay, I consider this morpheme to have no phonological content, and thus not present. Nothing rests on this assumption.

12. Parenthesized glides are epenthetic.

13. Note Kari's comment that the perfective paradigms are the most resistant ("the supreme test") to a phonological analysis (1976:167)

14. "Verb theme" and "verb base" are somewhat overlapping. They are defined in terms of the template. Both are related to notions of what constitutes a paradigm in the Athabaskan verb. *Verb base* usually refers to the classifier-stem combination, the verb constituent in the bipartite view. Although the morphology is productive, either many classifier-stem combinations are lexicalized or we do not yet understand the kinds of constraints imposed on the productivity by the aspectual properties on the morphemes. *Verb theme* usually refers to the classifier-stem combination and any other prefixes that combine to produce a meaning base in the verb. Although these are not formal terms, the insights they carry are essential to understanding the structure and meaning of the verbs. I refer the reader, as before, to the excellent discussion and examples in the Young and Morgan grammars.

15. The initial consonant of the <s> perfective has unusual phonology. Prefixes to it often show up in the onset of this syllable just as if it were empty, i.e., <h> + <sé> → <hé> (cf. <(y)ish>). The effects of this consonant are similar in many ways to the initial consonant in the so-called vowel initial stem <'ą́> 'eat'. Both consonants appear as the coronal fricative <s> in devoicing environment (edge of a word, after a voiceless consonant).

16. This is not strictly true, as forms like <'ajiyą> 'he's eating' show. However in this form the <'a> morpheme (3s) is what they call "thematic"—that is, it does not bind an argument of the verb (cf. <jiyą> 'he's eating it'). It is not clear that this is a correct characterization of this case. A full understanding of this phenomenon and co-occurrence restrictions remains to be worked out and must be related to quantification and argument structure.

17. There are dialect differences in Navajo. Some of them, such as this one, are probably best characterized as geographic; others, such as the loss of strong frication and coarticulation in the aspiration of consonants, are possibly best understood as

generational or sociological differences. The study of dialect differences is an important area of research in Navajo.

18.   Whether this is a dialect difference or whether there is inter- or intraspeaker variability is an open question. The point is that these forms exist as opposed to the invariability of the form in (30).

19.   'Move in a twisting or rolling manner, wind, tangle' (Young and Morgan 1987:324).

20.   Quantity insensitivity is a result of the fact of the constituent structure, not because of the phonology.

21.   Young and Morgan distinguish these from what they call the "Secondary Inflectional Determinants," which are the inflectional markers that "interact" with the primary ones. An example is the present of object marking in transitive verbs. The object marking is "secondary" because it is necessary if the verb is marked for transitivity in the primary prefixes—that is, by the causative or transitive classifiers.

22.   In these forms taken from Hargus and Tuttle (1995), I have used the symbols that they use, without changes. The forms are mainly from fieldnotes, as they note, and I believe we may assume they are written in broad phonetic transcription, in the IPA. They note "we have retranscribed data from our sources using standard phonetic symbols when it was clear to us how to do so" (first footnote in handout).

23.   Those sources listed without dates are from fieldnotes.

24.   In Young and Morgan (1987:330) "to act in a manner involving flatness and expansion, herd."

Bibliography

Bennet, J. F. 1987. Consonant Merger in Navajo: An Underspecified Analysis. *Studies in the Linguistic Sciences* 17(2):11-24.

Golla, V. K. 1970. Hupa Grammar. Ph.D. dissertation, University of California, Berkeley.

Hale, K. 1972. Navajo Linguistics. Unpublished manuscript, Massachusetts Institute of Technology.

Hale, K., and L. Honie. 1972. An Introduction to the Sound System of Navajo, Part I. Unpublished manuscript, Massachusetts Institute of Technology.

Halpern, A. 1992. Topics in the Placement and Morphology of Clitics. Ph.D. dissertation, Stanford University.

Hargus, S. 1985. The Lexical Phonology of Sekani. Ph.D. dissertation, University of California.

Hargus, S. 1995. Athabaskan Phonology. Talk given at the Athabaskan Morphosyntax Workshop, University of New Mexico.

Hargus, S., and S. Tuttle. 1995. Augmentation as Affixation. Paper presented at the Athabaskan Morphosyntax Workshop, University of New Mexico.

Hombert, J.-M. 1975. Phonetic Motivations for the Development of Tones from Postvocalic [h] and [ʔ]: Evidence from Contour Tone Perception. Report of the Phonology Laboratory 1:39–47.

Howren, R. 1971. A Formalization of the Athabaskan 'd-Effect'. *International Journal of American Linguistics* 39:96–114.

Jelinek, E. 1984. Empty Categories, Case and Configurationality. *Natural Language and Linguistic Theory* 2:39–76.

Kahn, D. 1976. Syllable-Based Generalizations in English Phonology. Ph.D. dissertation, Massachusetts Institute of Technology.

Kari, J. 1975. The Disjunct Boundary in the Navajo and Tanaina Verb Prefix Complexes. *International Journal of American Linguistics* 41.

Kari, J. 1976. *Navajo Verb Prefix Phonology.* New York: Garland.

Kari, J. 1989. Affix Positions and Zones in the Athabaskan Verb Complex: Ahtna and Navajo. *International Journal of American Linguistics* 55:424–454.

Kingston, J. 1990. Articulatory Binding. In J. Kingston and M. E. Beckman (eds.), *Papers in Laboratory Phonology*: Vol. 1: *Between the Grammar and Physics of Speech.* Cambridge: Cambridge University Press. 406–434.

Krauss, M. 1969. Proto-Athabaskan-Eyak and the Problem of Na-Dene: I. Phonology. *IJAL* 30:118–131.

Krauss, M. 1986. On the Classification in the Athabaskan, Eyak and Tlingit Verb. *Indiana University Publications in Anthropology and Linguistics Memoir,* Memoir 24.

Li, F.-K. 1946. Chipewyan. In C. Osgood (ed.), *Linguistic Structures of Native America.* Viking Fund Publications in Anthropology 6:76–90.

Leer, Jeff. 1979. *Proto-Athabaskan Verb Stem Variation.* (Alaska Native Language Center Research Papers, No. 4). Fairbanks: Alaska Native Language Center.

Leer, Jeff. 1982. *Navajo and Comparative Athabaskan Stem List.* Fairbanks: Alaska Native Language Center.

McDonough, J. 1990. Topics in the Phonology and Morphology of Navajo Verbs. Ph.D. dissertation, University of Massachusetts, Amherst.

McDonough, J. 1991. Consonant Harmony in Navajo. *Proceedings of West Coast Conference on Foreign Linguistics 10*, Stanford University Press. 121–136.

McDonough, J. 1995. Epenthesis in Navajo. In Jelenik, Saxon, and Rice (eds.), *Essays in Honor of Robert Young.* Albuquerque: University of New Mexico Press. 235–257.

McDonough, J. 1999a. Tone in Navajo. *Anthropological Linguistics* 41.

McDonough, J. 1999b. The d-Effect Syndrome in Navajo. Unpublished manuscript, University of Rochester.

McDonough, J. 1999c. Athabaskan Redux: Against the Position Class as a Morphological Category. *Morphologica.*

Morice, B. 1932. *The Carrier Language.* Vienna.

Randoja, T. K. 1989. The Phonology and Morphology of Halfway River Beaver. Ph.D. dissertation, University of Ottawa.

Rice, K. 1989. *A Grammar of Slave.* Berlin: Mouton de Gruyter.

Sapir, E., and H. Hoijer. 1967. *The Phonology and Morphology of the Navajo Language.* Berkeley: University of California Press.

Simpson, J., and M. Withgott. 1986. Pronominal Clitic Clusters and Templates. In H. Borer, ed.*Syntax and Semantics*: Vol. 19: *The Syntax of Pronominal Clitics.* Boston: Academic Press. 149–174.

Stanley, R. 1969. The Phonology of the Navajo Verb. Ph.D. dissertation, Massachusetts Institute of Technology.

Stump, G. 1991. On the Theoretical Status of Position Class Restrictions on Inflectional Affixes. *Yearbook of Morphology.* 211–241.

Thompson, C. 1993. The Areal Prefix *hË-* in Koyukon Athabaskan. *International Journal of American Linguistics* 59(3):315–334.

Tuttle, S. 1994. The Peg Prefix, the Foot and the Word Minimum: Evidence from Salcha Athabaskan. Unpublished manuscript, University of Washington.

Tuttle, S. 1998. Metrical and Tonal Structures in Tanana Athabaskan. Ph.D. dissertation, University of Washington.

Williams, E. 1994. *Thematic Structure*. Cambridge, MA: MIT Press.

Williams, E. 1996. Three Models of Morphology-Syntax Interface. Unpublished manuscript, Princeton University.

Wright, M. 1983. The CV Skeleton and Verb-Prefix Phonology in Navajo. In P Sells and C. Jones *Northeast Linguistic Society* 14:34–51.

Young, R., and W. Morgan. 1943. *The Navaho Language*. Salt Lake City, UT: United States Indian Service, Education Division.

Young, R., and W. Morgan. 1980. *The Navajo Language*. Albuquerque: University of New Mexico Press.

Young, R., and W. Morgan. 1987. *The Navajo Language*. Albuquerque: University of New Mexico Press.

Young, R., and W. Morgan. 1992. *An Analytic Lexicon of Navajo*. Albuquerque: University of New Mexico Press.

8

MONADIC VERBS
AND ARGUMENT STRUCTURE
IN AHTNA, SLAVE, AND NAVAJO

Keren Rice

Monadic verbs have been an important topic of research, both in linguistic theory in general (e.g., Perlmutter 1978; Rosen 1984; Grimshaw 1987, 1990; Van Valin 1990; Tenny 1994; Levin and Hovav Rappaport 1995) and in Athabaskan languages in particular (Hale and Platero 1996, Rice 1991). In this essay I focus on lexically monadic verbs in three Athabaskan languages, Ahtna, Slave, and Navajo. I concentrate in particular on how the syntactic position of nondiscourse participant subjects in these languages is determined. I make the following claims:

1. The subject of a monadic verb can appear in three positions at S-structure, external to the verb phrase, or in canonical subject position (A in (1)), internal to the verb phrase (B in (1)), and incorporated into the verb word (C in (1)).

(1)   IP

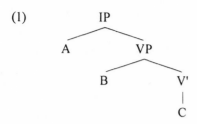

A   VP

B   V'
             |
             C

2. The surface position of a subject is determined by factors of sali-
    ency, agentivity, animacy, and humanness.

3. The position of the subject of a monadic verb need not be stipulated
    as part of the lexical entry of the verb, but is predictable based on
    the factors in (ii). Thus, a lexically encoded syntactic distinction be-
    tween two types of monadic verbs, or lexically encoded argument
    structure, is unnecessary.

The three languages under consideration, Ahtna, Slave, and Navajo, differ in
several ways, but lead us to a single overall conclusion: it is properties such as
agentivity and humanness that determine the syntactic position of the subject of
a monadic verb. Listing of argument structure, in the sense that the syntactic
position of a verbal argument is part of the lexical entry of the verb, does not
appear to be required in these languages.

8.1 Background

It has long been recognized, based on a number of different diagnostics, that
intransitive verbs fall into two basic classes. According to the Unaccusative Hypothesis as originally set forth by Perlmutter (1978) and defended by Rosen
(1984), there are two lexical classes of intransitive verbs. These two classes differ in their syntactic subcategorization properties, as shown in the schematic
lexical entries for the verbs given in (2) and (3). One class of verbs, often called
unergative verbs, have their sole argument external to the verb phrase (2a). Some
typical verbs of this type are included in (2b).

(2) a. unergative: NP [V]$_{VP}$

     b. walk, jump, swim, run, race, fly, gallop, dive, crawl, talk,
         shout, dance, work, cry, sing, spit, breathe

The second class of verbs, often termed unaccusative verbs, have their sole argument internal to the verb phrase, as in (3a); examples are given in (3b).

(3) a. unaccusative: [NP V]$_{VP}$

  b. break, crack, split, shatter, rip, tear, open, close, bend, drop, slide, move, sink, spin, shake, float, grow, spill, fall, burn, cook

The unergative and unaccusative verbs share in requiring a single argument; they differ in terms of their lexically listed argument structure, or the position of that argument. According to this hypothesis, the different patterning observed in the two classes is a consequence of their argument structure, or subcategorization frame. Under the Unaccusative Hypothesis, whatever semantic properties are shared by members of the class of unaccusative verbs or members of the class of unergative verbs are largely accidental, as it is syntax that is primary.

An alternative approach to the unaccusative/unergative distinction has been taken, namely a semantic approach; see Van Valin (1990). Under this approach, syntactic subcategorization frames are regarded as largely irrelevant, with the patterning of monadic verbs being predictable on semantic grounds. The relevant semantic properties include both thematic roles of undergoer and actor and aspectual information regarding telicity of the verb. Under this hypothesis, verbs with actor subjects might pattern one way and verbs with undergoer subjects a different way with respect to the diagnostics (see Van Valin 1990 for this terminology); atelic and telic predicates might pattern differently as well. See also Grimshaw (1990), Tenny (1994), Dowty (1991), Borer (1993), and Levin and Hovav Rappaport (1995) for arguments on the importance of aspect in monadic verb systems.

A third approach, argued for by Levin and Hovav Rappaport (1995), is to a large degree a reconciliation of the previous two approaches. Levin and Hovav Rappaport argue that the verb classes are semantically characterized and that they also have common syntactic properties.

In this chapter, I examine some possible unaccusative/unergative diagnostics in the Athabaskan languages Ahtna, Slave, and Navajo. I conclude that while there is evidence for the two types of surface syntactic structures shown in (2) and (3), the position of the noun internal or external to the verb phrase is predictable on semantic grounds. Further, the position of the noun with respect to the verb does not correlate with the unaccusative/unergative division, but rather with thematic properties of the subject. I further show that the kinds of asymmetries that might be expected if argument structure is part of the lexical entry are not found. The evidence presented offers no support for the claim that syntactic subcategorization must be included in the lexical entry of a monadic verb.

8.2 Terminology

Before turning to the main topic, a brief excursus on the use of several terms is in order. Consider first the pair of words *unergative* and *unaccusative*. I use these terms structurally, to refer to the structures in (2) and (3), respectively. Since work on the topic of intransitive structures has revealed a high degree of cross-linguistic overlap in terms of which class a verb belongs to, I will identify a verb as unaccusative or unergative based on findings in other languages. Thus, I assume that verbs such as *talk*, *spit*, *cry*, and *work* are unergative, while verbs such as *dry*, *freeze*, *boil*, and *grow* are unaccusative. When I refer to the Unaccusative Hypothesis, I mean the hypothesis that says that the syntactic position of a sole argument of a verb, or the argument structure of the verb, is specified in the lexical entry of that verb. It is this position that I argue against.

The second set of terms is *agent* and *patient*. I use these as very general terms: the agent is the one who initiates or brings about an event or who is the actor, while the patient undergoes the event or is affected by an event or state. "Agent" is similar to Van Valin's term "actor" and "patient" to his "undergoer."

Third, I use the term *subject* to refer simply to the single argument of a monadic verb with no implications as to syntactic position of that argument.

8.3   Evidence for the Position of Subjects: Ahtna

In this section, I examine evidence for the position of subjects in Ahtna, an Athabaskan language of Alaska. I argue that while subjects can have more than one position syntactically at S-structure, there is no need to consider the position of the subject of a monadic verb to be included as part of the lexical entry of that verb; rather its position is predictable.

8.3.1   Case Marking of Nonparticipant Pronouns: All Intransitives Show Subject Marking

One possible way that unergative and unaccusative verbs might be distinguished is in case marking of the subject: unergative verbs are predicted to have the same subject marking as transitive subjects, while aubject markers of unaccusative verbs might be of the same subject marking as objects of transitive verbs. In Ahtna, and in other Athabaskan languages as well, all subjects generally show identical case marking. The table in (4) summarizes subject morphology and the marking of a second argument of a transitive verb in Ahtna. All intransitive verbs show subject morphology.

(4)	Single argument of verb		Second argument of transitive verb (3 subject)	
Ø	3		y	3
k	3 plural human		b	3 topical
y	3 nonsalient		hw	3 plural human

Thus, the surface case of the subject of an intransitive verb is independent of its position. Case provides no evidence for monadic verbs having different argument structures.

8.3.2 Transitivity Alternations

It has been noticed that in a number of languages not all verbs participate in transitivity alternations, and it has sometimes been proposed that only unaccusative verbs take part in these alternations. Hale and Platero (1996) and Rice (1991) argue for Navajo and Slave, respectively, that the ability to enter into a morphological causative construction (marked by the causativizer *ł*) provides a diagnostic for unaccusativity/unergativity—only unaccusative verbs show a simple type of transitivity alternation. In this section I show that this is not the case in Ahtna: both unergative and unaccusative verbs can enter into the morphological causative construction. Given this, transitivity alternations do not provide evidence for two syntactic subcategorization frames for monadic verbs in this language.

I begin by discussing unaccusative verbs, or, to anticipate, verbs with patientive arguments, and then turn to unergative verbs, or verbs with agentive arguments. The morphological causative construction in Ahtna is marked by the presence of the valence-changing *ł*, one of the so-called classifiers found in the Athabaskan language family. This morpheme directly precedes the verb stem. Examples are set up as follows. The first line of each pair shows the lexical entry given in Kari (1990). The second line shows a verb word based on this lexical entry. The hyphen separates the stem, generally the final syllable of the verb, from the rest of the verb word. The causativizer, *ł*, is shown in boldface. The examples in (i) of each data set are intransitive, while those in (ii) are causative. All page numbers refer to Kari (1990).

(5)   Unaccusative verbs; verbs with patientive arguments (i—intransitive; ii—causative)

    a. i.   *G-Ø-ggan*   'become dry' (191–192)
            z-ggan   'It is dry.'
        ii. *c'etsen' ł-ggan*   'He is drying the meat.' (192)
            meat

    b. i.   *d-n-l-ghots*   'boil' (223)
            tnel-ghots   'It is boiling.'
        ii. *itneł-ghots*   'He boiled it.' (223)

    c. i.   *G-d-n-Ø-k'e'*   'become cool, tepid, cool off' (257)
            tsaey tnez-k'e'   'The tea cooled off.'
            tea
        ii. *itneł-k'e'*   'He cooled it off.' (257)

d. i.   *G-D-ten*   'freeze' (332)
        s-ten   'It froze, is frozen, he froze to death.'
  ii.   *dela' ł-ten*   'He froze his hand.' (332)
        reflexive.hand

e. i.   *G-Ø-t'aes*   'roast, fry, bake' (347)
        z-t'ae   'It is roasted, fried.'
  ii.   *yił-t'ae*   'He roasted it.' (347)

f. i.   *n-gh-l-ts'e'*   'freeze solid' (403)
        ngel-ts'e'   'It (animal) froze solid.'
  ii.   *ingił-ts'e'*   'He froze it.' (405)

g. i.   *G-D-caats*   'be rendered, liquefied' (110-111
        s-tcaats   'It was liquefied.'
  ii.   *yił-caats*   'He rendered it.' (111)

h. i.   *G-n-Ø/ł-yaa*   'grow, grow up, mature' (420)
        nez-yaan   'He grew up.'
  ii.   *sneł-yaan*   'He raised me.' (420)

i. i.   *G-Ø-c'el*   'tear, rip, split, peel' (124)
        uyinaltaeni z-c'eł   'His biceps got pulled.'
  ii.   *ighił-c'el*   'He tore it repeatedly.' (124)
        yił-c'eł   'He tore it once.' (124)

j. i.   *G-D-dloz*   'become wrinkled, softened by crum-
                           pling' (164)
        c'ezes gha-dloz   'The skin got crumpled.'
        skin
  ii.   *ighił-dloz*   'He softened it by crumpling.' (164)

k. i.   *G-D-ts'ic'*   'become smashed, squashed' (416)
        unaen' na-ts'i'   'His face became deeply wrinkled.'
        3.face
  ii.   *ingił-s'i'*   'He smashed them (berries).' (416)

l. i.   *d-D-let*   'smudge, smoking fire burns, smol-
                           der, burn down to ashes' (278)
        dad-let   'It was smoldering.'
  ii.   *idghi-łet*   'He burned it down to ashes.'

m. i.   *G-gh-Ø-naa*   'move, tremble, shake' (288)
        nen' ghighi-na'   'The earth was shaking.'
  ii.   *łts'ii ts'abaeli dgheł-naa* 'Wind is moving the trees.' (288)
        wind tree

There are also unaccusative verbs that do not appear to be able to enter into the causative construction.

(6)   *n-D-laat*   'Berries become ripe, ripen.' (161)
      gige nd-laat   'Berries are ripe.'
      berry

No causative form is given in Kari (1990), while causatives are generally listed for patientive-type verbs.

In Ahtna, unergative verbs, or verbs with agentive subjects, can also enter into the morphological causative construction.

(7)   a.   i.   *gh-D-naa*   'work' (288)
                 ghat-na'   'He was working.'
           ii.   *ighet-na*   'He is making him work.' (288)

      b.   i.   *Ø-tsaex*   'cry' (374)
                 ghi-tsaex   'He was crying.'
           ii.   *ighit-tsaex*   'He made her cry.' (274)

      c.   i.   *D-naan*   'drink O' (290)
                 c'et-naan   'He is drinking something.'
           ii.   *tuu ughet-naan'*   'I made him drink water.'

Kari does not indicate that many of these verbs can enter into the causative construction. In Koyukon, another Athabaskan language of Alaska, causatives of agentive verbs are quite common.

The facts from Ahtna suggest that the ability of a monadic verb to enter into transitivity alternations is not a diagnostic for the syntactic structure of that verb—there are unaccusatives that have a causative form and unaccusatives that do not have a causative form; there are unergatives that have a causative form and unergatives that do not appear to have a causative form. Thus the lexically encoded syntactic structure of a verb does not predict its ability to enter into transitivity alternations.

Are there then semantic factors that control which verbs can enter into transitivity alternations? It appears that there might be. Consider the following two verbs.

(8)   *gige' nd-laat*   'Low bush cranberries are ripe.' (161)
      berry

This verb, with a patientive subject, has no causative form.

(9)   *ighit-tsaex*   'He made her cry.' (274)

This verb has an agentive subject and allows a causative form.

In the first case, the ripening occurs on its own and cannot be caused—in a sense the berries themselves are the initiator of their own ripening.[1] In the second case, while the argument of 'cry' is the only one who can actually start the crying, an external causer may be involved. It appears that a closer investigation of the semantics of the causative construction may well reveal that patientive verbs that do not participate in transitivity alternations involve subjects that are both affected and affecting and that the arguments of agentive verbs that do participate in transitivity alternations can be viewed as noninitiators, or as affected by an external initiator. In any case, the transitivity alternations provide evidence that it is not syntactic structure that determines whether a verb will enter into these alternations—transitivity alternations do not exploit the difference between a subject internal to the verb phrase and one external to the verb phrase along the lines laid out by the Unaccusative Hypothesis.

8.3.3   Oblique object forms

So far I have shown that two potential diagnostics for the syntactic class of a monadic verb in Ahtna are inconclusive: case marking is not useful in distinguishing two classes, and transitivity alternations do not target just verbs that would have internal arguments; monadic verbs with external arguments are subject to transitivity alternations as well. Thus, so far we have seen no evidence for syntactically encoding these verb classes in Ahtna but rather evidence for semantic classes based on thematic properties of the argument of the verb. In this section, I examine a third possible diagnostic, the form of oblique object pronouns. This diagnostic is discussed in Rice (1989, 1991) for Slave and in Saxon and Rice (1993) for Ahtna and Koyukon.

In an Ahtna sentence with a third-person subject, an oblique object may have one of two forms; it may either be *y-* or *b-/u-* (phonological variants of the same morpheme; I will refer to it as *b-*). An initial hypothesis that receives some support is that the oblique object has the form *y-* when the verb is unergative and the form *b-* when the verb is unaccusative. I will show that this is not the case: *y-* is indeed often the oblique object form when the verb is unergative; however, *y-* may occur as an oblique object with any monadic verb whose single argument is human. While structural properties determine the form of the pronoun (see the discussion later in this section), these properties do not correlate with the structural unaccusative/unergative distinction.

The pronominal *y-* is generally used as a direct object when the subject is third person; this is the use termed "disjoint anaphor" by Saxon (1984).

(10)   *nayiɬ-tsiin* 'S/he made it again.' (291)
         3 made *y* again

It is also used as an oblique object when the subject is third person.

(11) *ya*   *ke-naes*   'S/he is talking about it/him/her.' (419)
      y.about talk

Finally, *y*- occurs as a subject under certain conditions. Semantically, *y*- is a subject when the subject is nonsalient; see Thompson (1989) and Saxon and Rice (1993). Structurally, Saxon and Rice (1993) argue that the choice of *y*- as a subject is syntactically represented as well: *y*- can be a subject when there is a clausemate NP which c-commands it; I return to this later. In the examples in (12), the c-commanding noun is a pronominal of the form *b*-. The *y*- subjects are in boldface and the *b*- oblique objects are underlined. In the glosses, the topical argument is italicized.

(12) a.   <u>*u'eł*</u>   **yayaał**   'S/he is walking with <u>him/her</u>.' (419)
           b.with   *y*.is walking

      b.   <u>*ba*</u>   *tayghighel*   'It fell in the water on <u>him</u>.' (217)
           b.on *y*.fell in water

      c.   <u>*biinał'aen*</u>   'It is looking at <u>him</u>.' (96)
           b.at *y* looks

Having surveyed the general distribution of *y*-, I now turn to a detailed examination of its distribution as an oblique object.

In general, when verbs have agentive human subjects, they occur with the pronoun *y*- as an oblique object.

(13) Human agentive subject: *y*- as oblique object

      a.   **ya** *ke-naes*   'She is talking about it/him/her.' (419)
           y.about talk

      b.   **ya** *at-naa*   'He is working on it.' (288)
           y.on work

Nonhuman animate agentive subjects can also appear with *y*- as oblique object.

(14) Nonhuman agentive subject: *y*- as oblique object

      a.   *ik'e dast-bets*   'It (a bird) landed on top of it.' (106)
           y.on up.pf.fluttered

      b.   *tikaani* **yuka** *tez-niic*   'A wolf reached for (scared)
           wolf *y*.for pf.reached   him/her.' (307)

With inanimate "agentive," or effector, subjects, the pronoun *b-* occurs as oblique object rather than *y-*.

(15) a.   *niget   uyughat-kay*   'Fear leapt into him/her (s/he got
            fear   *b.*into leapt   nervous).' (237)

      b.   *neniic   uyi   ghi-yaa* 'Happiness went into him (he became
            happiness *b.*into went   happy).' (422)

Saxon and Rice (1993) draw the following syntactic generalization about the distribution of *y-* and *b-* as oblique objects.

(16) *Structural account of the distribution of y-:* If a subject is external to the VP, then *y-* occurs as oblique object; if a subject is internal to the VP, then *b-* occurs as oblique object.

I will take this generalization that the choice of *y-* or *b-* as oblique object form is syntactically determined as an assumption. The two subject positions are shown in the structure in (17). When the subject is external, the oblique third person object is *y-*; when the subject is internal, the oblique third-person object is *b-*. This tree is simplified; see Saxon and Rice (1993) and Rice and Saxon (1994) for further details that are not directly relevant here.

(17)

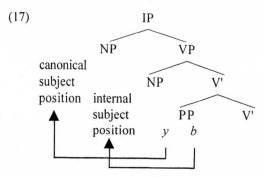

The question now arises of what subjects can be canonical, or occur external to the VP. The Unaccusative Hypothesis provides one possible account—subjects of unergative verbs are external to the verb phrase, while subjects of unaccusative verbs are internal to the verb phrase. In the following discussion I argue that this account of the distribution of subjects is not correct. Instead, I argue that it is semantic factors that determine the position in which a subject occurs in (17).

Saxon and Rice (1993) provide an initial hypothesis regarding the position of subject NPs. First, Saxon and Rice argue that subjects that are external to the verb phrase must be topical or salient. I will assume that all the examples that I give have salient subjects and thus disregard this factor for the moment; see also Saxon and Rice (1993) and Thompson (1989) for discussion. Second, Saxon and Rice claim that subjects in this position can be categorized by whether they are human or nonhuman. Topical human subjects must be canonical subjects, or external to the VP (13); topical nonhuman agents must also be canonical subjects (14). These criteria are summarized in (18).

(18) VP-external subject (canonical subject) position (Saxon and Rice 1993)
      Subjects in this position must be topical, or salient.
      Topical human subjects must be canonical subjects.
      Topical nonhuman agents must be canonical subjects.

So far I have shown that animate salient or topical agents occur with *y-* as their oblique object form, as in the examples in (13) and (14); I return to the examples in (15) later. First, however, consider monadic verbs with patientive arguments. Verbs with patientive subjects often have *b-* as their oblique object form. This can be seen in the examples in (19).

(19) Nonhuman patientive subjects: *b-*

    a.   *uggaaye' uyi nez-yaan*   'Its embryo grew inside it.' (420)
        *b.*embryo *b.*inside grew

    b.   *uk'e tay'de-ggaasi*   'skin stretcher, that on which skin is
        *b.*on something.dry.nom.   dried' (192)

    c.   *ut'aa   nace'en-t'esi*   'oven (in it something is roasted)'
        *b.*inside something.roast.nom (348)

    d.   *uk'enaa' ba   da-tsets*   'His working ability dried up on
        *b.*ability 3.for dry up   him.' (384)

    e.   *niłdooxetah   del   uts'inghes*   'Sometimes blood drips from it.'
        sometimes   blood *b.*from drip   (216)

Assuming the syntactic representation in (17), the presence of *b-* in these forms suggests that the arguments here are not in canonical subject position—that is, they are not external. Rather they are within the VP.

The data discussed so far show two types of verbs. The examples in (13) and (14) are unergatives with salient or topical agentive subjects, human or not, and those in (19) are unaccusatives with salient nonhuman patientive subjects.[2] Based on these data, the *y-/b-* test appears to provide a diagnostic for syntactic unaccusative/unergative classes. Specifically, it appears that unergative verbs license *y-* as an oblique object while unaccusative verbs license *b-* as an oblique object. If this were the case, then one would want to encode syntactic structure lexically in order to select the correct pronominal form. However, further investigation shows that the form of the oblique object does not in fact diagnose unaccusative/unergative structures.

I have so far not discussed unergative verbs with inanimate subjects or unaccusative verbs with human subjects. Consider first the forms in (13) and (14), unergative verbs with animate subjects. The oblique object pronoun that occurs is *y-*, as has been discussed. However, not all unergative verbs occur with *y-* as oblique object—the examples in (15) have unergative verbs with inanimate subjects. Here the oblique object has the form *b-*. These examples suggest a problem for the Unaccusative Hypothesis: unergative verbs with nonanimate subjects occur with *b-* as the oblique object while unergative verbs with animate subjects occur with *y-* as the oblique object. The unergative-unaccusative distinction does not appropriately capture the distribution of *b-* and *y-* as oblique object form since both can occur with unergative verbs.

Now consider unaccusative verbs with human subjects. Unaccusative verbs with nonhuman subjects occur with *b-* as oblique object, as in (19). Unaccusative verbs with human subjects display different patterning than either the verbs with agentive subjects or the verbs with nonhuman patientive subjects: they can occur with either *y-* or *b-* as oblique object. Several examples of *y-* are given in (20) and of *b-* in (21). Most of these verbs represent states rather than events.

(20)   Patientive verbs with human subjects may take *y-* as oblique object

      a.   *i'eł z-daa*   'He stays with him.' (133)
           y.with sit

      b.   *ic'aats'e' z-daa*   'He stays opposite from him.' (122)
           y.opposite sit

      c.   *ik'ez-taen*   'He is lying down on it.' (328)
           y.on lie

(21)   Patientive verbs with human subjects may take *b-* as oblique object

      a.   *udi-daa*   'He is sitting, touching him.' (64)
           b.sit

      b.   *u'iidze' z-daa*   'He stays hidden by it.' (92)
           b.hidden by sit

      c.   *uyighi-tsaan'*   He defecated into it.' (370)
           y.into defecate

As these forms show, one and the same verb can appear either with a *y-* oblique object form (20) or with a *b-* (21) oblique object form. These verbs have patient subjects; with agentive human subjects only *y-* is found. The statement on the distribution of *y-* thus requires rewording, as in (22).

(22) Agentive human subjects must be canonical subjects (13); human nona-
      gentive subjects may be canonical subjects (20, 21). Nonhuman nonagen-
      tive subjects may not be canonical subjects (19).

The form of the oblique object pronoun has ramifications for the Unaccusative Hypothesis. The distribution of oblique objects demonstrates that there are
indeed two positions for subjects, an external position and an internal position.
The arguments that appear as canonical subjects, or in external position, include
the subjects of unergatives but are not restricted to this class: human subjects of
unaccusatives can also appear in this position. Thus, while this test points to a
role for syntactic structure, it is not the role predicted by the Unaccusative Hypothesis. The argument structure that would be lexically associated with a monadic verb under this hypothesis does not determine which subjects are external
to the VP; rather factors of saliency or topicality, agentivity, humanness, and
animacy, factors which cross-cut the verb class distinction, do. No support is
found from the form of oblique object pronouns for the verbs themselves having
different syntactic subcategorization frames associated with them lexically—the
distribution of *y-* and *b-* is sensitive to semantic properties of the argument
rather than to argument structure of the verb.

8.3.4   An Aside on Aspect

Before examining to other possible criteria for distinguishing two lexical classes
of intransitive verbs, I would like to turn briefly to the relationship of situation
aspect and argument structure in Ahtna. As mentioned in section 8.1, it has
been argued that in many languages there are correlations between telicity or
boundedness and unaccusative/unergative properties. Van Valin (1990) and
Dowty (1991) both exploit these characteristics in their discussion of monadic
verb classes. Borer (1993) proposes that atelic verbs share a structural property:
their argument appears in the position of the functional projection that she calls
process. These verbs, she argues, show unergative properties. Telic verbs share
the property that their argument is in the specifier of the functional projection
which Borer calls event, or result; such verbs, Borer argues, show unaccusative
diagnostics. Arguments thus receive their interpretation by being in a particular
specifier position. Borer argues that there is a class of variable verbs which show
both unaccusative and unergative properties, and she proposes that these verbs
differ aspectually, and thus structurally. She reports that the Hebrew verb 'wilt'
falls in this class—when the aspect is telic it has unaccusative properties and
when it is atelic is has unergative properties. Because aspect can be an important
factor in determining the position of arguments of intransitive verbs in other
languages, I now turn, briefly, to the situation aspect system in Ahtna to examine whether situation aspect might play a role in determining the position of
verbal arguments in this language.
       It has long been recognized that event (i.e., nonstative) predicates can be di-

vided into three major classes based on parameters of telicity and duration (e.g., Vendler 1957, Smith 1991), achievements, activities, and accomplishments. The first of these are predicates that are telic but without duration; the second class is durative and atelic; and the final class is durative and telic. Different linguists use slightly different classes; this particular classification is appropriate for Ahtna; see Rice (in press) for detailed discussion using the terminology employed here and Kari (1979), Rice (1989), and Axelrod (1993) for discussion of a similar framework with different names. I will be concerned here only with activities and accomplishments.

Ahtna provides overt evidence for the situation aspect, or Aktionzart, classes of activities and accomplishments. One type of evidence is provided by the forms in (23): these show pairs of verbs where the first one is telic and the second nontelic in nature. Typical translations involve singular vs. plural, past as opposed to past progressive, or done as opposed to done repeatedly. The verbs in these pairs differ not only in their semantics, but also in two other ways. First, the stem form may differ between the telic and nontelic verbs. Second, the telic form occurs with a morpheme *s-*, which marks durativity and telicity, while the nontelic form has a morpheme *gh-* instead, which marks durativity and nontelicity. The presence of *gh-* is readily seen in the forms in (23); *s-* enters into phonological interactions and its presence is sometimes obscured.

(23) a. *s*:   *yiɬ-kaɬ*   'He chopped it once.' (233)
          gh: *ighiɬ-kaatl'*   'He was chopping it.' (233)

      b. *s*:   *yiz-taɬ*   'He shoved it once with his foot.' (323)
          gh: *ighi-tatl'*   'He shoved it repeatedly with his foot.' (323)

      c. *s*:   *ineɬ-tl'uul*   'He braided it (rope).' (366)
          gh: *inghiɬ-tl'uul*   'He braided them.' (366)

      d. *s*:   *inez-'aes*   'He strung them (beads).' (89)
          gh: *i'ngas-'aes*   'I strung something (beads) repeatedly.' (89)

In addition, there is a class of verbs in which number is inherently marked in the verb root. With these verbs, the singular forms pattern as accomplishments and appear with *s-* while the plural forms are activities and take *gh-*.

(24) *s*:   *izeɬ-ghaen* 'He killed it; he beat him up (singular object).' (213)
      s: *yiɬ-tsiin*   'He made it (singular object).' (386)
      gh: *i'ghi-ghaan* 'He made something, he killed something (plural).' (204)

Since situation aspect is overtly marked in Ahtna, a question arises as to whether it plays a role in determining the position of subjects in this language. The position of the subject appears to cross-cut aspect: subjects of telic predicates can be external, as evidenced by the occurrence of *y-* as oblique object, or internal, shown by the presence of *b-* as oblique object, and subjects of atelic predicates can also be either external (*y-*) or internal (*b-*). This can be seen in the following examples.

(25) situation aspect: *y* oblique object

i'eł z -daa	'He stays with him.' (133)	*s* telic
ic'aats'e' z -daa	'He stays opposite from him.' (122)	*s* telic
ik'ez -taen	'He is lying down on it.' (328)	*s* telic
itendze ghi -yaa	'He intercepted him.' (422)	*gh* atelic

(26) *b* oblique object

u'iidze' z-daa	'He stays hidden by it.' (92)	*s* telic
uyighi-tsaan'	'He defecated into it.' (370)	*gh* atelic
neniic uyi ghi-yaa	'Happiness went into him, he became happy.' (422)	*gh* atelic
nuuni c'oxe' uni dghi-yaa porcupine quill *b.*into went	'The porcupine quill became embedded in it.'	*gh* atelic

These forms show that telic verbs, as marked by *s-*, can occur with *y-* oblique object as well as with *b-* oblique object and atelic verbs, marked by *gh-*, with *b-* oblique object as well as with *y-* oblique object. This is not predicted if aspect is important in determining the position of a subject; the prediction rather would be that telic verbs would occur with *b-* and atelic verbs with *y-*.

Before dismissing the role of situation aspect entirely, however, one more factor should be considered. If we take into account only cases with human subjects that are not nonsalient, we find that agentive subjects must be external (13) while patientive subjects may be external (20, 21). This could be attributable to agentivity/patientivity; it could also be attributable to aspectual class: subjects of atelic verbs must be external, while subjects of telic verbs may be external. Factors of salience and humanness are clearly of great importance in Ahtna. With human subjects, agents and patients pattern in different ways, with agents being obligatorily external to the verb phrase and patients being only optionally so. Whether this difference in patterning is best attributable to properties of the argument (agent/patient) or whether it is best attributable to properties of the verb (atelic/telic) or to some combination of the two remains a question for further study.

8.3.5   Other Constructions Involving Subjects

I have argued that, based on tests of case marking, transitivity alternations, and aspect, Ahtna does not provide evidence for listing syntactic subcategorization frames as part of the lexical entry of a verb. It is relevant to raise one further issue with respect to this question. It could be argued that the types of surface properties that I have examined so far simply obscure the need for argument structure being lexically specified and that further tests will show the need for lexically specified subjects occurring in different relationships to the verb. Verb-phrase internal and ver*b*-phrase external positions, as assumed by the Unaccusative Hypothesis, provide only one possible way of differentiating two positions for subjects. It would be possible, for instance, to express the difference between unaccusative and unergative verbs by the position of an argument within the verb phrase; for instance, the subject of an unergative might be a daughter of VP and the subject of an unaccusative a daughter of V'. I will argue that this type of proposal offers no real solution to the problems that we have encountered for the Unaccusative Hypothesis; it simply displaces them by one level. The problems that arise for the Unaccusative Hypothesis can be seen by abstracting away from factors of saliency, and looking only at subjects that I have assumed are in position B in (17). In this case, we find no differences in patterning between the subjects of unergative verbs and the subjects of unaccusative verbs—both types of subjects can be nonsalient, both can be incorporated into the verb, both can enter into idioms.

First, consider nonsalient subjects, or those subjects marked morphologically by *y*- (see (12)). When a subject of an intransitive is not salient, unergative and unaccusative verbs pattern together in the form of both the subject and the oblique. Nonsalient third-person subjects have the form *y*- (see Thompson 1989 for detailed discussion of the semantics of *y*- subjects; see also Saxon and Rice 1993). When the subject is of the form *y*-, the oblique object is always of the form *b*-, whether the subject is a patient (27) or an agent (28). The *y*- subject and *b*- oblique object forms are boldfaced in (27) and (28).

(27)   Nonsalient subjects: subject marked by *y*- and oblique by *b*- in unaccusatives

   ba *tayghi-ghel*   'It fell in the water on him.' (217)
   b.on *y*.water fell

(28)   Nonsalient subjects: subject marked by *y*- and oblique by *b*- in unergatives

   u'*eł* **ya**-*yaał*   'S/he is walking with him/her.' (419)
   b.with *y*.walk

There is no evidence that these subjects occupy different positions with respect to the verb, as might be expected under the Unaccusative Hypothesis. Rather, both types of subjects are identical in patterning with respect to the oblique object form diagnostic.

Second, Ahtna allows incorporation of subjects into the verb. The semantic conditions of incorporation have not been examined in great detail in Ahtna. Axelrod (1990), in a detailed discussion of incorporation in Koyukon, another Athabaskan language, proposes that subject incorporation allows a noun to function in an atypical semantic relationship with a verb; in particular, incorporation allows agentive subjects without prototypical canonical subjects properties (nonvolitional, not highly potent; see Hopper and Thompson 1980 for details) to function as an agent. Ahtna allows nonprototypical subjects to be unincorporated, unlike Koyukon, but otherwise the conditions on incorporation appear to be quite similar between the two languages. What is important to see here is that both patientive and agentive subjects can be incorporated. In structural terms, subjects of unaccusative verbs can be incorporated, as is expected of subjects that are internal to the verb phrase; however, subjects of unergative verbs can also be incorporated, an unexpected property if these subjects are external to the verb phrase. See Saxon and Rice (1993) for detailed discussion.

The data in (29) illustrate that patientive, nonhuman subjects can be incorporated.

(29) Incorporated subjects: verb can be unaccusative/subject can be patientive or nonhuman

    a.   *ts'etenneł-ghotl'*   'The ice broke up.' (222)
            incorporate: *ten* 'ice'

    b.   *kełetde-'aa*   'Smoke is rising up.' (76)
            incorporate: *łet*   'smoke'

    c.   *da**xael**-z'an*   'A pack is up (on shelf).' (71)
            incorporate: *xael* 'pack'

The forms in (30) illustrate that agentive nonhuman subjects are available for incorporation as well.

(30) Incorporated subjects: verb can be unergative/subject can be agentive, nonhuman

    a.   *ta**del**-dlo'*   'Water is gurgling.' (324)
            incorporate: *ta* 'water'

    b.   *kanałidel-ghos*   'The dogs are howling now and then.' (207)
            incorporate: *łi* 'dog'
            stem: *dlo'* 'laugh'

In fact, even subjects of transitives can be incorporated in Ahtna, where the subject is agentive.

(31)   Incorporated subjects: verb can be transitive

    a.   *łiyiz-'ał*   'A dog bit him/her (once).' (280)
          dog.3object.bite
          incorporate: *łi* 'dog'

    b.   *nic'ałts'iidił-t'ak*   'The wind lifted it (e.g., feather) up.' (411)
          wind.3object.move up
          incorporate: *łts'ii* 'wind'

Noun incorporation provides no evidence that subjects bear different syntactic relationships to the verb as part of their lexical entry: all subjects can be incorporated regardless of whether they are subjects of lexically intransitive or transitive verbs; it is semantic properties associated with the verbal arguments that determine whether incorporation yields grammatical results or not.

Finally, subjects of both unaccusative and unergative verbs appear in idioms. Saxon and Rice (1993) point out that the occurrence of internal subjects in idioms is not surprising; however, the appearance of external subjects in idioms, like the incorporation of external subjects into the verb, is unusual. If these subjects all bear the same syntactic relationship to the verb, then the incorporation facts and facts about idioms are not so unusual.

(32)   Subject idioms: verb can be unaccusative; subject is patientive

    sciz'aani datdez-'aan   'I am excited'; lit. 'My heart is elevated.' (70)
    1sg.heart above.be located

(33)   Subject idioms: verb can be unergative; subject is agentive

    neniic uyighi-yaa   'He became happy'; lit. 'Happiness went into
    happiness b.into.sg go   him.' (422)

I am aware of no asymmetrical patterning between subjects of possible unaccusatives and subjects of possible unergatives when the subjects are internal to the verb phrase—both can be incorporated, both place the same requirements on oblique object form, both can enter into idioms. This evidence thus indicates that there are not asymmetries between internal subject types. While subjects can indeed be internal or external, as shown in (17), it is not syntactic properties of the verb or predicate that determine the possible positions of a subject but rather semantic properties of salience, agentivity, humanness, and animacy.

8.3.6   Noun/Verb Pairs

Hale and Platero (1996) argue that in Navajo, an additional unaccusative diagnostic exists. They propose that unergative verbs may pair with nouns while
unaccusative verbs do not. I will examine the facts of Navajo in section 8.4.2;
this statement is contradicted by pairs of nouns and unaccusative verbs in
Ahtna.

(34)   unergative

      sen   'spiritual power, medicine' *D-yen* 'be a shaman' (436)
      -yiits' 'breath, life, vapor'   *l-yiits'* 'breathe' (439)

(35)   unaccusative

      ten   'ice'   *D-ten* 'freeze' (332)
      łet   'smoke'   *d-D-łet* 'smudge, burn' (278)

8.3.7   Summary

I have argued that four possible diagnostics for assigning unaccusative and unergative verbs different syntactic structures do not provide evidence for these syntactic categories. First, case marking groups together the subjects of all intransitive verbs in Ahtna. Second, transitivity alternations do not correlate with unac-
cusative/unergative class but appear to be semantically determined. Third, the
pronoun *y-*, while licensed by an argument of an unergative verb, may also be
licensed by human arguments of unaccusative verbs: factors of saliency and humanness are important rather than syntactic subcategorization. Fourth, based on
a test proposed by Hale and Platero (1996), the lexical argument structure of a
verb is important in determining whether an intransitive has a noun pair; both
proposed argument structures have noun pairs. Finally, both unaccusative and
unergative verbs can occur with identical nonsalient subject marking, both allow
incorporation, and both enter into idiomatic constructions with the verb. Thus,
possible arguments for lexically listed argument structure do not provide support for the position that argument structure must be part of the lexical entry of
a verb. Rather the position of the subject appears to be predictable: it is a consequence of saliency, agentivity, and humanness rather than of syntactic class.
These properties are summarized in (36).

(36)   CHARACTERISTICS OF SUBJECT   POSITION OF SUBJECT

salient, human, agentive	external
salient, human, nonagentive	external
unmarked for saliency, human, agentive	external
nonhuman, agentive	external (animate)/internal (in-animate)/ incorporated
nonhuman, nonagentive	internal
nonsalient	internal

This analysis has consequences for lexical entries. Making a common assumption that lexical entries include only unpredictable information, syntactic subcategorization frames do not appear to be necessary in the lexical entries of monadic verbs in Ahtna. What needs to be said is that the verb is monadic—that is, it takes a single argument. Assuming that transitivity alternations are predictable on semantic grounds, no further information about argument structure must be included in the lexical entry. Verbal representations must also include information about thematic role: some take only agents, some take only patients, and some take either agents or patients.[3] Constituency with respect to the verb is simply irrelevant to determining the patterning of the verb.[4]

8.4   Beyond Ahtna—Slave and Navajo Revisited

I have argued that in Ahtna, argument structure is not basic to a verb. Instead, the position that an argument appears in is predictable from semantic factors. Further, it is not the case that unergative verbs take external subjects and unaccusative verbs take internal subjects because humanness as well as agentivity is important in determining subject position. There thus seems to be little basis for the syntactically encoded unaccusative/unergative distinction in Ahtna. However, other Athabaskan languages have been described as requiring unaccusative and unergative structures. In this section, I would like to briefly revisit Navajo and Slave to see if the evidence forces a structural account. I will begin with Slave.

8.4.1   Slave

Rice (1991) presents arguments for two classes of monadic verbs in Slave based on noun incorporation, transitivity alternations, impersonal passives, and oblique object forms. I examine each of these in turn.

8.4.1.1 Noun incorporation

Consider first the argument based on noun incorporation. Rice (1991) observes that unaccusative verbs can incorporate their subjects while unergative verbs cannot. Thus the examples in (37), with unaccusative verbs, are grammatical, while that in (38), with an unergative verb, is not. Examples are from Rice (1989) and Rice (1991).

(37) Noun incorporation: patientive subjects, or unaccusative subjects, can be incorporated

    a. *zhátthfi̜-zí*   'The heads are roasted.'
        incorporate: *tthí* 'head;' stem: *zí* 'roast, cook'

    b. *gozhíkǫ́da-wé*   'A fire starts (fire occurs in area).'
        incorporate: *kǫ́* 'fire;' stem: *wé* 'occur'

(38) Noun incorporation: agentive subjects, or unergative subjects, do not incorporate

    a. * *natłi̜déh-ja* 'The dog came back.'
        incorporate: *tłi̜* 'dog'; stem: *ja* 'sg. return, perfective'

    b. *tłi̜ nadéh-ja* 'The dog came back.'
        dog

Slave differs from Ahtna in this way: while Ahtna allows the incorporation of subjects of unergatives, Slave does not.

As Rice and Saxon (1994:175) point out, the argument that unergative verbs cannot appear with incorporated subjects fails, as there are verbs that appear to be unergative but can have incorporated subjects.

(39) Noun incorporation: unergatives can have incorporated subjects

    a. *k'etsii-tłah* 'The snow drifted.'
        incorporate: *tsih* 'drifted snow'; stem: *tłah* 'singular/dual go by land'

    b. *tárahxeníheʔó*   'raft comes ashore' (place name)
        incorporate: *xeníh* 'raft'; stem: *ʔó* 'go by water'

One possible account of these examples is that the verbs in question have dual lexical entries, one with the subject internal to the verb phrase (unaccusative) and one with it external to the verb phrase (unergative). However, this places an extra burden on the lexicon: it must include not only unpredictable information but also predictable information. Rice and Saxon (1994) suggest an alternative account, namely that the proper generalization here is that agents are not subject to incorporation, while patients are. Under this account, double lexical entries are not required.

8.4.1.2 Transitivity Alternations

Second, consider the argument based on causatives. Rice (1991) argues that in Slave the causativizer has a restricted domain, unlike in Ahtna: it can be added only to unaccusatives. The causativizer has the form [h] in Slave. The examples in (40) show unaccusative verbs participating in transitivity alternations.

(40) Transitivity alternations: unaccusative verbs participate

    a.   *zhátthíį-zí*   'The heads are roasted.'
           zhátthíįh-sí 'S/he roasted heads.'

    b.   *ré-zho*   'It grew.'
           reh-sho   'I raised it, grew it.'

Unergative verbs in Slave generally do not participate in transitivity alternations.

(41) Transitivity alternations: unergative verbs do not participate

    a. *yįtse*   'S/he cries.'
    b. * *seyįhtse*   'S/he made me cry.'

However, some verbs that might be considered to be unergative do participate in transitivity alternations, as in (42).

(42) Transitivity alternations: unergative verbs can participate

    a. *satsóné behchiné k'ína-tłah*   'The car goes around.'
          metal sled
    b. *satsóné behchiné k'ínah-tłah*   'S/he drove the car around.'

Verbs such as those in (42) present a particular problem: when these verbs have human subjects the subject is agentive, and transitivity alternations are not possible (see (41)). However, with nonhuman subjects, the subject is not agentive, but rather patientive, and transitivity alternations occur. One possibility with such a verb is to list two forms in the lexicon, one with an external subject (unergative) and one with an internal subject (unaccusative). However, as discussed, this places an extra burden on the lexicon. In this case, the position of the subject is redundant once properties of agentiveness and humanness of the subject are known.

As in Ahtna, the relevant generalization to determine which verbs enter into transitivity alternations does not appear to refer to structural position, but rather to the lack of agentivity or control: verbs with nonagentive subjects are subject to causativization in Slave while those with agentive subjects are not. The conditions on causativization in Slave are thus a subset of those in Ahtna.

8.4.1.3 Impersonal Passives

One argument for the Unaccusative Hypothesis comes from the patterning of impersonal passives. Perlmutter (1978) argues that unergatives may have impersonal passives associated with them, but unaccusatives do not. Rice (1991) provides some evidence supporting this distinction in Slave: unergative verbs may have impersonal passive forms.

(43) a. *yets' ę́ yahti* 'S/he preaches to her/him.'
     *y.*to preach

   b. *bets' ę́ yati* 'There is preaching to him/her.'
      *b.*to preach

(44) a. *dagohwe* 'They dance.'

   b. *dagowe* 'dance (it is danced)'

(45) a. *ʔehkw'i* *ʔadi* 'S/he speaks truly.'
      truth   speak

   b. *ʔehkw'i* *ʔagodi* 'It is spoken truly.' (go–expletive subject)
      truth   it is spoken

However, there are verbs that would be classed as unaccusatives that can form impersonal passives as well.

(46) a. *yek* *'édezhǫ* 'I know him/her/it.' (oblique object *y-*)
      *y.*of 1sg.know

   b. *mek* *'édejǫ* 'It is known.'

While the conditions under which impersonal passives can occur are not clear, the correct division does not seem to be based on lexically specified argument structure.

8.4.1.4   The Distribution of Oblique Object Pronouns

The next argument is based on the distribution of *y-* and *b-* as oblique objects with third-person subject monadic verbs. As in Ahtna, with clearly unergative verbs with agentive subjects, the oblique form is *y-*. All page references are to Rice (1989).

(47)   Verbs with third-person human agentive subjects take *y-* as oblique object

    a.   *ʔamá*   *yek'é*   *ʔa-já*   'Mother went after him/her.' (1008)
        mother   *y*.after   went

    b.   *yeká*   *dukǫde-da*   'She is looking for him.' (1008)
        y.for   look

    c.   *yets'*   *ę́rá-di*   'She helps him.' (1008)
        y.to   help

Monadic verbs with nonhuman agentive subjects occur with *b-*, as shown in (48).

(48)   Verbs with nonhuman agentive subjects take *b-*
    mehchįé   *metee*   *áh-tɬa*   'A truck ran over him/her.' (289)
    truck   *b*.across   went

Further, monadic verbs with nonhuman nonagentive subjects occur with *b-*, as in (49).

(49)   Verbs with nonhuman nonagentive subjects take *b-*

    a.   *bįtl'ada-wé*   'It fell from his/her hand.' (1008)
        b.hand.from fall

    b.   *tsę bek'e yį-ɬǫ́*   'There was lots of dirt on it.'
        dirt *b*.on many   (1008)

    c.   *ts'o bek'e whe-ʔǫ*   'A fly is on it.' (1008)
        fly *b*.on

    d.   *tthik'íi*   *megohthę déh-k'é*   'The gun shot him.'
        gun   *b*.against   shot

    e.   *mendaá yie thę́ yáedí-yoh*   'Stars shine in his/her eyes.'
        b.eye   in   star distributive shine   (1008)

Monadic verb with human nonagentive subjects may occur with *b-*.

(50)   Verbs with human nonagentive subjects may take *b-*

     Mary   *bets'ę?óné ?adéh-shá*   'Mary is bigger than he is.' (1008)
           3.comparative be bigger

However, monadic verbs with human nonagentive subjects may also occur with *y-*.

(51)   Verbs with human nonagentive subjects may take *y-*

    a.   *yeghǫ ?etered-lį*   'S/he is sorry for him/her.' (270)
    b.   *yįtl'ada-wé*   'She/he fell from his/her hand.' (1009)

To summarize, the distribution of *y-* and *b-* in Slave is shown in (52).

(52)   Human agentive subjects take *y-*.
      Nonhuman agentive subjects take *b-*.
      Nonhuman nonagentive subjects take *b-*.
      Human nonagentive subjects may take *b-* or *y-*.

Consider the prediction of the Unaccusative Hypothesis (Rice 1991). One would expect that unergative verbs would occur with *y-* as oblique object and unaccusative verbs with *b-* as oblique object. This hypothesis accounts well for some of these forms, namely those in (47) and (49, 50), where there is a correlation between unergativity and the use of *y-* as oblique object and unaccusativity and the use of *b-* as oblique object. However, the form in (48) suggests that a nonhuman agentive subject can take *b-* as oblique object, and the examples in (51) show that a human nonagentive subject can take *y-* as oblique object. Thus, the internal/external subject hypothesis fails to account for all the data. In discussing forms such as those in (51), Rice (1989:1009) suggests that if a human subject of an unaccusative verb can be interpreted as agentive, or if the action can be regarded as volitional or controlled, then the pronoun *y-* can be used as oblique object. This then is consistent with the semantic hypothesis that humanness and agentivity are important rather than argument structure.

Thus in Slave human agentive subjects are external, nonhuman agentive subjects are internal. Further, while nonhuman patientive subjects are internal, human patientive subjects are variable in their position. Clearly it is factors of agentivity and humanness that are important in determining argument position rather than purely syntactic factors. The high degree of overlap between agentivity and subject of unergative makes it difficult to separate out the two hypotheses, but the evidence points to agentivity and humanness being the factors that determine whether a subject can be external or not.

8.4.2   Navajo

I now examine the status of the Unaccusative Hypothesis with respect to Navajo. Hale and Platero (1996) present two types of arguments for a structural account of the monadic verb classes. While the structures proposed are slightly different from those given in (2) and (3), the claim that argument structure is basic, or part of the lexical entry, is shared in their analysis.

8.4.2.1   Transitivity Alternations

The major argument that Hale and Platero present is based on the morphology of transitivity alternations: unaccusatives participate in these alternations but unergatives do not enter into simple causative constructions marked just by the presence of the causativizer *ł*. Some of their examples of causatives based on unaccusatives are given in (53) and of causatives based on unergatives in (54).

(53)   Transitivity alternations: unaccusatives show simple transitivity alternations

    a.   *tóshjeeh*   *si-ts'il*   'The barrel shattered, broke to pieces.'
        barrel   shattered

        łeets'aa'   *sé-ł-ts'il*   'I shattered the dish.'
        dish   1sg.cause.shatter

    b.   *tin yí-yį́į'*   'The ice melted.'
        ice melted

        yas yí-ł-hį́į'   'I melted the snow.'
        snow 1sg.cause.melt

(54)   Transitivity alternations unergative verbs show a complex causative construction

    a.   *'awéé'*   *naa-ghá*   'The baby is walking around.'
        baby   walk around

        'awéé'   *na-b-iish-ł-á*   'I am walking the baby around.'
        baby   *b*.cause.walk around

    b.   *'awéé'*   *yi-dloh*   'The baby is laughing.'
        baby   laugh

        'awéé'   *bi-y-eesh-dloh*   'I am making the baby laugh.'
        baby   *b*.cause.laugh

In the final form, the presence of the *ł* is obscured by phonological requirements. Hale and Platero (1996) argue that the examples in (53) and (54) provide evidence for the Unaccusativity Hypothesis: unaccusative verbs can be causativized simply through the use of *ł*, but unergative verbs, on the other hand, require what Hale and Platero (1996) call complex transitivization, requiring morphological material, the *b-* in the forms in (54), in addition to the causativizer.

While the complex transitivization structure is found with some unergative verbs, it does not seem that it is found with all such verbs. Assuming that the following verbs are unergative, they appear with the simple causative. (Whether these verbs are unergative or not is not easy to determine. They are of the class mentioned in the discussion of Slave—with a human subject, the verb has unergative diagnostics, but with a nonhuman subject it has unaccusative diagnostics.) The examples come either from Young and Morgan (1987) (YM) or Young, Morgan, and Midgette (1992) (YMM).

(55) Unergative verbs can appear with the simple causative

    a. *náá-bał*   'S/he is whirling around.' (YMM 48)
        náásh-bał 'I am twirling, whirling O around.'

    b. *'aníí-cháá'*   'I fled away out of sight.' (YMM 77)
        'anííł-cháá' 'I chased O away out of sight' (78)

And the complex transitive structure seems to be allowed with some unaccusative verbs.

(56) Some unaccusative verbs occur in the complex causative construction

    a. *'aneez-dá* 'Something sat down.' (YM 116)
        binish-daah 'I sit O down, seat O, give O a seat, make O sit down.'

    b. *shii-jéé'*   'We are lying.' (YM 263)
        bishééł-jéé'   'I keep pl. O.'
        naa'ahóóhai tádiingo bishééł-jéé' 'I keep 30 chickens.'

These facts suggest that the type of causative structure that an intransitive takes is not completely predictable. What determines the choice of causative construction is not clear, but it is not simply the structural relationship between the verb and its single argument.

8.4.2.2 Noun/Verb Pairs

Hale and Platero propose a second argument for two different syntactic structures for intransitives—at least some unergative verbs have nominal counterparts. They provide the verb/noun stems in (57).

(57) At least some unergative verbs have nominal counterparts

Verb	Noun		
dloh	*dlo*	'laugh'	(YMM 156)
wosh	*-wosh*	'sleep'	(YMM 660)
yih	*-yih*	'breathe, breath'	(YMM 702)
yol	*-yol*	'inhale/breathe, breath'	(YMM 723, 728)
za'	*-za'*	'belch'	(YMM 731)
zheeh	*-zhéé'*	'spit'	(YMM 770)

However, at least some unaccusative verbs also have nominal counterparts, as the examples in (58) show.

(58) At least some unaccusative verbs have nominal counterparts

Verb		Noun		
łid	'burn'	*łid*	'smoke'	(YMM 370)
tin	'freeze'	*tin*	'ice'	(YMM 509)
zéí	'crumble'	*séí*	'sand'	(YMM 739)
zhǫǫd	'be(come)'	*zhǫ'*	'levity, fun thing'	(YMM 795)

This diagnostic, then, is inconclusive as both monadic verb types can have nominal counterparts.

8.4.2.3 Oblique Object Pronouns

Much has been written about the form of object pronouns in Navajo (e.g., Hale 1973, Perkins 1978, Speas 1990, Willie 1991, Young and Morgan 1987), and this is an exceedingly complex area to which I cannot do justice. Factors such as topicality enter in, and I will attempt to abstract away from these here by ignoring the word order that gives *b-* as an object. I will simply remark here that the *y/b* split does not appear to correlate with unergative/unaccusative structures. Rather, *y-* is found when a subject is agentive and when a subject is human; *b-* can occur when the subject is nonhuman. When the subject of a monadic verb is agentive, an oblique object has the form *y-*.

(59) Human or nonhuman agentive subject, *y-* as oblique object

    a.   *'ashkii   níbaal   yíyah niizį́*
        boy   tent   *y.*under stand
        'The boy is standing under the tent.'   (YM 257)

    b.   *łį́į'   naa'ahóóhai   yik'i ch'élwod*
        horse chicken   *y.*on
        'The horse ran over the chicken.'   (YM 28)

    c. *łééchąą'í'*   *ańt'i'*   *yigháa'na'*
       dog   fence   y.through crawl
       'The dog crawled through the fence.'   (YM 42)

If the subject can be interpreted as agentive or as a controller, even though the verb would be unaccusative by the transitivity alternations test, it can also appear with *y*- as oblique object.

(60)   Inanimate agentive subject: *y*- as oblique object

     nástsáán   *tsé*   *yik'i ch'ínímááz*
     log   rock   y.on
     'The log rolled over the rock.' (28)

Young and Morgan (1987:28) suggest that *y*- "connotes the fact that the noun first mentioned is the subject of the sentence, and that the second noun (if any) is the object of the postposition. If this order relationship does not obtain, the pronoun prefix on the postposition is the 3rd person *bi*- form." They thus predict that, abstracting from topicality, only the *y*- form will occur as an oblique.

Despite Young and Morgan's claim, there are occasions which do not appear to involve topicality where *b*- can appear as an oblique object. When the subject of a monadic verb is patientive, an oblique object may have the form *y*- or *b*-. The following data all involve locative verbs. If the subject is human, the oblique object has the form *y*-, as in (61).

(61)   Human subject: *y*- as oblique object

    a. *shádi*   *dóó*   *shideezhí*   *bik'idah'asdáhí níneezí-gi*
       1s.older sister and   1s.younger sister sofa

                 yikáá'   *dah siké*
                 y.on   up 2.sit
       'My big sister and my little sister are sitting on the sofa.' (689)

    b. *'ashkii*   *tsé*   *yik'i*   *dah*   *neezdá*
       boy   rock   y.on   up   sit
       'The boy sat down on the rock.' (28)

However, *b*- is possible if the subject is nonhuman, as in (62).

(62)   Nonhuman, nonagentive subject: *b*- as oblique object

    a. *bikáá'adáni*   *bikáa'gi*   *tó*   *siką́*
       table   b.on locative   water lie (something in open container)
       'There's water on the table.' (686)

b. *shi'éétsoh   bik'idah 'asdáhí   bikáa'gi   siłtsooz*
    1sg.coat   chair   *b*.on.locative   lie (clothlike object)
    'My coat is lying on the chair.' (687)

c. *biníhííyį́*
    biní 'into it, penetrating it' + *hííyį́* 'water extends'
    'It (water) extends into it (to form a gulf or inlet).' (233)

d. *biní'íígháázh*
    'It gnawed into it, eroded it (wind, water, acid into soil or rock).'

The sentence in (62b) is particularly interesting, as topicality of the oblique object does not seem to be an issue here, given the word order.

The examples in (59) through (62) illustrate that while unergative verbs take *y-* as oblique object form, unaccusative verbs can take either *y-* or *b-*, depending on properties of the subject. Again, we do not find structure playing an important role in predicting patterning. Rather, verbs with agentive subjects take *y-* as oblique object form; verbs with patientive subjects take *y-* or *b-*, depending on properties of the subject. As in Ahtna, thematic properties of the subject rather than properties of the verb appear to be what is relevant in determining surface position of the subject. The tests that I have found to differentiate between two surface positions for subjects do not demand two lexical classes of intransitives based on syntactic structure; rather, they suggest a single type of lexical entry with surface syntactic position being predictable.

8.5 Conclusions

I have argued that a number of diagnostics that one might expect to correlate with unaccusative/unergative structures do not in fact yield this particular distinction; instead semantic factors are important in determining the syntactic position of the subject. Table 8.1 summarizes the major factors involved in causativity, the *y-*/*b-* distribution, and incorporation in the three languages discussed. If these conclusions are correct, they have several consequences. Most important, none of the diagnostics used provide any evidence for syntactic information about the position of arguments being included in the lexicon, as the position of a subject is predictable. As a consequence, whether a subject appears internally or externally is not related to the syntactic class of the verb but rather to semantic properties associated with the argument. In these three Athabaskan languages, at least, it appears that a semantic hypothesis provides the better account of the patterning of monadic verbs, with apparent syntactic generalizations being a result of the strong semantic congruence among the verbs within an intransitive class. A second consequence of this analysis concerns the types of factors that do determine the surface position of the subject. Two types of factors are identified in the literature, qualities of the argument and qualities of the verb form. In Athabaskan languages, qualities of the argument appear to be more important in

TABLE 8.1 *Summary of Major Factors*

	Ahtna	Slave	Navajo
Causatives	Most verbs can be causativized; if a verb cannot be causativized, it may be because it is incompatible with an external causer.	A verb with a non-agentive subject can be causativized.	Conditions not clear, but does not seem to correlate with unaccusativity.
y- as oblique object	*y*- occurs as oblique if the subject is salient, animate, and agentive; *y*- may occur as oblique if the subject is salient, human, and patientive.	*y*- occurs as oblique if the subject is salient, human, and agentive; *y*- may occur as oblique if the subject is salient, human, and patientive.	*y*- occurs as oblique if the subject is salient and agentive or interpretable as agentive; *y*- occurs as oblique if the subject is salient, human, and patientive.
Incorporation	Nonhuman agents and patients can be incorporated.	Nonanimate agents and patients can be incorporated.	No incorporation.

determining subject position, with saliency, humanness, animacy, and agentivity playing a role—salient agentive humans are always canonical, or external, subjects; nonsalient subjects are always noncanonical, or internal, subjects. The languages differ in terms of just what combinations of these properties allow nouns to be canonical. Aspect, if it is relevant at all, crosscuts this: only once saliency is extracted and only once human subjects are considered does a difference between the patterning of telic and nontelic predicates become apparent.

The conclusion that argument structure is not part of the lexical entry supports claims made by others in recent work. Cummins (1996) and Ghomeshi and Massam (1994) argue that syntactic structure is not listed in the lexicon, but rather the syntactic position of nouns is determined by a wide range of factors. Whether argument structure is never listed for verbs, as Cummins and Ghomeshi and Massam conclude, or whether the diagnostics used here simply fail to demonstrate the need for such information being in the lexicon remains an open question.

Notes

I would like to thank Leslie Saxon and Ted Fernald for their help with this chapter. Thanks also to the audience at the Athabaskan Conference on Syntax and Semantics and to Ted Fernald for providing me with an opportunity to pursue this topic. This work was partially funded by a Killam Research Fellowship.

1. The verb in (24) has *d* voice/valence. This morpheme is a marker middle voice (see Arce-Arenalas, Axelrod, and Fox 1994, Thompson 1989, and Thompson 1996) marking low elaboration of participants. It is possible that this verb actually has two semantic arguments assigned to a single noun. If the causativizer can be used only with verbs in which the agent need not be interpreted as an initiator (e.g., 'cry'), it may be that the type of subject of this verb precludes its appearing with the causativizer. I leave this for further investigation.

2. I have included the examples in (15) for completeness; they suggest that in addition to a distinction between human/nonhuman, a distinction between animate and inanimate is in order; I will not go into this here in any detail.

3. Presumably this final class can be unspecified for thematic role.

4. This account allows verbs like 'work' to have a single lexical entry; when the subject is agentive it is necessarily external if it is salient; when it is patientive and nonhuman, it is internal to the verb phrase.

References

Arce-Arenales, Manuel, Melissa Axelrod, and Barbara Fox. 1994. Active Voice and Middle Diathesis: A Cross-Linguistic Perspective. In Barbara Fox and Paul Hopper (eds.). *Voice: Form and Function.* Amsterdam:Benjamins. 1–21.

Axelrod, Melissa. 1990. Incorporation in Koyukon Athapaskan. *International Journal of American Linguistics* 56(2):179–195.

Axelrod, Melissa. 1993. *The Semantics of Time: Aspectual Categorization in Koyukon Athabaskan.* Studies in the Anthropology of North America Series. Lincoln: University of Nebraska Press.

Borer, Hagit. 1993. *The Projection of Arguments.* Occasional Papers in Linguistics, University of Massachusetts, Amherst.

Cummins, Sarah. 1996. Meaning and Mapping. Ph.D. dissertation, University of Toronto.

Dowty, David. 1991. Thematic Proto-roles and Argument Selection. *Language* 67:547–619.

Ghomeshi, Jila, and Diane Massam. 1994. Lexical/Syntactic Relations without Projection. *Linguistic Analysis* 24:175–217.

Grimshaw, Jane. 1987. Unaccusatives—An Overview. In *Proceedings of the North East Linguistics Society* 17:244–259. GLSA, University of Massachusetts, Amherst.

Grimshaw, Jane. 1990. *Argument Structure.* Cambridge, Mass.: MIT Press.

Hale, Kenneth. 1973. A Note on Subject-Object Inversion in Navajo. In R. B. Kachru, et al. (eds.). *Issues in Linguistics: Papers in Honor of Henry and Rene Kahane,* 300–309. Champaign-Urbana: University of Illinois Press.

Hale, Kenneth, and Paul Platero. 1996. Navajo Reflections of a General Theory of Lexical Argument Structure. In E. Jelinek, S. Midgette, K. Rice, and L. Saxon (eds.). *Papers in Honor of Robert Young.* Albuquerque: University of New Mexico Press.

Hopper, Paul, and Sandra Thompson. 1980. Transitivity in Grammar and Discourse. *Language* 56:251–299.

Kari, James. 1979. *Athabaskan Verb Theme Categories: Ahtna.* Fairbanks: Alaska Native Language Center.

Kari, James. 1990. *Ahtna Athabaskan Dictionary.* Fairbanks: Alaska Native Language Center.

Levin, Beth, and Malka Hovav Rappaport. 1995. *Unaccusativity: At the Syntax-Lexical Semantics Interface.* Cambridge, Mass.: MIT Press.

Perkins, Ellavina. 1978. The Role of Word Order and Scope in the Interpretation of Navajo Sentences. Ph.D. dissertation, University of Arizona, Tucson.

Perlmutter, David. 1978. Impersonal Passives and the Unaccusative Hypothesis. In *Proceedings of the Fourth Annual Meeting of the Berkeley Linguistics Society,* 157–189. Berkeley: Berkeley Linguistics Society, University of California.

Rice, Keren. 1989. *A Grammar of Slave.* Berlin: Mouton de Gruyter.

Rice, Keren. 1991. Intransitives in Slave (Northern Athapaskan): Arguments for Unaccusatives. *International Journal of American Linguistics* 57:51–69.

Rice, Keren. In press. *Morpheme Order and Semantic Scope: Word Formation in the Athapaskan Verb.* Cambridge: Cambridge University Press.

Rice, Keren, and Leslie Saxon. 1994. The Subject Positions in Athapaskan Languages. In H. Harley and C. Phillips (eds.). *The Morphology-Syntax Connection.* (MIT Working Papers in Linguistics, No. 22), 173–195. Cambridge, Mass.: MIT Press.

Rosen, Carol. 1984. The Interface between Semantic Roles and Initial Grammatical Relations. In D. Perlmutter and C. Rosen (eds.), *Studies in Relational Grammar,* Vol. 2, 38–77. Chicago: University of Chicago Press.

Saxon, Leslie. 1984. Disjoint Anaphora and the Binding Theory. In *Proceedings of the West Coast Conference on Formal Linguistics* 3, 242–251.

Saxon, Leslie, and Keren Rice. 1993. On Subject-Verb Constituency: Evidence from Athapaskan Languages. In *Proceedings of the West Coast Conference on Formal Linguistics* 11, 434–450.

Smith, Carlota. 1991. *The Parameter of Aspect.* Dordrecht: Reidel.

Speas, Margaret. 1990. *Phrase Structure in Natural Language.* Dordrecht: Kluwer.

Tenny, Carol. 1994. *Aspectual Roles and the Syntax-Semantics Interface.* Dordrecht: Kluwer.

Thompson, Chad. 1989. Voice and Obviation in Athabaskan and Other Languages. Ph.D. dissertation, University of Oregon.

Thompson, Chad. 1996. The Na-Dene Middle Voice: An Impersonal Source of the D-Element. *International Journal of American Linguistics* 62:351–378.

Van Valin, Robert. 1990. Semantic parameters of split intransitivity. *Language* 66:221–260.

Vendler, Zeno. 1957. Verbs and Times. *Philosophical Review* 56:143–160.

Willie, MaryAnn. 1991. Pronouns and Obviation in Navajo. Ph.D. dissertation, University of Arizona.

Young, Robert, and William Morgan. 1987. *The Navajo Language.* Revised edition. Albuquerque: University of New Mexico Press.

Young, Robert, William Morgan, and Sarah Midgette. 1992. *Analytical Lexicon of Navajo.* Albuquerque: University of New Mexico Press.

9

THE SEMANTICS OF
THE NAVAJO VERB BASE

Carlota S. Smith

The Navajo verb poses problems for semantic analysis that do not arise with simpler verb forms. The verb base of Navajo contains several types of morpheme: there are verb roots expressed in different stems sets, classifiers, thematic prefixes, and derivational prefixes. It is difficult to identify the roles played by each morpheme, because there are many interacting factors. Semantic analyses of the Navajo verb have tended to treat morphemes of the same morphological and positional classes as similar; but they are not necessarily the same semantically. To address the question of semantic interpretation, the morphemes of the verb base must be analyzed from a lexical-semantic point of view.

I suggest in this article an approach to the Navajo verb which depends on close lexical analysis of specific morphemes. Armed with a principled analytic approach, we may arrive at an understanding of the individual parts and their contribution to the meaning of the whole. My goal is to characterize the event structure of Navajo as expressed by the verb bases of the language. This characterization will help us to better understand the Navajo verb bases.

I'll begin by considering the lexical conceptual structure of verbs generally. I present an information-based approach, using the method of close lexical analysis, and a format for representing the meanings of verbs. Section 9.2 applies the approach to some verb bases of Navajo, focusing on verb stems and derivational prefixes. Section 9.3 shows in some detail how the framework handles a fairly well-understood group of derivational prefixes known as the Subaspects. Section 9.4 comments on the contribution to verb meaning of thematic prefixes and the traditional aspectual categories; Section 9.5 concludes with a few general remarks about the format for lexical representation of verbs.

9.1   An Information-Based Approach to Lexical Analysis

In order to develop a semantic account of verbs it is necessary to understand the information they convey. The information-based approach to lexical conceptual structure makes clear the relationship between meanings and the contribution of particular morphemes.

The leading idea that I want to pursue is the simple and quite traditional one that verbs encode several types of information. Recent work in linguistics elucidates this idea with an emphasis on the internal structure of events; in what follows I adapt some of this work to the lexical semantics of Navajo verbs.[1] I'll distinguish three types of information: *event structure* articulates the internal structure of the situation (the term includes events and states) denoted by a verb base; *argument structure* identifies the participants in the situation indicated by the verb base; and *qualia structure* sets out the particulars of that situation. The representation for a given verb will state all three as separate tier, in such a way as to bring out the relations between them. The tripartite lexical representations are partly inspired by the work of Croft (1987), Jackendoff (1990), and Pustejovsky (1991, 1995).

The lexical conceptual structure of a typical English verb unpacks information which is expressed in portmanteau fashion by a single morpheme. Detailed lexical analysis of the basic form involves decomposition into primitives. The primitives are abstractions which allow us to represent the information conveyed by the morpheme. Simple, monomorphemic verbs appear in many languages, such as English, French, and Chinese. (I consider only the bare verb stem here, ignoring conjugational morphemes which give information about tense and aspectual viewpoint.) In some other languages, verbs typically have more than one morpheme: Russian, for instance, has relatively complex verb morphology (Forsyth 1970, Smith 1991).

Navajo does not have a direct counterpart to the simple surface verb. Both the verb root and verb stem are quite abstract, while the full verbal complex contains additional affixes and thus other information. The verb base is the unit which is closest semantically to the simple verb of English. Young and Morgan comment that "the verb base constitutes the skeleton of a lexical form: one in which lexical meaning is apparent, but which still lacks essential markers" (1987:140).[2] The "verb base" is an abstract unit consisting of the verb stem, classifier, thematic prefixes, and derivational prefixes. The surface verbal complex has, in addition, pronouns and conjugational prefixes which express aspectual viewpoint, futurity, and other notions. I'll assume that the verb base is the level at which verb meaning is expressed in Navajo. This discussion focuses on the verb base.

I begin by introducing the three tiers of the lexical conceptual structure of verbs. Situations are events and states that vary in indefinitely many ways, yet we particularize them according to a few general notions. The particulars that identify a given situation constitute its "qualia structure." To state these particulars we need a set of basic properties, primitives which can give information about a wide range of situations. I will use the primitives listed in (1), following Leonard Talmy (1985).

(1)   Figure, Motion, Ground, Path, Cause, Manner, State

I have added an additional primitive to the list, that of final or resultant State. The resultant State is a particular of telic events, which result in a change of state.

These primitives organize situations in terms of spatial location and motion. They are intended to apply to both events and states. All events have literal or metaphorical motion; telic events have literal or metaphorical changes of location/state. States, too, have literal or metaphorical locations: they are maintained rather than changed. The approach is based on the localist theory of Gruber (1965) and others. As Jackendoff puts it, "the basic insight . . . is that the formalism for encoding concepts of spatial location and motion, suitably abstracted, can be generalized to many other semantic fields" (1990:25). Examples of the parallelism between the spatial and other semantic fields include possession (*The inheritance went to Philip*), ascription of properties (*The light changed from green to red*), and scheduling (*The meeting was changed from Monday to Tuesday)*; the examples are Jackendoff's.

We can identify in every situation a principal object, or Figure, using the primitives of (1). The Figure is the center of a situation in two senses. Events involve motion or change of state, and it is always the Figure that moves or changes.[3] In Statives, a property is ascribed to the Figure. The second sense in which the Figure is central is that the other components of a situation pertain to it. The Figure may traverse a path toward a Goal, or from a Source; it may move in a certain Manner. If Ground is specified, it indicates the orientation of the Figure to its surroundings; Path gives the direction of motion traveled; Cause, the agent that brings about the motion or change of state.

Verbs or verb bases may use some or all of the set of primitives. Cause or agent is specified by many transitive verbs, unspecified in many intransitives and passives: in English, compare transitive *break* as in *John broke the glass* to intransitive *break* as in *The glass broke*, or passive *break*, as in *The glass was broken*. The lexical representation of transitive *break* will specify an Agent participant, but the representations of the other two verbs will not. Again, the English verb *run* specifies manner of motion, but the verb *go* does not. The qualia structure representation for a given verb base will contain only the primitives it specifies.

Languages differ in the expression of these primitives, Talmy argues (1985). The main vehicles of expression are the basic verb form itself, the verb, verb base or root, and grammatically related "satellites"—independent morphemes such as affixes, particles, prepositional phrases, and other complements. Talmy distinguishes three major patterns of expression that are predominant in different languages. In the first pattern, the verb tends to express Motion and Manner, while other information is specified by particles or other satellite forms. English and many Indo-European languages are predominantly of this pattern, Talmy suggests. The second pattern expresses Motion and Path in the verb; other information is specified by complements and satellite forms. Romance, Semitic, and Polynesian languages tend to have this as a major pattern. It is the third expressive pattern which interests us here.

In the third major pattern, the verb or verb root expresses the primitives of Figure and Motion, while Ground, Path, and Manner are conveyed by independent forms. Navajo has many verb bases of this pattern, as does the Hokan language Atsugewi (Talmy 1985, 1991).[4]

The expression of Figure and Motion is particularly clear in the "motion verbs" of Navajo, a large and important class.[5] The meanings of Navajo verb roots of motion include the type and number of objects that move, and often the kind of motion. There are different verbal roots for handling, propulsion, independent action, action by conveyance. As Young, Morgan, and Midgette (henceforth YMM) put it,

> The roots that describe locomotion define not only the manner of movement but, for some root categories, the physical attributes or number attaching to the subject or object as well . . . verbs that involve the abrupt movement of an object (toss, bounce, drop) and those that describe the abrupt independent movement of an object through space (fly, fall) classify subject or object on the basis of shape, texture, mass, number, animacy and other features. (1992:1098)

In Navajo, the arguments associated with the verb base appear as pronouns in the verb composite, with optional nouns in the sentence. The arguments must accord semantically with the verb base that underlies a given verb composite.

The examples of (2) illustrate with verb composites of two Navajo roots; each stem denotes a type of object and a kind of motion.

(2) Navajo stem: Figure + Motion; prefixes: Ground, Path, Manner

   a. *'ahéénishyeed* 'Subj. runs around in a circle'; *'adaashyeed* 'S descends', *ha'alyeed* 'unspecified S climbs up', *kíishyeed* 'S runs up an incline'

   b. *yilk'oł* 'a wave, ripple arrives, comes rolling'; *'iliik'ooł* 'wave, ripple rolls away out of sight' (prefix *'a*); *ch'élk'ooł* 'wave, ripple rolls horizontally out' (prefix *ch'í*)

The classification of verb stems according to type of object and type of motion is a well-known feature of Navajo; it is thoroughly documented in Young and Morgan 1987 (henceforth YM) and YMM. I'll return to the discussion of verb bases and prefixes later; now I briefly introduce the other components of lexical conceptual structure.

Event structure characterizes situations according to the internal temporal properties of dynamism, telicity, and duration. The classification is an aspectual one. There are several such classifications, e.g., Vendler (1957), Dowty (1979), Mourelatos (1978), Smith (1991); the one presented here follows Smith (1991) with some different terminology. The distinction between events and states is due to the property of dynamism: events are dynamic, with successive stages which take time; states are static and homogenous. Events are subclassified according to the properties of telicity and duration. Telic events, or Transitions, involve a change of state, goal, or outcome. Such events have a natural final endpoint, which occurs when the goal is reached. Atelic events are Processes. They consist simply of successive stages with no result or outcome: they can end at any time. Events of both types may be durative or instantaneous. Example (3) illustrates the major classes of situation with English examples.[6]

(3)   *Event Structure: Types of situation*

    Process event (atelic)
        Durative: push a cart, sing songs, stroll in the park
        Instantaneous: cough, flap a wing, knock

    Transition event (telic):
        Durative: walk to school, open the door, build a house
        Instantaneous: arrive, break a glass

    State: know the answer, be tall

The present discussion deals only with events.

The internal structure of events can be modeled with the temporal features of telicity and duration. Processes (atelic events) consist of stages that follow each other in time. Transitions are more complex. What is essential to a Transition (telic event) is a change of state: the minimal requirements are the process of change and the resultant state. Durative events have successive stages, while instantaneous events have only one stage. The diagrams in (4) show the internal structure of Process and Transition events in the format of Pustejovsky (1991).

(4)   Durative:

    a.   Process   b.   Transition
        John walked around.   Mary closed the door.

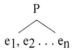

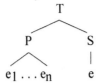

    Instantaneous:

    c.   Process   d.   Transition
        John walked around.   Mary closed the door.

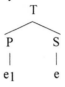

The Instantaneous events have single stages. For simplicity, I will use the notation of (5) to represent events, abstracting away from the property of duration. Both Process and Transitions are events, E; they differ in internal structure as indicated.

(5) $E = P$: e_1 = Process $E = T$: e_1 = Process
              e_2 = State

But duration will be required in a full account: the feature of duration has syntactic reflexes in the Navajo verb base (Smith 1991, 1996a).

    Argument structure: the verb or verb base gives information about the participants which are associated with a given event. An event may have one or more participants, or arguments. Each argument is associated with a particular semantic role, known as a "thematic role" (Jackendoff 1972). Thematic roles include Agent, Theme, and others, as indicated in (6).

(6)   Argument Structure: Agent, Theme, Location, Instrument, etc.

The meaning of a thematic role can be intuitively grasped by considering the types of events in which it appears. For instance, the transitive English verb *open* requires two participants, as in *Mary opened the window:* an Agent, which causes an opening event; and a Theme (the Figure) which undergoes the opening. The intransitive verb *open* has only one participant, as in *The window opened*; the verb does not directly involve an agent, although such a role may be implied.

Thematic roles are associated with different parts of event structure. For instance, in a Transition event involving agency, the agent is associated with bringing about a change of state, but not necessarily with the change itself. For some verbs the entity which undergoes the change is also the agent, as with path verbs such as *walk* or *run*; the change is one of location. The entity undergoing the change may be a Theme, as with the direct objects of *open* and *put*. Thematic roles and event structure are discussed in Croft (1987), Grimshaw (1990), Dowty (1991), Smith (1991), and Pustejovsky (1991).

The arguments of a verb are thus related to the event which it denotes in different ways, determined by the structure of the event. The representation of verb meaning should show this. It should also show how the subevents of event structure are associated with the particulars of the event.

The lexical meaning of a verb base includes information about event structure, argument structure, and qualia structure. The representation for a verb or verb base has three tiers, corresponding to the three kinds of information. The specification of qualia structure includes features from the other two tiers, so that qualia structure is the locus for stating relations between the kinds of information. I will use a single unified representation, following the basic outlines of Pustejovsky (1991); my account departs from his in some respects, especially in qualia structure.[7]

I begin with an example of a simple English verb. Example (7) gives the representation for transitive *close*, as in *Mary closed the door*. The Figure in this sentence is *the door* since it is the entity that undergoes a change of state.

(7)   Lexical representation for the transitive verb *close*

$$\text{EVENT} = \text{T:} \quad e_1 = \text{Process} \quad \text{ARG:} \quad \text{Arg}_1 := [1] \text{ Agent}$$
$$e_2 = \text{State} \qquad\qquad \text{Arg}_2 := [2] \text{ Theme}$$

QUALIA:
   Cause [1]
   Figure = [2]
   Motion (e_1)
   State = (e_2) closed

The event structure for *close* indicates that the event denoted is a Transition, with two subevents, e_1 and e_2; the argument structure indicates two arguments and their thematic roles, [1] and [2]. These notations allow links to qualia structure. In qualia structure, both subevents and arguments are associated with particular primitives. Motion and final State realize the subevents of the Transition, and the arguments realize Cause and Figure. Recall the convention that only primitives that are relevant to a given verb form appear in the lexical representation for that form. Ground and Manner do not appear in (7), since the verb *close* gives no information about them.

All Navajo verb bases contain more than one morpheme: even maximally simple verb bases have a classifier (not necessarily overt) and belong to a given stem set. Classifiers convey whether a verb base is intransitive, transitive, or passive, and sometimes other information. Stem sets are associated with the morphological categories known traditionally as aspectual; some of these categories clearly convey semantic information, others may have less semantic content.[8] Generally, a decomposition analysis of the verb stem is appropriate. For instance, the verb composites presented in (1) have verb stems which convey information about Figure and Action, following the pattern discussed at the beginning of this section. Many derivational prefixes also convey information that requires decomposition into primitives.

Adapting the representation to the Navajo verb base requires a provision for the information conveyed by each morpheme. The representations will include notations that show how information is parceled out among the prefixes and verb stem, including decomposition where appropriate. Eventually the morphemes of the verb stem will also be included as separate units of information, but at this stage the verb stem is treated as a single unit.

I present in (8) a representation of the Navajo verb base that underlies the surface form *yílk'ooł*. This is a simple verb base, with no derivational prefixes. The verb denotes a telic event of literal motion, with the arrival as natural final endpoint. Here and below, Navajo verb forms are cited in the Imperfective unless otherwise noted, following the practice of YM and YMM.

(8)   *yílk'ooł* 'A wave is arriving, comes rolling.'

EVENT = T: e_1 = Process   ARG: Arg_1 : = [1] wave, flowing matter
               e_2 = State

QUALIA:
   Figure = [1]
   Motion
   Path   } (e_1)
   State = (e_2) arrive

The representation identifies the components of meaning and relates them to each other, as in the English example given. The event is a Transition; the verb has one argument. The subevents and arguments are identified with particulars of qualia structure. The verb base has no prefixes, so that in this case the analysis is a decompositional one.

I would like to comment briefly on the methodology of close lexical analysis before going on to discuss more complex verb bases. For verbs in a language like English, one investigates the syntactic alternations that a verb allows—dative shift, resultatives, middle constructions, for instance. Also relevant are the co-occurrence possibilities of a verb with certain key adverbials. The analyst looks at the alternations and asks which factors of meaning vary and which remain constant. For Navajo, one studies the morphological alternations which are available for a given verb stem, in particular the derivational prefixes with which the stem may appear. The aim is to find a common meaning that inheres in all of the cases. Similarly, for derivational prefixes one considers the stems and alternations in which they participate. This is essentially what YMM present in their distillations of root/stem meanings, classifier meanings, thematic prefix, and aspectual category meanings.

9.2   Some Derivational Prefixes of Navajo

In this section I discuss several derivational prefixes. Basing the interpretations on the characterizations of YM and YMM, I ask what information a prefix contributes to the different levels of lexical meaning. The analysis involves comparisons of the verb bases with which a given prefix appears and comparisons of that prefix with different verb bases. I will assume that the derivational prefixes have consistent semantic meanings, using the interpretations of YM and YMM. I have not had access to the judgments of native speakers while doing this work, so the particular analyses must be taken as tentative.

In this preliminary study I focus on derivational prefixes and treat verb stems as units. Other factors are ignored or neutralized. Verb stem sets are associated with particular categories, known as aspectual in the literature. To neutralize this factor, I hold it constant. The examples are all of the Momentaneous category of stem set. This category is widely agreed to be varied and heterogeneous, and probably does not make a consistent contribution to meaning. Despite its semantic name, the Momentaneous category has little if any semantic content (see Smith 1991 and Axelrod 1993 on the corresponding category in Koyukon). I ignore thematic prefixes, which are closely related to verb roots and often have idiosyncratic meanings. I also ignore conjugational morphemes. These morphemes indicate Mode in the verb composite. They vary in form; whether the different forms contribute to lexical meaning is an open question.[9] Finally, I do not attempt to determine the thematic roles of arguments but simply note their contribution to qualia structure. The thematic role of a given argument probably follows from its place in event structure and qualia structure, as noted previously.

The prefixes are presented with typical verb stems; for each example, I give a tripartite lexical representation which specifies the contribution of stem and prefix.

Consider first the prefix '*a*, glossed as 'away out of sight,' which appears typically with verb stems of literal motion. (9a) presents a form which has this prefix and the same verb stem as the example (8) (*yílk'ooł*).

(9a)   '*iilk'ooł* 'wave, ripple rolls away out of sight' (prefix '*a*)

The event is a Transition, and there is a single argument, as in (8). The prefix does not affect either event structure nor argumentstructure. Rather, it specifies particulars of the Path, Ground, and resultant State; with the addition of this prefix, the verb base denotes a different event ('wave arrives' is the event of (8)). In our terms, the prefix contributes to the qualia structure of the verb base. (9b) gives the lexical representation for the verb base underlying *'iilk'ooł*.

(9b) Lexical representation for the verb base of *'iilk'ooł*

$$\text{EVENT} = \text{T:}\quad e_1 = \text{Process}\qquad \text{ARG: Arg}_1\text{: } = [1]\text{ wave, flowing matter}$$
$$e_2 = \text{State}$$

QUALIA:
Figure = [1]
Motion = rolls, ripples (e_1)
Path
State (e_2) $\Big\}$ *'a* (away out of sight)

The prefix meaning is given here and in the following examples, for perspicuity. I assume that the predictable meaning of a derivational morpheme would not appear in each lexical entry but would be listed once in the lexicon.

Another prefix, *ch'i*, specifies type and direction of motion: 'motion horizontally out'. *Ch'i* typically appears with verbs of literal motion. The prefix contributes information about Path, Manner, and final State; these are particulars of an event, and are stated in qualia structure. Example (10) illustrates a surface form and the lexical representation of the verb base, with the verb stem of the preceding example:

(10) *ch'élk'ooł* 'flowing matter (wave) rolls horizontally out' (prefix *ch'í*)

$$\text{EVENT} = \text{T:}\quad e_1 = \text{Process}\qquad \text{ARG: Arg}_1\text{: } = [1]\text{ flowing matter}$$
$$e_2 = \text{State}$$

QUALIA:
Figure = [1]
Motion (e_1)
Path
Manner $\Big\}$ *ch'í* (out horizontally)
State (e_2)

These prefixes are quite productive: they appear with many verb stems, generally with the meanings ascribed to them here. To illustrate, I give some additional examples of bases with prefixes *'a* and *ch'i*; O denotes Object (animate or inanimate).

(11) Consistent cases with derivational prefixes

> a. *'iishyeed*   'run away out of sight'
> b. *'iists'ǫǫd*   'stretch away out of sight'
> c. *'iistįįh*   'carry O away out of sight'
> d. *ch'éshyeed*   'run out horizontally'
> e. *ch'ínísts'ǫǫd*   'stretch out horizontally'
> f. *ch'íníshtįįh*   'carry O out horizontally'

There are many other productive prefixes of this same general type. They appear with motion verbs, they specify type and/or direction of motion, and they are relatively consistent in meaning.

Occasionally a prefix does not make its predicted contribution to the meaning of the verb base. In such cases the meaning of the base is not compositional but must be stated separately; it must also be learned separately, I assume. Example (12) illustrates such cases for the same two prefixes.

(12) Inconsistent cases with derivational prefixes

> a. *'iidlóóh* (with prefix *'a*) 'laugh and laugh', 'laugh oneself to death';
>   lit., 'laugh away out of sight'
>
> b. *ch'ínásh'nííł* (with prefix *ch'í* + *ná*) 'release plural O', 'set O free';
>   lit., 'let out again horizontally'

These verb bases have particular meanings which differ significantly from their literal meanings. I assume that for verb forms like these, the particular meaning is stated in the lexical entry for the verb base. I will have nothing more to say about special cases like this but will concentrate on forms in which a derivational prefix has its consistent, predictable meaning.

Now consider a verb base in which the derivational prefix, *ts'a*, affects all three tiers of lexical conceptual structure. The verb stem is the same as in (8)–(10). The prefix is postpositional, introducing an argument.

(13a) *bits'álk'ooł* 'wave rolls away from O' (prefix *ts'á*)

The event denoted by the verb base underlying (13a) is a Process: the event of rolling away has no clear final endpoint. Recall that the event denoted by the maximally simple (8) is a Transition. The difference between (8) and (13a) is due to the prefix *ts'á*, which adds to qualia structure by indicating the Path and its relation to the Ground. Example (13b) gives the lexical representation of the verb base underlying (13a).

(13b) Lexical representation for the verb base of *bits'álk'ool*

EVENT = P: e₁ = Process   ARG: Arg₁: = [1] flowing matter
                                     Arg₂: = [2] object

QUALIA:
    Figure = [1]
    Motion (e₁)
    Path   *ts'a*
    Ground [2]

The second argument functions as part of the Ground: it provides the locus from which the first argument moves.

Five additional examples follow that indicate more fully the range of this framework for lexical representation. The examples consist of verb bases with derivational prefixes, some with postpositions. The representations are constructed along the same lines as those given previously. I comment briefly on each example.

The verb stem underlying (14) is transitive; the base has the prefix *ada*. The first argument is Cause, and the second argument is Figure. The prefix specifies Path, Ground, and State, in the way that is now familiar.

(14) *'adaashteeh* 'I take animate object down from a height.' (prefix *ada*)

EVENT = T: e₁ = Process   ARG: Arg₁: = [1]
            e₂ = State   Arg₂: = [2] animate object

QUALIA:
    Cause = [1]
    Figure = [2]
    Motion (e₁)
    Path   ⎫
    Ground ⎬ *ada* (down from a height)
    State   ⎭

Both prefix and verb stem require decomposition, in this case.

The next example presents a Process event with two arguments. This is an event of metaphorical motion; the second argument functions as part of the Ground.

(15) *bíkádéé'íí'* 'subject looks for someone' (thematic prefix *dí*, prefix *ka*)

EVENT = P: e_1 = Process   ARG: Arg_1: = [1]
                                      Arg_2: = [2] animate object

QUALIA:
  Figure = [1]
  Motion (e_1)
  Path ⎱
  Ground [2] ⎰ *kadí*: *dí* + *ka* (for)

The event of (15) is similar to (13), although the latter is more directly a motion event. This verb base specifies that the object of the search is a person, unlike the roughly corresponding English verb *seek*.

The next examples give additional cases of how derivational prefixes specify the qualia structure of an event: the first is a Transition, the second a Process.

(16) *wó'ąabéézh* 'O boils over, foams over' (prefix *wó'a*)

EVENT = T: e_1 = Process   ARG: Arg_1: = [1]
           e_2 = State

QUALIA:
  Figure = [1]
  Motion (e_1)
  Path ⎱
  State (e_2) ⎰ *wó'a* (over an edge)

(17) *tá'díshį́įh* 'O eats around here and there' (prefix *tá'dí*)

EVENT = P: e_1 = Process   ARG: Arg_1: = [1]

QUALIA:
  Figure = [1]
  Motion (e_1)
  Ground ⎱
  Path ⎰ *tá'dí* (here and there)

It is the prefix that makes (16) a Transition: the same verb theme appears in other verb bases, both Process (atelic) and Transition (telic) bases. The prefix also contributes to the event type of (17): again, the verb theme appears in both telic and atelic bases.

The next example involves a lending event, a Transition with three arguments. The final State is within the scope of the prefix. At the final state the object O is in the possession of the recipient, as specified in the representation.

(18) *ba'nishtįįh* 'Subject lends animate O to someone.' (postposition *a*')

      EVENT = T: e_1 = Process   ARG: Arg_1: = [1] agent
                    e_2 = State Arg_2: = [2] animate O
                                              Arg_3: = [3]

      QUALIA:
        Cause = [1]
        Figure = [2]
        Motion = (e_1)
        Path
                      }   *a*' (lend)
        Ground
        State (e_2) [2] at [3]

The examples show how a wide range of events can be analyzed with the primitives that are relevant to events involving motion and location. This verb base has a motion root, $[tą́]_1$, which 'describes a handling movement . . . by manual contact' and has many extended meanings (YMM:473); the prefix contributes the key notion of lending.

    The framework of analysis thus applies nicely to a variety of cases. The pattern identified by Talmy holds: the verb stems tend to denote Figure and Motion, and other information is given by the derivational prefixes. The notion of Figure is associated with motion or change of state at a relatively abstract level of event structure. Strikingly, the Figure cannot be identified with a syntactic position or thematic role. Consider the Figure participant in three of the examples above. In (7), *Mary closed the door*, 'the door' is Figure because it undergoes a change of state; the Figure is syntactic object and argument 2, a theme. In (15), roughly 'Subject looks for someone', the Figure is the syntactic subject, argument1, an agent. In (18), roughly, 'Subject lends animate object to someone', the Figure is the object that is lent because it traverses a path and changes its metaphorical location; the Figure is syntactic object, argument2, a theme.[10]

9.3 The Subaspectual Prefixes

I would like now to present an analysis of the derivational prefixes known as subaspects in the literature.[11] These prefixes appear quite freely with many verb bases and also combine with each other. As the label *aspect* suggests, their contribution to meaning is to specify the internal structure of events. The Subaspects vary considerably. Analyzing the Subaspects in this framework enables us to find and represent their similarities and differences. As we shall see, they function at different levels of lexical representation.

    There are six prefixes in this class: the Reversionary *ná*, the Prolongative *dini*, the Semeliterative *náá*, the Seriative *hi*, the Inceptives, and the Terminative. The characterizations used here are those of YM and YMM. I discuss the contribution of each to the meaning of a verb base and how the meaning should be represented in tripartite lexical structure.

I begin with the Reversionary, which appears with certain verb bases of Transition events.[12] The prefix *ná* gives the information that the event constitutes a return to a previous state, as the glosses of the b examples indicate.

(19) Reversionary: return to previous state; prefix *ná*

     1a.   *hatin*   'area freezes'
     1b.   *nááhatin*   'area freezes again'

     2a.   *k'éshdǫǫh*   'I straighten it, as a nail.'
     2b.   *k'ínáshdǫǫh* 'I restraighten it.'

Does this information affect event structure, argument structure, or qualia structure? Since neither the type of event nor the participants are involved, it is clear that qualia structure is affected. The prefix provides information about the final State of Transition verb bases, as indicated in (20):

(20) Reversionary:

     Qualia: State: *ná* . . . : (*ná*: 'return to previous state')

To show how the Reversionary fits into lexical structure, I give the representation for (19-1b):

(21) *nááhatin* 'area freezes again' (with prefix *ná*)

     EVENT = T: e_1 = Process   ARG: Arg_1: = [1]
                e_2 = State

     QUALIA:
       Figure = [1]
       Motion = (e_1)
       State (e_2) frozen: *ná* (return to previous state)

The Reversionary prefix has scope over the final State of the Transition event.

    The Prolongative is another Subaspect that appears with verb bases of Transition events. Signaled by the prefix *dini* and the related prefixes *dinii, ńdíníí*, and *nikidíníí*, the Prolongative indicates that the final state of a Transition event continues. Example (22) illustrates; the viewpoint is Perfective (notated perf) in these examples.

(22) Prolongative

    a.   *chidí yiih dinolwod*
        car into-it prolong-perf-it-run into
        'The car ran into it and remained (stuck).'

    b.   *yah 'adinidááh*
        into-enclosed-space away-prolong-perf-he-go
        'He went inside and stayed.'

    c.   *diniishgęęzh*
        prolong-it-perf-I-stare
        'I fixed my gaze on it.'

Again, the information is part of qualia structure: neither the structure of the event nor the participants are affected. Like the Reversionary, the prefix specifies particulars of the resultant state of a Transition.

(23) Qualia: State: *dini* (continues)

The Prolongative prefix has scope over the final state of a Transition event. For an extensive discussion of the Prologative and its interaction with the other subaspectual prefixes, see Smith (1999b).

    The Semeliterative *náá*, another subaspectual prefix, indicates that an event is a single repetition of a previous event. The prefix is found in verb bases of Process and Transition events, as in (24).

(24) Semeliterative

    a.   *bits'ánáánálk'ool*   'wave rolls away again from O' (Process)
    b.   *k'ínáshdǫǫh*   'I straighten it again.' (Transition)

The Semeliterative also appears with stative verb bases, indicating that a state has obtained before, and with certain number prefixes. The prefix contributes to qualia structure.

    The Semeliterative prefix has scope over all the particulars of an event, since it is not associated with any particular primitive. Therefore it appears at the global level of qualia structure, as in (25).

(25) Qualia: E = *náá* (single repetition)

I now turn to the Seriative, a more complex case.

    The Seriative prefix *hi* appears in events of two types. It "marks verbal action as inherently segmented or as successive, involving 3+ subjects, objects, or actions" (YMM:877). I refer to these as events with Seriative stages (inherently segmented action in YMM) and Seriative events (successive action in YMM). Example (26) illustrates the latter type:

(26) Seriative events

    a.   *tóshjeeh 'ahééníłmááz*
        barrel in a circle-it-perf-I-roll
        'I rolled the barrel around in a circle.'

    b.   *tóshjeeh 'ahééhéłmááz*
        barrel in a circle-ser-it-perf-I-roll
        'I roll the barrel around in a succession of circles.'

    c.   *naaltsoos ch'íníjaa'*
        book out-them-perf-I-carry
        'I carried the books out (in one load).'

    d.   *naaltsoos ch'éhéjaa'*
        book out-ser-them-perf-I-carry
        'I carried the books out one after another.'

The sentences in a and c denote single events ("action" in YM's terms), while the sentences in b and d have the Seriative morpheme and denote successive events. The nature of the subevents is given by the verb base without the Seriative. Thus (26b) denotes a series of events of rolling a barrel around in a circle; (26d) denotes a series of events of carrying out a book. The other type of Seriative event is illustrated in (27):

(27) Events with seriative stages

    a.   *tsídii yah 'ahóócha'*
        bird into-an-enclosure away-ser-impf-it-hopping
        'The bird is hopping in.'

    b.   *hishghaał*
        ser-impf-I-move
        'I am wriggling.'

In these verb bases the Seriative morpheme is an essential component: it gives the particulars of the motions of wriggling or hopping. Verb bases with related, nonsegmental meanings (such as a single hop or wriggle) are available for some verb themes of inherently segmented motion. Such bases tend to have other lexically specific categories rather than the presence or absence of the Seriative morpheme.[13]

Now consider the lexical representations of the two meanings. Seriative events are conceptualized as multiple events consisting of a series of subevents.

Example (28) models such events such as those of (26b) and (26d), which are both Transitions:

(28)   Seriative event: Transition

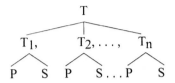

In the representation of this type of situation, the Seriative morpheme has the global Transitive event in its scope.[14]

Events with seriative stages have inherently segmented action such as hopping and wriggling. They are conceptualized as single events. The event of (27a) is a Transition consisting of a Process and State: the bird hops in (to some place). The Process consists of a series of stages, each stage a hop. The event of (27b) is a Process which consists of stages, each stage a wriggle. The structures are a durative Transition and a durative Process respectively, as presented in (4) and repeated here as (29a–b).

(29)   a.   T   b.   P

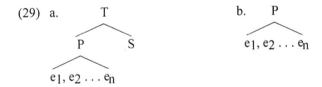

In these situations the stages of the Process are seriative. They consist of a series of distinct and successive motions which together make up a particular type of motion. To see this, compare hopping in and wriggling with processes of other types. Some processes have varied stages, such as building a house; others do not have discernible stages, such as enjoying a movie or pushing a cart. Inherently segmented processes like this are known as iterative or repetitive in the linguistics literature (Forsyth 1970).

The two types of Seriative events, then, involve segmentation at different levels of structure. Seriative events consist of distinct Transition subevents. In a tripartite representation, the Seriative morpheme is at the top level of event structure, as in (30):

(30)   Seriative event

EVENT: Seriative (T)   ARGUMENT

QUALIA

Further specification of the internal structure will follow the model of (28). Events with seriative stages, in contrast, are single events. The Seriative morpheme appears in qualia structure, specifying that the component of Action has distinct segments. Example (31) illustrates for a Transition event:

(31)   Transition with Seriative Stages

     EVENT= T: e_1 = Process   ARGUMENT
                 e_2 = State

    QUALIA:
     Figure
     Seriative (Motion)

Summarizing, both types of Seriative events are triggered by the Seriative morpheme. The morpheme appears at a different level of structure for each type.

This treatment of lexical event structure departs somewhat from other lexical approaches, such as those of Grimshaw (1990) and Pustejovsky (1991). Lexical event structure is sometimes presented as a very general classification which essentially coincides with the aspectual situation types.[15] I suggest rather that the lexical event structure of a language should include features that play a lexical role in that language, including features that are signaled morphologically. The representations given follow this line of reasoning. The Seriative feature appears in the event structure of seriative events.

The Inceptive and the Terminative are also subaspect prefixes. They focus the endpoints of an event, presenting beginnings and endings as events in themselves. The essential function of the Inceptive and the Terminative is to narrow the presentation of an event to part of the event. Their semantic contribution is thus somewhat different from the other prefixes discussed, which are lexical in nature. Lexical morphemes contribute to specifying a particular kind of event. The Inceptive and the Terminative do not give such particulars. I refer to morphemes like the Inceptive and the Terminative as "superlexical" because their only semantic contribution is the narrow view; they have also been called "aspectual" and "procedural" in the literature (Forsyth 1970; Smith 1993, 1995).[16]

Beginnings and endings are Transition events: they involve changes into or out of an event. Thus, verb bases with Inceptive and Terminative morphemes denote Transitions. Navajo has several such prefixes; several are given in (32).

(32)   Inceptives and Terminatives

    a.   *niki: tsinaa'eełgóó niki'nííkǫǫ́'*
       boat-toward start-it-perf-I-swim
       'I started to swim to the boat.'

b.   *nii: bilasáana bi'niiyą́ę́ą́ę́'*
apple it-start-Perf-I-eat
'I started to eat the apple.'

c.   *ni: diyogí niníłł'ǫ́*
rug finish-it-Perf-I-weave
'I finished weaving the rug.'

d.   *ni: nihonítą́ą́l*
finish-Perf-I-sing a song
'I finished singing a song.'

There are subtle differences between these morphemes, discussed in Young and Morgan (1988). Here I will consider only the nature of their contribution to the verb base.

Inceptives and Terminatives consist of a process and change of state, like other Transition events. But they differ from most Transitions. Generally, a Transition event involves a change from a situation of rest to another situation of rest, the latter with a change of state; the event consists of the change. What distinguishes the Inceptive from this standard is the final state. The final state of an Inceptive is an internal stage of an ongoing event. In Navajo, the ongoing event is denoted by the other morphemes of the verb base. For instance, the sentence (32a) presents a change from a situation of rest to an event of swimming to the boat, repeated and modeled in (33):

(33)   Inceptive: *tsinaa'eełgóó niki'níłkǫ́ǫ́'* (I started to swim to the boat.)

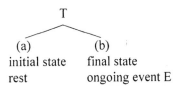

The Inceptive has a final state that differs from the final state of other Transitions.

The distinguishing feature of the Terminative is the initial state: the change is not from rest, but from an internal stage of an ongoing event, namely the one denoted by the other morphemes of the verb base. Thus (32d) presents a change from an ongoing singing event to a final state at which there is no singing, modeled in (34):

(34) Terminative: *nihonítááł* (I finished singing a song.)

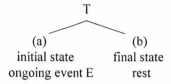

(a)   (b)
initial state   final state
ongoing event E   rest

The Terminative has an initial state that differs from the initial state of most Transitions. A different analysis of the Terminative is considered in Smith (1999b).

The superlexical Inceptive and Terminative morphemes denote narrow-view events with the structures of (33) and (34). The events have complex, derived event structures. The final State of an Inceptive is an ongoing event E, where E is the event denoted by the verb base without the inceptive morpheme. The initial State of an Terminative verb base is an ongoing event E, where E is the event denoted by the verb base without the Terminative. Without the inceptive and terminative, the events of the relevant verb bases are standard Transitions or Processes.

In tripartite structure Inceptives and Terminatives appear at the level of event structure. They trigger derived structures which consist of two subevents. The event focused is the beginning or ending; the complement is the event which begins or ends. The contribution of these superlexical morphemes to the verb base are given here:

(35) Inceptive

EVENT: $E1 = T =$ $e_1 =$ Process (inception)
                    $e_2 =$ event E2

(36) Terminative

EVENT: $E1 = T =$ $e_1 =$ event E2
                    $e_2 =$ state (termination)

This general notion of derived event structure holds for other superlexical morphemes, which focus an internal interval of an event.

The Subaspects can combine with each other in various ways. For instance, YM note the "inceptive prolongative." These combinations and their interpretations are predicted by the account given here, according to the scope of a given subaspectual morphemes in lexical representation.

9.4   Extending the Analysis

9.4.1   Thematic Prefixes

Thematic prefixes have narrow, idiosyncratic meanings and appear only with a narrow class of bases.[17] They often require particular classifiers. The root [k'ol], for instance, is glossed as 'undulate' in YMM; it appears with nonneuter bases in two conditions. With the L classifier, it underlies themes with bases of movement of waves in water, or (heat) in air; with the thematic prefix *ni* and the L classifier, it underlies themes involving blinking the eyes. There are twelve bases of the first type, illustrated by (37a), and two of the second, illustrated by (37b).

(37)   a.   *yílk'ool* 'wave arrives, comes rolling'

      b.   *nishk'ol* 'blink the eyes repeatedly'; lit., 'move the eyes terminatively, in an undulating fashion'

Evidently, the thematic prefix may make a significant difference in the meaning of the verb base. In some cases the classifiers themselves have a thematic role with a given root/stem, according to YMM.

    Thematic prefixes have a wide range of meanings, including the specification of a component of an event, such as vision, fire, darkness, arms and legs, stomach; a general type of event, such as dwindling, suffering, examining, relinquishment, absorption of moisture; a general area, such as pain, scolding, etc.; see YM, YMM for examples and comments. Certain prefixes make a predictable contribution to meaning. The thematic prefix *di*, for instance, indicates that an event involves fire. This prefix appears in many verb bases that denote fire events. (38) illustrates: (a) has the root [k'áéáé'], (b) has the root [náád], (c) has the root [nóód], (d) has the root [lid]. In some examples *di* appears with derivational prefixes, as noted.

(38)   a.   *'adi: 'a* (away, out of sight) + *di*
        adik'ą́ąh 'Fire spreads, moves away out of sight.'

     b   *hadi: ha* (up, out vertically) + *di*
        hadinaad 'Fire flares up.'

     c.   *didi: di* (Position 1a) + *di* (Position 6b)—both involving fire
        'ąą didinood 'S (e.g., fire) spreads.'

     d.   *dilid* 'S is burning, smoldering.'

This prefix is relatively productive and might be treated as a derivational prefix in lexical representations. Some thematic prefixes appear with only a few verb roots and can be simply listed with those roots. Other prefixes are more idiosyncratic.

Sometimes a thematic prefix appears only with certain verb bases of a given verb root, yet all the bases of that root have the relevant meaning. One such prefix is *ná*, which occurs in certain bases of the root ['ah$_2$], having to do with skinning or butchering of animals; it appears with the barred L classifier. There are eleven verb bases associated with this root, according to YMM; four appear with the thematic prefix, the others do not. One example of each type is given here; (39b) has the thematic prefix.

(39) a.   *yish'ah* 'I in the process of skinning, butchering O.' (Cursive)

  b.   *násh'ah* 'I skin, butcher, O.'

The root/stem carries the essential meaning, with *ná* an optional component.[18] There may be subtle difference in the bases with and without *ná*.

9.4.2 *Aspectual Categories*

The lexical semantics of the morphological categories known traditionally as aspectual—Verb Lexeme Categories, or VLCs—are also susceptible to analysis in this framework. Here I can only indicate a tentative analysis in summary form.

VLCs are discontinuous morphological categories which combine with the verb theme to form the verb base. All event verb bases in Navajo realize one of these categories. Example (40) presents the skeletons of five different VLC verb bases formed with the root ['AH$_1$], denoting movement of a flat object (YMM 1992:6). Actual verb bases that realize these VLC skeletons may have other prefixes as well.

(40) ['áád], [na ... 'ah], ['ad], [yi ... 'ad], ['ał]

The VLC categories are recognizable by patterns of root/stem variation; some also have distinctive prefixes, and some occur with particular viewpoint morphemes.

The essential point is that the VLCs make different contributions to verb base meaning. This is evident when their meanings are stated in the tripartite representational format used in this chapter. The meanings of VLCs appear at different levels and components of lexical structure. Most VLCs appear at qualia structure or event structure; there are two that may be formal categories only, with no consistent meaning.

Some VLC categories are clearly lexical, giving information about the Figure, Motion, or Path, associated with an event. These include the Distributive, the Diversative, the Repetitive, and the Reversative. Other VLCs, namely the Conclusive and the Durative, give information about duration. In our framework, these properties are stated at the tier of qualia structure. All Transitional verb bases involve changes of state, or Transition events. Thus the Transitional VLC pertains to event structure. However, I am not sure whether the Transitional VLC can be said to trigger a Transition; perhaps not. There are many Transition events of other VLC categories.

The Cursive is unique among VLCs in structure and in semantic function. Structurally, the Cursive is mutually dependent with the Progressive Mode. Semantically it always presents an interval of an event. The Cursive triggers a derived event structure, on the pattern of the Inceptive and Terminative prefixes discussed previously. The Cursive is therefore a superlexical morpheme, stated at event structure.

The remaining VLCs are the Momentaneous and the Semelfactive. They are heterogeneous semantically. They probably do not make a consistent contribution to the meaning of the verb base and should be regarded as morphological categories without semantic content, at least in the modern language.

This analysis is outlined in Smith (1996a), though without lexical representations. The representational format developed in this article can be fruitful for the study of VLCs as for the other categories of the Navajo verb base.

9.5 Concluding Remarks

The tripartite format for lexical representation has been equal to the tasks set out at the beginning of this article. The format has made it possible to distinguish different types of information conveyed by the morphemes of the Navajo verb base, to relate information about one level to the others, and to better understand the event structure of Navajo. We have seen that the Figure of an event may be realized in different syntactic relations and different thematic roles. With a more fully developed account of the argument structure level it will be possible to consider carefully the question of how event structure, argument structure, and qualia structure are related.

This work suggests at least one constraint on the tripartite format of representation. The constraint involves the relations between the tiers of argument structure and qualia structure. We may wish to require that argument structure be directly related to qualia structure. Representations with Arguments which did not appear in qualia structure would be ill formed. Since the particulars of qualia structure include the components of event structure (e_1, e_2, State), this requirement would in effect pertain to all levels of the representation. Further development may suggest other constraints and predictions concerning lexical structure and its representation.

Notes

I would like to thank Ted Fernald for insightful and meticulous comments on an earlier version of this article. I also thank Lisa Green, Manfred Krifka, Gil Rappaport, and Steve Wechsler for helpful discussion of the earlier version.

1. I draw primarily on work in lexical semantics of Talmy (1985, 1991), Pinker (1989), Jackendoff (1972, 1990), Levin and Rappaport-Hovav (1995); and on work in event structure of Vendler (1957), Dowty (1979), Smith (1991).

2. In the discussion of Navajo morphology I rely on the characterizations of Young and Morgan (1980), Young and Morgan (1987), and Young, Morgan, and Midgette (1992).

The verb composite consists of a verbal unit with a series of prefixes and other forms; the prefixes have fixed positions, both hierarchical and sequential. Following Young and Morgan (1987), three levels of the verb composite are distinguished. The first is the verb theme, which contains the verb root and classifier. At the next level is the verb base, where the verb root is realized concretely as a set of stems. The base consists of a verb stem, often with prefixes conveying lexical, adverbial, and thematic concepts, including plurality. The next level includes the pronominal and conjugational prefixes, which are hierarchically outside the verb base. The hierarchical structure is this:

Verb Theme: $_{Theme}$[classifier [root/stem]]
Verb Base: $_{Base}$[prefixes . . . $_{Theme}$[classifier+root/stem]]
Verb Composite: $_{VComp}$[pronom & conjug prefixes [base]]

The linear order of the prefixes differs from their hierarchical order. I assume that they are added in hierarchical rather than linear order, following Speas (1986:228).

Young and Morgan identify derivational prefixes according to their position in the verb base. Kari (1989) and McDonough (1996) offer different approaches.

3. This approach may be compared to that of Grimshaw (1990). Grimshaw also discusses the relation of participants to events. In her analysis, the Agent is identified as the most prominent participant in an event.

4. Talmy concentrates on Atsugewi exemplars of the Motion+Figure type. For instance, he cites "verb roots of Motion with conflated Figure: *-lup-* small shiny spherical object to move, be located; *-ɬ* smallish planar object to move, be located; *-caq-* slimy lumpish object to move/be located . . ."; Talmy gives many other examples in his article.

Most languages have a dominant tendency or pattern but are not absolutely consistent. English has some verbs that depart from the general tendency and incorporate Path, e.g., *enter, exit, pass, rise, descend,* and *return,* Talmy notes. Similarly, not all Navajo verbs are of the Motion+Figure type even though this is the predominant pattern.

5. In Navajo and Athabaskan linguistics, verb roots are traditionally identified as either motion or nonmotion roots, according the prefixes with which they appear and other factors (Kari 1990). This traditional use of the term *motion* is partly semantic and partly depends on morphological criteria. It is not the same as the primitive concept of motion introduced previously, and used in the lexical representations of this article.

6. Vendler's (1957) classification of events (and many others) distinguishes events with and without duration as distinct types. Durative Processes are "Activities," Durative Transitions are "Accomplishments," instantaneous Transitions are "Achievements." For Vendler, instantaneous Processes are a special type of Achievement; Smith (1991) puts them in a separate category of "Semelfactive."

7. Qualia structure is quite different in Pustejovsky's work: for him, "four basic roles constitute the qualia structure for a lexical item . . . (they are) Constitutive—Material, Weight, Parts; Formal—Orientation, Magnitude, Shape, Dimensionality, Color, Position; Telic—Purpose, Functions; Agentive—Creator, Artifact, Natural Kind, Causal Chain" (1995: 85–86).

There are some differences between Postejovsky's account of event structure and this one. My treatment of derived events differs. I will suggest later that the lexical Event structures of a language should be closely related to those event structures which are grammaticized in that language, either overtly or covertly (see the discussion of situation types in Smith 1991, 1993, 1995).

8. I refer to these categories as Verb Lexeme Categories, or VLCs, so as not to prejudice the question of whether they are semantically aspectual (Smith 1991, 1996a). VLCs are discussed briefly at the end of this article.

9. Mode morphemes may also contribute to meaning. There are some dependencies of form between the shape of the mode morpheme, the VLC, particular derivational prefixes, and particular verb stems and bases. Whether they signal consistent meanings is under debate; see Young and Morgan (1987), Smith (1991), Axelrod (1993), Midgette (1996), and Rice (1996).

10. The Figure can probably be identified with Theme. This identification can only be maintained if dual thematic roles are allowed. This would account for cases where the Agent causes some change of state to itself, and can thus be seen as Theme: in other words, where a single argument has the two roles of Agent and Theme.

11. The Subaspects are distinct from the Aspectual categories, or VLCs. As Young and Morgan point out, they differ morphologically from the Aspectual categories: they do not have associated stem sets; they combine with each other and with the Aspectual categories.

12. The Reversionary, like most of the subaspects, appears only with certain VLCs.

13. The contrasts often involve different aspectual verb lexeme categories (VLCs). For instance, some verb roots have a contrast between a single-stage event in the Semelfactive VLC and an event with seriative stages in a different VLC. In the case of breathing, where the normal case involves multiple breaths, the more basic form has the Repetitive VLC and the form with the prefix *hi* has the VLC known as Momentaneous:

a.   *ńdísdzih* 'breathe' (Repetitive)

b.   *'adahisdziih* 'to draw in a series of breaths' (w prefix *hi*)

14. The Seriative does not have scope over the higher-level Process node. If it scoped the Process node of a Transition, the situation would involve a repetition of an entire Process before a change of state. If the Seriative scoped a Process node alone, the situation would be a multiple-event series of Processes. I am not sure that there are such events; perhaps a habitual pattern of Processes could be conceptualized in this way.

15. The aspectual situation types of a given language are covert grammatical categories with a characteristic set of syntactic and semantic properties such as Activity and Accomplishment (Smith 1991). The situation types are realized by a verb and its arguments in a sentence. The aspectual feature of a given verb makes an essential contribution to the meaning of a sentence, however. Although telic events are distinguishable in Navajo, they do not constitute a separate situation type in this sense (Smith 1991, 1996a).

16. Discussing the Russian system, for instance, Forsyth calls certain morphemes "procedural" because they "leave unaltered the basic meaning of the original verb." In contrast, other morphemes "modify the meaning of a verb to produce a lexical derivative

. . . a new verb denoting a type of action different from that denoted by the original verb" (1970:19). Compare these forms of the basic Russian verb in *a*:

a.   *govorit'* (speak)
b.   *zagavorit'* (begin to speak)
c.   *ugovorit'* (persuade)

The prefix of *zagovorit'* is a procedural morpheme while the prefix of *ugovorit'* is lexical because it contributes to a verb denoting a different sort of situation.

17. Kari, discussing the related Athabaskan language Ahtna, treats thematic prefixes as part of the verb theme: "Thematic prefixes are part of the structure of the verb theme ...(they) cannot be explained as...a productive derivational or inflectional process" (1990:46). Axelrod considers thematic prefixes among the 'qualifier' prefixes in her analysis of Koyukon, another Athabaskan language (1993:14).

18. The forms with thematic *ná* appear in Momentaneous and Conclusive VLCs; the Cursive bases do not have it, nor do some of the Momentaneous forms.

References

Axelrod, Melissa. 1993. *The Semantics of Time: Aspectual Categorization in Koyukon Athabaskan*. Lincoln: University of Nebraska Press.

Croft, William. 1987. Categories and Relations in Syntax: The Clause-Level Organization of Information. Ph.D. dissertation, Stanford University.

Dowty, David. 1979. *Word Meaning and Montague Grammar*. Dordrecht: Kluwer.

Dowty, David. 1991. Thematic Proto-roles and Argument Selection. *Language*, 67:547–619.

Forsyth, John. 1970. *A Grammar of Aspect: Usage and Meaning in the Russian Verb*. Cambridge: Cambridge University Press.

Grimshaw, Jane. 1990. *Argument Structure*. Cambridge, Mass.: MIT Press.

Gruber, Jeffrey. 1965. Studies in Lexical Relations. Ph.D. dissertation, Massachusetts Institute of Technology.

Jackendoff, Ray. 1972. *Semantic Interpretation in Generative Grammar*. Cambridge, Mass.: MIT Press.

Jackendoff, Ray. 1990. *Semantic Structures*. Cambridge, Mass.: MIT Press.

Kari, James. 1989. Affix Positions and Zones in the Athabaskan Verb Complex: Ahtna and Navajo. *International Journal of American Linguistics*, 55:424–454.

Kari, James. 1990. *Ahtna Athabaskan Dictionary*. Fairbanks: Alaska Native Language Center.

Levin, Beth, and Malka Rappaport-Hovav. 1995. *Unaccusativity*. Cambridge, Mass.: MIT Press.

McDonough, Joyce. 1996. Epenthesis in Navajo. In E. Jelinek, S. Midgette, K. Rice, and L. Saxon (eds.), *Essays in Honor of Robert Young*. Albuquerque: University of New Mexico Press.

Midgette, Sally. 1996. Lexical Aspect in Navajo: The Telic Property. In E. Jelinek, S. Midgette, K. Rice, and L. Saxon (eds.), *Essays in Honor of Robert Young*. Albuquerque: University of New Mexico Press.

Mourelatos, Alexander. 1978. Events, Processes, and States. *Linguistics and Philosophy*, 2:415–434.

Pinker, Steven. 1989. *Learnability and Cognition*. Cambridge, Mass.: MIT Press.

Pustejovsky, James. 1991. The Syntax of Event Structure. *Cognition*, 41:47–81.

Pustejovsky, James. 1995. *The Generative Lexicon.* Cambridge, Mass.: MIT Press.

Smith, Carlota. 1991. *The Parameter of Aspect.* Dordrecht: Kluwer.

Smith, Carlota S. 1993/1995. The Range of Aspectual Situation Types: Derived Categories and a Bounding Paradox. In Bertinetti (ed.), *Proceedings of the Workshop on Tense and Aspect.* Turin: Rosenberg and Sellier.

Smith, Carlota. 1996a. Aspectual Categories in Navajo. *International Journal of American Linguistics,* 62:227–263.

Smith, Carlota. 1999a. Activities? States or Events? *Linguistics and Philosophy.*

Smith, Carlota. 1999b. The Navajo Prolongative and Lexical Structure. Coyote Papers. Tuscon, Arizona.

Speas, Margaret. 1986. Adjunctions and Predictions in Syntax. Ph.D. dissertation, Massachusetts Institute of Technology.

Talmy, Leonard. 1985. Lexicalization Patterns: Semantic Structure in Lexical Forms. In T. Shopen (ed.), *Language Typology and Syntactic Description,* Vol. 3. Cambridge: Cambridge University Press.

Talmy, Leonard. 1991. *Path to Realization: A Typology of Event Integration.* (Buffalo Papers in Linguistics, No. 1). Buffalo: State University of New York.

Vendler, Zeno. 1957. Verbs and Times. *Philosophical Review.* 56, 143-160.

Young, Robert, and William Morgan. 1980. *The Navajo Language.* Albuquerque: University of New Mexico Press.

Young, Robert, and William Morgan. 1987. *The Navajo Language.* Rev. Ed. Albuquerque: University of New Mexico Press.

Young, Robert, and William Morgan. 1988. Inception in the Navajo Verb. Unpublished manuscript.

Young, Robert, William Morgan, and Sarah Midgette. 1992. *An Analytical Lexicon of Navajo.* Albuquerque: University of New Mexico Press.

10

ICONICITY AND WORD ORDER IN KOYUKON ATHABASKAN

Chad L. Thompson

Koyukon and other Athabaskan languages are often described as being SOV languages. However, it is also well understood that Athabaskan languages sometimes allow deviations from this word order. Subject Object Inversion (SOI) in Navajo and other Athabaskan languages is a famous example of such deviation. Koyukon, an Athabaskan language spoken in the interior of Alaska, does not generally allow SOI, but it is not unusual for one to find postverbal constituents or adjuncts in texts. The present paper looks at such constituents, discusses the problems they pose for theories of iconicity, and, with support from a quantified analysis and from psycholinguistic evidence, suggests explanations for their usage.

Functional linguistics has far from ignored the problem of word order. Several recent volumes have been published on the subject (Payne 1992, Tomlin 1986, Yokoyama 1986, inter alia). In addition, psycholinguists have examined word order, providing a cognitive basis for functional claims (see Gernsbacher 1990 for a summary of such work). In addition to describing the textual function of postverbal NPs, this chapter will ground these functions in cognitively valid principles. Kibrik (1994) criticizes many of the text-based studies as being little more than descriptive, and points out that Givón himself states that explanations for such things as word order must not be "about the text," but "about the mind" (Givón 1992: 317).

Noun phrases, postpositional phrases, adverbials, and complements can be found after the verb. This chapter primarily discusses postverbal NPs. Below are two examples of such NP constituents taken from traditional myths (*Kk'edonts'ednee*) told by Catherine Attla. In these and the other examples here, I have made the minor changes necessarily to get from the older orthography used in Attla (1983, 1989), Pilot (1975), inter alia to the orthography presently in use.

(1) *Dehoon gheel   tl'ee   ho'oodedets'eeyh,   go   kk'es.*
    and   really   still   s/he.pinch.her/himself   DEM   alder
    'The alder was still pinching herself.' (Attla 1989: 166)

(2) *Dehoon heyeetlyeł,   go   noghuye.*
    while   3p.grabbed.3s   DEM   frog
    'and they grabbed the frog' (Attla 1983:8)

The context of (1) is that culture hero/trickster Raven has just been killed and his "wives," or tree spirit helpers, are mutilating themselves in mourning. The alder pinches herself and bleeds, which gives the alder its reddish color. The context of (2) is that some young boys see, grab, torment, and dismember a frog. A young orphan boy puts the frog back together and buries it. Later, the frog appears to him as an old woman and helps him to lead a good life.

In section 10.1, I give further examples of the various types of postverbal constituents. In section 10.2, I present the methods and results of my textual analysis. Finally, section 10.3 is a discussion of the theoretical issues involved with iconicity and syntax, iconicity being any nonarbitrary relationship between form and meaning or form and function. Furthermore, in section 10.3, I attempt to reconcile the contradictions between the Koyukon data and predictions made by particular principles of iconicity.

First, however, it is necessary to talk briefly about preposing, or SOI, in Koyukon. As stated above, it is rare, but it does happen. It is found in sentences involving the transitive verb, *deyeeloh* 'get, kill' (examples (3) and (4)). I have also found two instances of SOI in Jetté (both 1908:349), one of which is reproduced in (5) in the modern orthography, and in one example in the Koyukon Junior Dictionary (Jones 1983), which is shown in (6). Because the use of SOI is so rare in Koyukon, not enough data are available to discuss its function. It will not be discussed any further in this chapter. The *ye-/be-* alternation, on the other hand, is clearly present in Koyukon and is discussed in Thompson (1989).

(3) *John too   deyeeloh.* (also *John too debeeloh*)
    John water   got
    'The water got John' (i.e., 'John drowned')

(4) *John kkuł dibeeloh.* (also *John kkuł deyeeloh*)
     John cold got
     'A cold got John' (i.e., 'John caught a cold')

(5) *mekk'e kkun' denaa ghe'oł.*
     after.3s fire   man s.walking
     'A man of fire is going after him.' (Jetté 1908:316)

(6) *sołt'aanh sis   dzaabedegheełgheł.*
     woman   bear startled
     'The woman was startled by the bear.' (Jones 1983:161)

10.1 Postposing in Koyukon

10.1.1 Postposing in Other Athabaskan Languages

Postverbal constituents have been reported for other Athabaskan languages. For example, Golla (1985:16–18) reports flexible word order for Hupa, including the use of postverbal nouns. He does not discuss the function or pragmatics of such various word orders but clearly explains how the verb morphology allows flexible word order. In (7) below, the fourth-person subject prefix, *ch'i-*, indicates a human subject, so all of the sentences mean 'John saw the dog':

(7) a. *John   no:k'ine:yo:t ch'iłtsa:n.*
         John   dog   saw

     b. *No:k'ine:yo:t ch'iłtsa:n John.*

     c. *John ch'iłtsa:n no:k'ine:yo:t.*

     d. *No:k'ine:yo:t John ch'iłtsa:n.*

         'John saw the dog.'

  Rice (1989:1003–1004, 1191–1196) discusses the presence of postverbal elements in Slave. She does not, however, report any postverbal nouns or simple NPs. Postverbal relative clauses do appear as is seen in (8). In addition, Slave has postverbal PPs and subject complements, as is shown in (9).

(8) a. *John lį [ʔeyi ts'ǫ́dani kayįhk'a yįlé   i]   wehk'é.*
         John dog the   child   3.bit   PAST COMP 3.shot

     b. *John lį   wehk'é [ʔeyi ts'ǫ́dani kayįhk'a yįlé   i].*
         John dog shot   the   child   3.bit   PAST COMP
         'John shot the dog that bit the child.' (Rice 1989:1327)

(9) a. *yundáa   nóodéht'e   ndu   ts'é̞.*
         ahead   paddle.across   island   to
         'he paddled across to the island' (Rice 1989:1191)

     b. *kegǫ́fa   líbalá   líts'e'a   gha.*
         is.difficult canvas   one.folds   COMP
         'It is hard to fold canvas.' (Rice 1989:1195)

Rice says, "Extraposed postpositional phrases give extra information not crucial to the discourse; the material simply offers further explanation" (1989:1193). Such an explanation squares well with the pragmatic order principle discussed in section 10.3 below, but, as we will see, the data in Koyukon do not entirely.

10.1.2 Types of Postverbal Arguments

As stated above, NPs, PPs, adverbial clauses, and complement clauses can be postposed in Koyukon. Of the NPs, simple NPs, relative clauses (with or without a head), and conjoined NPs may be postposed.

10.1.2.1 Postverbal NPs

10.1.2.1.1 Simple NPs

Examples (10)–(12) demonstrate the presence of simple NPs occurring postverbally. In (10) and (11), the postverbal noun is preceded by the demonstrative *go* 'this.' As will be shown in section 10.2, this demonstrative is present in the vast majority of postverbal NPs. The postverbal noun in (12) is preceded by the definite article *eey.* Also in (12), the postverbal NP appears within a quotation. This example is included to demonstrate that postposing does appear in direct quotations, even though such discourse is excluded from the statistical study done in section 10.2.

(10) *Huyeł gheel   beyeenhooldlet   go   tsook'aale.*
      And.then   3s.became.angry   DEM   old.woman
      'And then the old woman became angry.' (Attla 1983:20)

(11) *Huyeł   gheel   buhudeneenaayh go   bedzeyh.*
      and   really   they.die   DEM   caribou
      'All the caribou would die.' (Attla 1989:52)

(12)   *'Anaa!*   *Haats'ehooneege*   *ts'e*   *setl'onon'oyh*   *eey*
       don't   gently   COMP   give.back.to.me   DET
             setlaatleele',   *'yełnee.*
             my axe   3s.told.3s
       '"Don't! Just give my axe back to me gently," he told him.' (Attla
       1989:22)

10.1.2.1.2   Postverbal Relative Clauses and Nominalized Verbs

Examples (13) and (14) show postverbal relative clauses. In (13), the postverbal
clause is headless, while its place in the preverbal clause is filled with the independent third-person singular pronoun, *ɏdenh.* In (14), the relative clause appears postverbally, while its head appears preverbally.

(13)   *dehoon gheel ɏdenh*   *yeen'*   *yeh*   *ledo,*   *go*   *de'ot*   *okko*
       while   3s   only   house   stay   DEM   3s.wife   for
             neeyo-nenh
             come-REL
       'while only the one who had come for his wife remained in the house'
       (Attla 1989: 100)

(14)   *Kk'ɏdaa*   *yɏh*   *delenh*   *no'eedeghaanh*   *gheelhee,*
       now   so   3.bro.-in-law   3.carried.3.back   truly
             go   *bɏhdeegheeneeg-enh.*
             DEM   had.been.injured-REL
       'and then the Northern Lights Man carried back his brother in law who
       had been injured' (Attla 1989:362)

10.1.2.1.3   Postverbal Conjoined NPs

Examples (15)–(17) are examples of postverbal conjoined NPs. Conjunction in
Koyukon is done with *yeł,* which is also the associative postposition 'with'.
Examples (15) and (16) are interesting in that the postverbal conjoined NPs are
represented preverbally by a more general, nonconjoined NP—*nee'eedeneege*
'clothing' in (15) and *baabe* 'food' in (16). Example (16) is further interesting in
that the subject of the sentence, *go sołt'aanh* 'this woman', appears in addition
to the conjoined direct object.

(15)   *Bɏgh nee'eedeneege*   *eghonh,*   *gets*   *yeł*
       clothing   make   mittens   and
             yooghe   *kkaaken*   *yeł.*
             there   boots   and
       'She was making a lot of clothing, mittens and boots.' (Attla 1989:266)

(16) *Ts'ʉh nonłe kk'ʉdaa baabe neeneelo, go sołt'aanh*
    so   there now   food   laid.out DEM woman
               saanyee nelaan ggunh yeł.
               summer meat   dried and
    'The girl laid out some food, including dried meat from the summer.' (Attla 1989:56)

(17) *Ał edezeldetl k'etsaan' edezeldetl kk'eeyh tl'otsets yeł.*
    boughs 3.hit.self grass   3.hit.self birch rotten   and
    'He hit himself with spruce boughs. He hit himself with grass and rotted out birch.' (Attla 1983: 96)

10.1.2.2 Postverbal Postpositional Phrases

Examples (18) and (19) show postverbal postpositional phrases. Such postposing will only be discussed briefly here.

(18) *Naangge tonosaadletlet, go bedeeggude yeł.*
    up   3.rushed   DEM ice.chisel with
    'He rushed up the bank with his ice chisel.' (Attla 1989:202)

(19) *Yoogh taaghe nek'ets'edelet kk'e dehut'aanh huyeł, gełtl aahaa*
    there   water poke   like   act   and gaff with
    'He acted like someone poking around in the water with a gaff hook.' (Attla 1989:250)

10.1.2.3 Postverbal Adverbial and Complement Clauses

Examples (20) through (22) show postverbal adverbial clauses. Examples (23) and (24) show postverbal complements. Notice that the postverbal clauses in (20), (21), and (23) are preceded by the demonstrative *go*.

(20) *Dehoon degge taaldo' go nelget ts'en'.*
    while   up   sat   DEM 3.afraid SUB
    'She started to sit up [=did not sleep] out of fear.' (Pilot 1975:10)

(21) *ts'ʉh naaltaanh, go debeeznee ts'en'*
    so   lie.down DEM be.told   SUB
    'So he went to bed as he had been told.' (Attla 1989:24)

(22) *Kk'ʉdaa honoyegheełtlaatl teghenoltenh łonh ts'en'.*
    now   chop.out   frozen.in   oh   SUB
    'He had to chop it out of the ice because it had frozen in.' (Attla 1989:36)

(23) *Yoogh   kk'ʉdaa   dzaan   nek'eheghaałeno',   go   yenk'eedet'oł.*
      here   now   day   working   DEM   cutting.fish
      'People had been working all day, cutting fish.' (Attla 1989:72)

(24) *Tłaa   eey   dotaaghsneeł   dehugh soo' deseyoh.*
      hey   that   I.don't.know.why   happened.to.me
      'I don't know why this happened to me.' (Attla 1989:76)

(25) *Ts'ʉh   gheel   de'ot t'edle'taanh   go   nedoł   kk'aa.*
      so   3.wife   put.on.back   DEM   be.heavy   for
      'He put his wife on his back to make himself heavy.'

10.1.3   Are Postverbal Elements 'Afterthoughts?'

It is possible that postverbal elements in Koyukon are so-called afterthoughts, disfluencies which are necessary because of what Chafe (1987:40) calls premature closures. If this possibility is true, it would make no sense to try to determine the pragmatic function or cognitive base for the postverbal NPs in Koyukon.

I am assuming that postverbal elements are not disfluencies on the basis of the four following facts:

(a)   The Catherine Attla texts which form the basis for most of the analysis were edited by Catherine Attla and Eliza Jones. Disfluencies were removed before publication.

(b)   Postverbal elements are equally as common in published texts of other narrators (e.g., Pilot 1975; Jetté 1908, 1909) as they are in Attla's texts.

(c)   Postverbal NPs occur frequently enough in texts to make their status as disfluencies questionable.

(d)   In several instances lines with postverbal NPs not on the original taped recording were added during the editing process (e.g., Attla 1989:90, line 5, and 152, line 5)

10.1.4   The Degree of Integration of Postverbal Elements into the Clause

It is an important question as to whether or not postverbal words are part of the clause which they follow. Unfortunately, the evidence is contradictory. Example (26) supports the idea that postverbal NPs belong to the clauses whose verbs they follow. The reflexive possessive prefix *hede-* is used, indicating that the possessor is coreferential with the subject of the clause.

(26) *Ts'ʉh ehdenh   yaan'   nok'ehodon'   hede-to'   yeł.*
    So   3p   only   3p.ate   3s-father and
    'Only she and her father ate.' (Attla 1989: 58)

In examples (27) through (29), on the other hand, the postverbal NP appears not after the clause to which it logically belongs but after a quotative verb following the clause in question. In (27) there are three verbs between the postverbal NP and what would be its preverbal position.

(27) *Neełkk'aats'e   yo   enaałdeł   eetl'ekk   beeznee   go   tl'ooł.*
    both.sides   sky   snap   3.heard   it.is.said DEM rope
    'It is said that he heard the rope snap back and hit the sky on both sides.' (Attla 1989:68)

(28) *Uhts'e   heghe'en heł   dooghe hu ode heł   k'eyełonaa*
    that   reason   to this day   do.not.eat.
                         beeznee   go   denaałekk'eze.
                         they.say DEM cranberries
    'That is the reason that, to this day, bears do not eat cranberries.' (Attla 1989:130)

(29) *hełde   k'etaatlmaats   meezenee   go   sołt'aanh*
    and   started.boiling it.is.said DEM woman
    'It is said that the woman started boiling it.' (Jette 1909:468)

It is possible for a postverbal NP to follow a different coreferential NP. For example, see (30). Jetté's punctuation is reproduced in this example, although his orthography is not. Notice the two coreferential NPs following the verb. In addition to the comma between them, both are preceded by the demonstrative *go* 'this.'

(30) *Yeełkek,   łonh!   go   me'ot,   go   nenel'een'   eldlaadenh.*
    3.take.3   oh   DEM 3.wife DEM stickman   became.REL
    'His wife who had become a stickman took it.' (Jetté 1908: 316)

Examples (16) and (30) have two postverbal NPs. In (31), two postverbal NPs also appear. They do not corefer, however, as they do in (30). In (30), the first postverbal NP is the subject of the clause; the second NP, *kk'oyedenaa'oyee* 'which he was carrying' is a relative clause alienated from its head *le'on* 'stone' which appears to the left of the verb. Again, Jetté's punctuation has been repeated, while the orthography has been changed to the contemporary orthography.

(31) *Ts'eyehuts'e*   *le'on*   *deets'aaggeyee*   *lekk'ulee*   *ts'aadenaanee'onh*
      and then   stone   narrow.REL   white.REL   took.out
                  go   *keele,*   *kk'oyedenaa'oyee*
                  DEM   boy   carry.around.REL
      'And then he took out a small white stone which he was carrying.' (Jetté
      1908:310)

Together, these data suggest an ambiguous syntactic status for postverbal
elements. The use of the possessive reflexive prefix in (25) indicates that such
NPs belong to the clause which they follow, but the subsequent data presented
suggest otherwise. Because of this ambiguous status, postverbal elements may
best be called *postverbal adjuncts*.

10.1.5   Postverbal NPs and Continuity

More will be said about topic continuity in the following sections, but first it
must be said that postverbal NPs may indicate a switch in subject or topic, but
not necessarily. For example, the postverbal subject in (32b) is the eagle man,
while in (32c) it is *be'ot* 'his wife'. The context of this passage is that early in
the story a woman is abducted by the eagle man. The woman's husband searches
desperately for her and is eventually aided by a powerful spirit woman. The man
makes his way to the eagle man's village. His entering of the eagle man's house
and seeing his wife for the first time since the abduction is related in (32).

(32) a.   *Kk'ʉdaa*   *yet*   *hedaaheneedaatl.*
           now   inside   they.went

      b.   *degheel*   *nonee*   *yoodeggu*   *zo*   *dots'eldo,*   *denaa*   *kuh.*
           -           upriver   up   -   sit.above   man   big

      c.   *Tł'ogho*   *bets'en*   *doyeeldo,*   *go*   *be'ot.*
           really   by.3s   sit.above,   DEM   his.wife

      d.   *Yeey!*   *Nedaa aanee hʉn*   *yetaatl-'aanh.*
           oh.dear   there   3.INC.see

      e.   *ło'ts'eyʉh*   *go*   *denaa*   *doghulaah?*
           but   DEM   man   Q.do

           'They [the people of the village] went in. [A] big man [the eagle man]
           was sitting above, against the back [downriver] wall. His wife was
           sitting right next to him [the eagle man] ... Oh dear! There she was,
           but what could he do to the eagle man?' (Attla 1989:98)

Contrasting with (32), there is no shift in topic in (33). The postverbal NP in
(33a) refers to the same rock man as the postverbal NP in (33d). In the story
from which the passage was taken, Raven is making people after recreating the

world. He first makes people out of rock. They are immortal but do not have good minds.

(33) a. *Dehoon   notołdlelaa   go   denaa.*
      while   not.die   DEM   man

   b. *Dehoon   behɥyo'   koon   edetɥghe   detołt'aa'aa.*
      while   his.mind   also   RFL.among   not.be
      (his mind would not be right)

   c. *go   le'on   nelaanh*
      DEM   rock   be

   d. *Ts'ɥh   gheel   eeydee   etltseenh   eehu tlaahoo'*
      so   thus   that   make   in.vain
            ts'ednee,   le'on   denaa.
            it.is.said   rock   man

   'This man, then would never die. And in addition, his mind would not be right, because he was rock. So, it's said that that's what he made the first time, a rock man.' (Attla 1983:134)

10.2   Textual Analysis

Three functions that can determine the morphological and syntactic treatment of nominals in a text are (1) predictability, (2) importance, and (3) thematic structure (Givón 1983). *Predictability* refers to the degree to which a referent is established and expected (i.e., accessible) in discourse. Givón (1985:196) and others have pointed out that, on a scale of most predictable to least predictable: zero anaphora > unstressed pronouns/verb agreement > stressed pronouns > full NPs > modified full NPs. *Importance*, in contrast, refers to the degree to which a referent is a major character in the discourse. *Thematic structure* refers to the structuring of the discourse into units such as paragraphs and episodes.

Givón (1983) has developed methods for indirectly measuring predictability and importance. Predictability can be so measured by determining the referential distance of a referent. A referent's referential distance is the number of clauses preceding the referent before which a coreferential argument is found. For example, the referential distance of postverbal NP in (32d) is 1, because a coreferential argument appears in the preceding clause. No referent is assigned a referential distance above 20. If an argument is new, or if it has not been referred to for 20 or more clauses, its referential distance is 20. Importance is determined indirectly by the cataphoric measurement of persistence. A referent's persistence is the number of clauses out of the subsequent 10 in which a coreferential argument is found.

10.2.1   Comparing Postverbal and Preverbal NPs

Determining a hypothesis for postverbal NPs in Koyukon is problematic. The pragmatic order principle of linear order (Givón1995:55), that more important as well as less predictable information would appear first in a string, would suggest that preverbal NPs would have a greater persistence than postverbal ones. Preliminary data in Thompson (1991) contradict this, however. Furthermore, in other languages, postverbal NPs are more important than preverbal ones (for Cayuga, Ngandi, and Coos, see Mithun 1987; for spoken French, see Lambrecht 1987). I will explain the apparent contradiction between the data and the prediction on importance from the Pragmatic Order Principle in the next section.

Before proceeding, however, some basic information must be given: (1) the frequency of postverbal NPs relative to preverbal ones and (2) the syntactic roles of the NPs in both constructions. Postverbal NPs are far less frequent than preverbal ones. Between pages 52 and 62 in Attla (1989; six pages of text), four instances of postverbal NPs can be found, while 45 preverbal NPs are there. In order to find 100 instances of preverbal NPs, I looked at 21 pages of text in Attla (1989) and at the two stories in Pilot (1975), while to get 100 tokens of postverbal NPs, I had to look at all of Attla (1989), all of Attla (1983), and Pilot (1975).

The number of occurrences of the various syntactic roles can be seen in Table 10.1. Notice that postverbal NPs are more likely to be subjects (81%) than anything else and that direct objects are three times as likely to be preverbal than postverbal.

10.2.1.1   Importance

We will now move on to the relative importance and predictability of preverbal and postverbal NPs. On the basis of previous work, the hypothesis for persistence is:

(34)   *Hypothesis 1:* Postverbal NPs will have a greater persistence than preverbal NPs.

TABLE 10.1.   *Syntactic Roles of Preverbal and Postverbal NPs*

	Preverbal	Postverbal
Subj. Intrans	32	64
Subj. Trans	4	17
Direct Object	34	11
Locative Noun	13	0
Possessor	8	3
Oblique	9	5
Total	100	100

TABLE 10.2. *Persistence of Preverbal and Postverbal NP*

	n	Mean	Median
Preverbal	100	1.27	1
Postverbal	100	4.41	4

To test Hypothesis 1, the persistence of 100 postverbal NPs and of 100 preverbal NPs in Attla (1983, 1989) and Pilot (1975) was measured. The mean and median scores for persistence are given in Table 10.2. Notice that postverbal NPs are four times as persistent as preverbal ones. These data would support Hypothesis 1.

A different measurement of importance, one that focuses on generic rather than textual importance, is to measure the percentage of a particular type of referent (pre- or postverbal in the present study) which is human, or as is necessary for traditional Koyukon myths, personified. I would hypothesize:

(35) *Hypothesis 2:* A greater percentage of postverbal NPs than of preverbal NPs are human or personified.

The percentages of preverbal and postverbal human NPs are given in Table 10.3. These data support Hypothesis 2.

10.2.1.2 Predictability

The Pragmatic Principle of Linear Order also predicts that less predictable information will come first in a string. Givón (1983:19) claims that more continuous topics tend to be coded by right dislocation, while less continuous topics are coded by left dislocation. On the basis of this prediction, the hypothesis for referential distance is:

(36) *Hypothesis 3:* Postverbal NPs will be more predictable than preverbal NPs.

The mean and median referential distances for 100 preverbal and 100 postverbal NPs are given in Table 10.4. These results support Hypothesis 3.

TABLE 10.3. *Percentage of Human or Personified Referents*

	n	Human	Nonhuman
Preverbal	100	21	79
Postverbal	100	86	14

TABLE 10.4. *Referential Distance of Preverbal and Postverbal NPs*

	n	Mean	Median
Preverbal	100	13.01	20
Postverbal	100	3.88	1

10.2.1.3   Definiteness

It is possible that definiteness may be involved in the use of postverbal NPs. Li and Thompson (1975) have claimed that postverbal NPs are normally interpreted as being definite and preverbal NPs as definite (although Givón 1992 and Sun and Givón 1985 claim the determining factor in preposing NPs is contrastiveness). Slavic languages apparently behave similarly (see Yokoyama 1986). See the Chinese below:

(37) a. *Ren lai le.*
          people come ASP
          'The people have come.'

      b. *Lai ren le.*
          come people ASP
          'Some people have come.'

For other languages, the opposite is true. For example, see the Ojibwa data from Tomlin and Rhodes (1992). For definiteness and Papago word order see Payne (1987).

(38) a. *Mookman nglii-mkaan.*
          knife I-found-it
          'I found a knife.'

      b. *Nglii-mkaan mookmaan.*
          I-found-it knife
          'I found the knife.'

Both definite and indefinite nouns can occur in Koyukon, but the vast majority of postverbal NPs are definite (99 out of 100 in my sample). Furthermore, most postverbal NPs are preceded by the definite, proximate demonstrative *go* 'this'. Koyukon does not require definite NPs to be preceded by any article or demonstrative indicating definiteness, but it does have definite determiners, the two most common being *go* and the determiner *eey(ee)* 'the, that.' The averages in table 10.4 above indicate that indefinite NPs tend to precede the verb in Koyukon, while postverbal NPs tend to be quite predictable. There is a strong tendency for postverbal NPs to be preceded by go. In Table 10.5 we see this tendency.

TABLE 10.5.   *The Presence of Go in Preverbal and Postverbal NPs*

	n	*go*	*no go*
Preverbal	100	9	91
Postverbal	100	94	6

10.2.2   Comparing Postverbal NPs and Pronominal Arguments

10.2.2.1   Thematic Structure

Postverbal NPs are surprisingly predictable for full NPs. They are predictable enough to be coded by pronouns, and one is left to wonder why they are not so coded. A possible explanation may be found by referring to information structure. Information at the beginning of a thematic unit (i.e., a paragraph or episode) may be coded differently than that in the middle or the end. In fact, a referent at the beginning of a thematic unit in English and other languages is more likely to be coded by a full NP than by a pronoun. Tomlin (1987:475) states, 'Individuals will use full nouns on first mention after an episode boundary; individuals will use pronouns to sustain reference during an episode.' Although Tomlin does not specifically address postverbal and preverbal NPs, appeal to thematic structure may explain their use in Koyukon. One might hypothesize (39a) on the basis of his findings. Cooreman (1992) claims that, in Chamorro, the paragraph initial position favors Subject-Verb word order, while clauses with Verb-Subject order and passives appear more in paragraph medial and final positions. This finding would also lead us to hypothesize (39b):

(39) a.   *Hypothesis 4a*: A greater percentage of postverbal NPs will occur in paragraph initial position than will pronominal arguments.

     b.   *Hypothesis 4b*: A greater percentage of preverbal NPs will occur in paragraph initial position than will postverbal NPs.

The hypotheses in (39) are not supported by the data. As can be seen in Table 10.6, preverbal and postverbal NPs occur in roughly the same percentage of paragraph initial, medial, and final positions. Pronominal arguments occur in the paragraph initial position in a slightly lower percentage than the full NPs do, but this difference is not statistically significant ($p < .7$ by the chi-square test). For the present study, the paragraphing in Attla (1983, 1989) was accepted. Defining paragraphs in a different manner or looking at different thematic units may lead to different conclusions, but for now the data would suggest that thematic structure does not play a role in the use of postverbal NPs.

TABLE 10.6.   *Position of Nominals in Paragraphs*

	n	Initial	Medial	Final
Preverbal	50	12	30	13
Postverbal	50	13	30	12
Pronominal	50	8	37	5

10.2.2.2   Potential Ambiguity

The choice between pronoun and postverbal NP is still unclear. Both code continuous topics (see Thompson 1989 for predictability of pronouns). Thematic structure apparently plays no role in the choice. One possibility is that of potential interference or ambiguity. If a compatible but not coreferential referent appears in the preceding clause, it may necessitate the use of a full NP instead of a pronoun. Because preverbal NPs are mostly new information, it makes little sense to measure potential inference with them. The question, then, is whether there is a difference between postverbal NPs and pronominal arguments. One would hypothesize as follows:

(40)   *Hypothesis 5*: A greater percentage of postverbal NPs will have potential interference than will pronominal arguments.

Table 10.7 shows the percentage of preverbal, postverbal, and pronominal arguments for which a noncoreferential, semantically compatible argument can be found in the preceding clause. (I have not used the method employed by the authors of Givón 1983 in which potential interference is calculated as 1 or 2).

The results shown in Table 10.7 are mixed. On the one hand, they indicate a strong tendency for postverbal NPs to be potentially ambiguous. On the other hand, there is no tendency for pronominal arguments to lack such ambiguity. One cannot claim, then, that potential ambiguity, as measured here, "triggers" or "causes" postverbal NPs, but one can claim that there is a definite correlation between postverbal NPs and referential ambiguity.

TABLE 10.7.   *Potentially Ambiguous Referents in the Preceding Clause*

	n	PA	Percentage
Postverbal	50	48	96%
Pronominal	50	27	54%

TABLE 10.8. *The Duration of Pauses in Milliseconds*

	n	Mean	Median
V PP	23	984.1	1000
V NP	41	356.41	135.01
NP V	38	208.77	65.17

10.2.3. Comparing Postverbal NPs with Postverbal PPs

Possibly, claims made about postverbal NPs should also take into account other postverbal elements, such as postpositional phrases. I will leave this subject open to further research, but for now it is important to point out that there is some evidence suggesting that postverbal NPs and postverbal PPs are two different populations: there is a significantly longer pause between a final verb and a prepositional phrase than between a final verb and a noun phrase, especially in the median duration. The mean and median pauses are shown in table 10.8. Also included are the mean and median duration of pause between a preverbal NP and a verb. The pause before a postverbal NP is much closer to the pause after a preverbal NP than it is to the pause before a postverbal PP.

10.3   Analysis

To summarize the results of the analysis presented in section 10.2, it can be said that postverbal NPs in Koyukon tend to be highly predictable in terms of referential distance but not in terms of potential ambiguity, that postverbal NPs are mostly definite and mostly human, that they are associated with topical participants, and that they are more likely to be subjects than preverbal NPs. Preverbal NPs, on the other hand, code less predictable and less important participants. In this section the relevance of the Koyukon data to iconic and cognitive principles will be examined.

10.3.1   Iconicity

The principle of iconicity most relevant to the present study is the Pragmatic Principle of Linear Order. This principle, as worded by Givón (1995) is given in (41):

(41) Pragmatic principle of linear order:

    a. More important or more urgent information tends to be placed first in the string.

    b. Less accessible or less predictable information tends to be placed first in the string. (Givón 1995: 55)

The same principle has been identified by others but worded slightly differently. Mithun, for example, states that the most "newsworthy" information tends to be presented first in languages with pragmatically controlled word order (1987, 1992).

The data from Koyukon are, in part, consistent with the Pragmatic Order Principle. There is a very strong tendency to present new and less predictable information before the verb. This tendency is consistent with (41b). However, preverbal NPs are less important in the discourse than postverbal ones. This tendency is inconsistent with (41a).

The second principle of iconicity relevant to the present study is the proximity principle. Givón words this principle as shown in (42):

(42) The proximity principle:

    a. Entities that are closer together functionally, conceptually, or cognitively will be placed closer together at the code level, i.e. temporally or spatially.

    b. Functional operators will be place closest, temporally or spatially at the code level, to the conceptual unit to which they are most relevant. (Givón 1992: 51)

The Koyukon data is somewhat out of line with (42a). Relative clauses can be separated from their heads (see (14)) and conjoined NPs can be split up (see (17)). Furthermore, postverbal elements in general are isolated from the clause to which they logically belong.

It should be pointed out that violations of principles of iconicity are, in and of themselves, not problematic. Language operates under competing motivations (see Haiman 1983 and the papers in Haiman 1985), and one iconic or cognitive principle may override another. The problem, then, is discovering the reason that Koyukon violates principles (41) and (42).

10.3.2 *Activation*

Psycholinguists view the short-term memory involved in text processing to be governed by the notion of activation. Memory cells are activated, suppressed, or enhanced by incoming information (Gernsbacher 1990:2). Chafe (1987) claims that, after the initial pause of a new intonation unit, three changes in the activation state can take place: (1) an inactive concept can become active, (2) a semi-active concept can become active, and (3) an active concept can become semi-active.

It has been observed that the content words or participants mentioned first in a sentence are more activated than those mentioned later in the clause (Chang 1980; Gernsbacher 1990; Gernsbacher and Hargreaves 1988, 1992; inter alia). Gernsbacher has termed this advantage, The Advantage of First Mention (AFM) (Gernsbacher 1990:10).

Listeners and readers also take longer to process or activate first-mentioned items (Gernsbacher 1990:8–9). This fact has been demonstrated by reaction time experiments (Cairns and Kamerman 1975, Foss 1969, inter alia) and by measuring the N400 brain wave, which is larger than average upon encountering the first content word of a sentence (Kutas, van Petten, and Besson 1988). The N400 brain wave is also associated items that are less expected in the text and words that are less familiar. Gernsbacher (1990) and Gernsbacher and Hargreaves (1992) believe that such facts support their claim that language comprehension is a structure-building activity and that the first content words of a sentence help the addressee lay a foundation for the rest of the sentence.

Counteracting the AFM is the fact that participants in the most recently mentioned clause are more activated than those in previous clauses. Gernsbacher (1990) and Gernsbacher and Hargreaves (1992) call this advantage the Advantage of Clause Recency (ACR). Their experiments show, however, that ACR diminishes over time. During presentation of a second clause, ACR takes precedent over AFM. After 150 milliseconds, their effect is about the same. After 1400 milliseconds, AFM takes precedence over ACR.

These facts have ramifications for the analysis of postverbal NPs in Koyukon. Before discussing these facts, however, we will look at the psycholinguistic evidence for activation and anaphora. Relevant to this fact is what Gernsbacher (1990) calls the 'Explicitness Principle.' This principle is given in (43):

(43)   Explicitness Principle:

The more explicit the concept, the more likely it is to trigger the suppression of other concepts; when used anaphorically, the more likely it is to enhance its referent. (Gernsbacher 1990:133)

In other words, anaphoric pronouns would be less likely to enhance the activation of their referents and suppress other referents than would anaphoric nouns. The facts support this claim. For example, Corbett and Chang (1983) found, in terms of reaction time, Zero Anaphors < Pronouns < Repeated Nouns. Gernsbacher (1989) found that pronouns maintain activation of their antecedents, but do not increase it, whereas anaphoric nouns enhance the activation of their antecedents.

10.3.3   The Function of Postverbal NPs

Three questions need to be answered with regard to postverbal NPs in Koyukon: (1) What governs the choice of using a postverbal NP over a preverbal one? (2) What governs the choice of using a postverbal NP over a pronominal prefix? and (3) What function do nonnominal postverbal elements serve in Koyukon? Aside from these questions is the broader typological question as to why some languages appear to use postverbal elements in roughly the same manner as Koyukon, while others, Slavic languages in particular, appear to behave in exactly the opposite manner.

10.3.3.1   What governs the choice of using a postverbal NP over a preverbal one?

The Koyukon data strongly suggest that new information is given preverbally while old, predictable information is given postverbally. This fact supports (41b). It also is in line with the psycholinguistic evidence. Both new information and first-mentioned information is given more attention in terms of processing time and N400 brain wave activity than other information. The question of importance is a bit more problematic. The Koyukon data clearly are not in line with (41a).

I would suspect that the pragmatic principle of linear order, as defined by Givón, is too broad. The principle of the competing motivations of isomorphism (Haiman 1983) and economy also have some relevance to this problem. The need for economy in a code will lead to a more syntactically defined word order in language. The need for isomorphism and iconicity will lead to a more pragmatically defined word order.

There are also two competing principles of iconicity: isomorphism and polysemy. Isomorphism is driven by the need for clarity in code, polysemy is driven by the need for economy of code. See (44):

(44)   a.   Isomorphism: Each function (and meaning) will be coded in a manner distinct from all other functions (and meanings).

b.   Polysemy: Whenever possible, a function (or meaning) will be coded in the same or similar manner as a similar function.

Givón's concept of urgency and Mithun's concept of newsworthiness imply both importance and unpredictability. I would suggest that these functions can be coded in different manners in different languages. A language such as Koyukon puts unpredictable, unimportant information preverbally (but does not prepose it), and predictable, important information postverbally. On the other hand, in English, clefting (e.g., 'It's eggplant that I love.') and preposing ('Eggplant, I love.') occur with concepts that are both important and unpredictable.

If postverbal NPs are, to some extent, outside the clause to which they logically belong, Gernsbacher's Advantage of Clause Recency may have some relevance. The ACR principle would predict that postverbal NPs will have a short-term advantage over preverbal NPs. Because postverbal NPs code cataphorically important information, the activation of these NPs would be maintained by subsequent references.

There is an additional possible reason for the choice of placing an NP postverbally. It may be for the purpose of foregrounding whatever new information appears preverbally, or in the verb. By placing the NP at the back of the clause, the speaker, in a sense, backgrounds its referent and foregrounds what precedes it. Remember that addressees take more time to process first mentioned and unexpected information than other information. The referents of postverbal NPs are already established and expected. Being so, they would not require extra processing time, whereas new information would.

10.3.3.2 What governs the choice of using a postverbal NP over a pronominal prefix?

It is clear that postverbal NPs, while having a relatively low referential distance, are more likely to have potential interference than are referents coded by pronominal prefixes alone. The Koyukon data, together with the psycholinguistic evidence summarized by Gernsbacher's Explicitness Principle, would suggest two things: (1) postverbal NPs are more likely to enhance the activation of their referents than are pronominals and (2) postverbal NPs are more likely to suppress the activation of other referents than are pronominals.

The Explicitness Principle together with the Advantage of Clause Recency would predict that postverbal NPs, while coding old information, signal to the addressee that the referents of these NPs should be enhanced and others suppressed. To use Chafe's (1987) terminology, postverbal NPs would reactivate their referents.

10.3.3.3 What function do nonnominal postverbal elements serve in Koyukon?

I have paid little attention to postverbal prepositional phrases, other postverbal adverbials, and postverbal complements. While not as common as postverbal NPs, they do occur. The function of such constituents is more difficult to measure with the methods used here. The data on duration of pause, as shown previously, suggest that postverbal PPs are different from postverbal NPs. I suspect that postverbal NPs share certain functions with postverbal PPs and so, because of the principle of economy (polysemy), they are both postverbal, but because of the principle of isomorphism, there is a difference in the duration of pauses. The principal functional difference between postverbal NPs and PPs is that the NPs tend to code old information while the PPs tend to code new information

Here, I suggest only three principles that govern nonnominal postverbal elements; these are based on my non-quantified analysis of the data (see (45)). More work clearly needs to be done.

(45) a. Nonnominal postverbal elements contain background information.

b. Nonnominal postverbal elements focus attention on what appears verbally or preverbally.

c. Nonnominal postverbal elements contain information which narrows information already contained in the clause.

TABLE 10.9. *The Narrowing Function of Postverbal Elements*

Preverbal (General)	Postverbal (Specific)
Pronominal	Full NP
Head	Relative Clause
Generic Noun	Specific Conjunction

My prediction in (45c) may apply to postverbal nominals as well. The data in (15) and (16) show how a postverbal conjoined phrase can narrow a more general nominal given in the main clause. In fact, the fact that a postverbal NP appears in the verb as a pronominal may be interpreted as a type of narrowing as well, in which case (45b) would also apply to postverbal NPs. See table 10.9.

The concept of narrowing is relevant to Gernsbacher's Explicitness Principle. Preverbal pronominals, being less explicit, can be narrowed by postverbal nouns and thereby enhanced. It would make no sense to narrow something preverbally and then make it more general postverbally.

The concept of narrowing is also relevant to that of backgrounding and fore-grounding. By placing a more general argument in the preverbal clause, or in the verb, different and new information is highlighted—other participants, the verb itself, important adverbials, amd so on. The enhancement provided by the post-verbal, specific element does not occur until after new, important information has been introduced. Hopper (1987) claims that, in Malay narrative, preverbal NPs orient the discourse toward the noun, while postverbal NPs orient it toward the verb. In his words, "Verb-initial clauses narrate, noun-initial clauses de-scribe" (1987:471). His statement may be broadened to say that whatever comes first in a clause orients the discourse toward that element.

10.4 Conclusion

We return to the question as to why Koyukon appears to violate part of the Pragmatic Principle Of Linear Order as stated in (41). The answer is this:

(46) a. Preverbal NPs are in their normal, unmarked position. Koyukon does not normally prepose them.

    b. The participants coded by postverbal NPs are already activated. The increased attention demanded by having them appear first in the clause is necessary.

    c. Postposing old information foregrounds new, preverbal and verbal in-formation.

In short, postposing in Koyukon allows for the enhancement of the participants coded by postverbal NPs as well as the increased attention needed by the hearer to process new, preverbal or verbal information.

The answer to the question as to why postverbal material in Koyukon violates the proximity principle is similar. Postverbal material is isolated from the rest of the clause because it is meant to be processed in a manner different from preverbal or verbal material. Similarly, in other languages, clefting, preposing, or even placing contrastive stress on an item signals cognitive as well as syntactic or structural isolation.

References

Attla, Catherine. 1983. *Sitsiy yugh noholnik ts'in': As My Grandfather Told It.* Fairbanks: Alaska Native Language Center and Yukon Koyukon School District.

Attla, Catherine. 1989. *Bakk'aatugh ts'uhuhniy: Stories We Live By.* Fairbanks: Alaska Native Language Center and Yukon Koyukon School District.

Cairns, H. S., and J. Kamerman. 1975. Lexical Information Processing during Sentence Comprehension. *Journal of Verbal Learning and Verbal Behavior* 14:170-179.

Chafe, Wallace. 1987. Cognitive Constraints on Information Flow. In Russell Tomlin (ed.), *Coherence and Grounding in Discourse*, 21–51. Amsterdam: John Benjamins.

Chang, F. R. 1980. Active Memory Processes in Visual Sentence Comprehension: Clause Effects and Pronominal Reference. *Memory and Cognition* 8:58–64.

Corbett, A. T., and F. R. Chang. 1983. Pronoun Disambiguation: Accessing the Subjective Lexicon. *Memory and Cognition* 2:130–138.

Cooreman, Ann. 1992. The pragmatics of word order variation in Chamorro narrative text. In Doris Payne (ed.), *Pragmatics of Word Order Flexibility*, 243–263. Amsterdam: John Benjamins.

Foss, D. J. 1969. Decision Processes during Sentence Comprehension: Effects of Lexical Item Difficulty and Position upon Decision Times. *Journal of Verbal Learning and Verbal Behavior* 8:457–462.

Gernsbacher, Morton Ann. 1990. *Language Comprehension as Structure Building.* Hillsdale, N.J.: Lawrence Erlbaum.

Gernsbacher, Morton, and David Hargreaves. 1988. Accessing Sentence Participants: The Advantage of First Mention. *Journal of Memory and Language* 27:699–717.

Gernsbacher, Morton and David Hargreaves. 1992. The Privilege of Primacy: Experimental Data and Cognitive Explanations. In Doris Payne (ed.), *Pragmatics of Word Order Flexibility*, 83–116. Amsterdam: John Benjamins.

Givón, T. (ed.). 1983. *Topic Continuity in Discourse.* Amsterdam: John Benjamins.

Givón, T. 1985. Iconicity, Isomorphism, and Non-Arbitrary Coding in Syntax. In John Haiman (ed.), *Iconicity in Syntax*, 187–219. Amsterdam: John Benjamins.

Givón. T. 1992. On Interpreting Text-Distributional Correlations: Some Methodological Issues. In Doris Payne (ed.), *Pragmatics of Word Order Flexibility*, 305–320. Amsterdam: John Benjamins.

Givón, T. 1995. Isomorphism in the Grammatical Code: Cognitive and Biological Considerations. In Raffaele Simone (ed.), *Iconicity in Language*, 47–76. Amsterdam: John Benjamins.

Golla, Victor. 1985. *A Short Practical Grammar of Hupa.* Hoopa: Hoopa Valley Tribe.

Haiman, John. 1983. Iconic and Economic Motivation. *Language* 59:781–819.

Haiman, John. 1985. *Iconicity in Syntax.* Amsterdam: John Benjamins.

Hopper, Paul. 1987. Stability and Change in VN/NV Alternating Languages: A Study in Pragmatics and Linguistic Typology. In Jef Vershueren and Marcella Bertuccelli-Papi (eds.), *The pragmatic perspective,* 455–476. Amsterdam: John Benjamins.

Jetté, Jules. 1908. On Ten'a Folk-lore. *Journal of the Royal Anthropological Institute.* 38: 298–305.

Jetté, Jules. 1909. On Ten'a Folk-lore. *Journal of the Royal Anthropological Institute.* 39: 460–505.

Jones, Eliza. 1983. *Junior Dictionary for Central Koyukon Athabaskan: Dinaakkanaaga ts'inh huyoza.* Anchorage: National Bilingual Materials Development Center.

Kibrik, Andrej. 1994. Review of Pragmatics of Word Order Flexibility, ed. by Doris Payne. *Studies in Language* 19:223–237.

Kutas, M., C. van Petten, and M. Besson. 1988. Event-related Potential Asymmetries during the Reading of Sentences. *Electroencephalography and Clinical Neurophysiology* 69:218–233.

Lambrecht, Knud. 1987. On the Status of SVO Sentences in French Discourse. In Russell Tomlin (ed.), *Coherence and Grounding in Discourse,* 217–261. Amsterdam: John Benjamins.

Li, Charles N. and S. Thompson. 1975. The Semantic Functions of Word Order: A Case Study in Mandarin. In C.N. Li (ed.), *Word Order and Word Change, 163–195.* Austin: University of Texas Press.

Mithun, Marianne. 1987. Is basic word order universal? In Russell Tomlin (ed.), *Coherence and Grounding in Discourse,* 281–328. Amsterdam: John Benjamins.

Mithun, Marianne. 1992. Is Basic Word Order Universal? In Doris Payne (ed.), *Pragmatics of Word Order Flexibility,* 15–61. Amsterdam: John Benjamins.

Payne, Doris. 1987. Information Structure in Papago Narrative Discourse. *Language* 63:783–804.

Payne, Doris (ed.). 1992. *Pragmatics of Word Order Flexibility.* Amsterdam: John Benjamins.

Pilot, Sally. 1975. *I. Donooghnotok'idaatlno / II. Gaadook.* Fairbanks: Alaska Native Language Center.

Rice, Keren. 1989. *A Grammar of Slave.* Berlin: Mouton de Gruyter.

Sun, C.-F., and T. Givón. 1985. On the So-called SOV Word-order in Mandarin Chinese: A Quantified Text Study and its Implications. *Language* 61:329–351.

Thompson, Chad. 1989. Pronouns and Voice in Koyukon Athabaskan: A Text-based Study. *International Journal of American Linguistics* 55:1–24.

Thompson, Chad. 1991. The Low Topicality Prefix *k'i-* in Koyukon. *Studies in Language* 15:59–84.

Tomlin, Russell. 1986. *Basic Word Order: Functional Principles.* London: Croon Helm.

Tomlin, Russell. 1987. Linguistic Reflections of Cognitive Events. In Russell Tomlin (ed.), *Coherence and Grounding in Discourse,* 455–479. Amsterdam: John Benjamins.

Tomlin, Russell and Richard Rhodes. 1992. An Introduction to Information Distribution in Ojibwa. In Doris Payne (ed.), *Pragmatics of Word Order Flexibility*, 117–135. Amsterdam: John Benjamins.

Yokoyama, Olga. 1986. *Discourse and Word Order*. Amsterdam: John Benjamins.

11

NAVAJO AS A DISCOURSE
CONFIGURATIONAL LANGUAGE

MaryAnn Willie and Eloise Jelinek

Baker (1996) defines "polysynthetic" languages as requiring registration of argument structure in the verbal morphology. The goal of this paper is to define the semantic features that underlie this typological propery, as manifested in Navajo. We argue that Navajo is a discourse configurational language, where nominals are adjuncts ordered according to the topic/focus articulation of the clause, while incorporated pronominal arguments in the verb-sentence carry the grammatical relations. We show that some properties of anaphora and focus in Navajo provide crucial evidence on argument structure in the language. We identify strong vs. weak pronouns in Navajo, the syntax of the nominals, and the role of the Direct/Inverse voice alternation in determining word order and the topic/focus articulation of the clause.

11.1   Weak and Strong Pronouns

Pronouns have two distinct and complementary functions in universal grammar: as discourse anaphors and as deictic elements. *Weak pronouns* are discourse anaphors, backgrounded information, and exclude focus; *strong deictic pronouns* have inherent focus. In many languages, "weak" versus "strong" pronouns can be differentiated adequately on the basis of stress, intonation, or other focus devices that may be analyzed separately from the pronouns as a lexical set. However, there is a large class of languages where these two functions of pronouns are represented in distinct pronominal paradigms that have very different morphological and syntactic properties, making it necessary to recognize two distinct closed-class categories in the grammar, the weak versus strong pronouns. In some languages, weak pronouns alternate with strong pronouns in argument positions, according to whether the use of the pronoun is anaphoric or deictic. The Yaqui examples in (1) illustrate this familiar contrast (Escalante, 1990).

(1) a. *'apo'ik=ne   viča-k*
         him=I   see-PERF
         'I saw *him*.' (strong object pronoun has focus)

     b. *'inepo   'a-viča-k*
         I   him-see-PERF
         '*I* saw him.'   (strong subject pronoun has focus)

Yaqui is an SOV language with case-marked NP arguments (including freestanding pronouns) and a limited inventory of clitics. Clitic "doubling" is not required, and there is no subject-verb agreement. In (1a), the freestanding object pronoun has been fronted for focus, and the backgrounded subject is a second position clitic, which may attach to any word. In (1b) the freestanding subject pronoun has focus, and there is an object prefix on the verb. In Yaqui, speakers follow discourse dynamics in choosing between freestanding strong versus incorporated weak pronouns (Jelinek and Escalante, 1991). Yaqui also has noun incorporation, as in (2b), which removes an indefinite noun from focus.

(2) a. *maaso-ta=ne   'aamu*
         deer-ACC=1sNOM   hunt:IMPF
         'I'm hunting a *deer*.' (Object NP has focus)

     b. *maaso-'aamu=ne*
         deer-hunt:IMPF=1sNOM
         'I'm deer-hunting.'   (Focus on activity)

In (2a), the ACC marked object NP is fronted for focus, and the subject clitic is backgrounded. In (2b), the activity has focus, and the incorporated noun cannot receive contrastive focus. While incorporation "subtracts" focus, making contrastive focus impossible, adding an independent lexical item makes it possible.

Partee (1987) argued that NPs in English do not correspond to a single semantic type, but show "type-shifting" across their various uses. Compare the uses of the word "dogs" in example (3):

(3)   a. The dogs ran away.   Referential
       b. Fido and Spot are dogs.   Predicational
       c. Dogs are loyal companions.   Quantificational; Generic

Kiss (1998) identifies the important contrast between two kinds of focus. There is "information" focus (the ordinary default focus that marks new information) vs. "identificational" focus, which is quantificational in nature: it picks out some subset from a presupposed set of individuals. This contrastive identificational focus is marked in English by heavy stress and an intonation peak.

(4) Contrastive (Quantificational) Focus

     a. The DOGS ran away.   (not i.e., the cats)
     b. Fido and Spot are DOGS.
     c. DOGS are loyal companions.

     d. It was the DOGS that ran away.
     e. It was YOU that ran away.
     f. YOU ran away.

By using contrastive or "identificational" focus, the speaker is picking out some individual (or subset) rather than some others of a familiar set. Kiss notes that this contrastive focus is often expressed across languages by a "cleft" construction, as shown in (4d,e). In English, any element in an A-position, including pronouns (4e,f), can receive contrastive focus.

In pronominal argument languages, there is a more constrained mapping between argument structure and focus structure. The incorporated pronouns are discourse anaphors, whose reference is fixed by NPs occuring earlier in the discourse. As we saw with the Yaqui examples, incorporated and encliticized elements cannot receive contrastive focus; this applies to the pronominal arguments in polysynthetic languages. In these languages, contrastive focus is *excluded* from elements in A-positions (the weak pronouns), and confined to freestanding lexical items—NPs (including the strong pronouns). In Navajo, strong pronouns are adjuncts that do not mark a grammatical relation by morphological shape or syntactic position. Consider first an intransitive sentence, as in (5).

(5)   a.   *yáshti'*   b.   *shí yáshti'*
             1sNOM-speak   I   1sNOM-speak
             'I am speaking.'   '*I* am (the one who is) speaking.'

In (5a), the incorporated first singular nominative pronoun is backgrounded and cannot receive contrastive focus; the freestanding strong pronoun is added for this function in (5b). The problem of analysis is to distinguish this co-occurence of weak and strong pronouns from an agreement system. Example (6) shows a transitive sentence:

(6)   *nisisdlągd*
        2sACC-1sNOM-believed
        Focus-Topic-V
        'I believed you.'

Both the pronominal arguments in (6) are presuppositional, established in the discourse. Of the two, the subject pronoun *I* is topical, and the patient pronoun *you*, which is leftmost in the word, has focus as part of the new information that is the communicative burden of the sentence. This is the "default" focus structure of the Navajo verb-sentence. Neither of the incorporated pronominal arguments can receive contrastive stress; a strong pronoun must be added. This strong pronoun appears immediately before the verb, in the focus position, regardless of the grammatical relation of the corresponding weak pronoun.

(7) a. *ni*   *nisisdlągd*
         YOU   2sACC-1sNOM-believed
         '*You* are the one I believed.'

     b. *shí*   *nisisdlągd*
         I   2sACC-1sNOM-believed
         '*I* am the one who believed you.'

In (7a) the strong pronoun immediately preceding the verb-sentence refers to the subject; in (7b), to the object. Adding two strong pronouns is unacceptable.

(8)   *## shí ni nisisdlągd*

Focus is a dynamic system, and the focus structure of a sentence may be altered by a number of grammatical devices, including word order, intonation, focus particles, etc. (Hajičova, Partee, and Sgall, 1995). Adding a strong or contrastive pronoun alters the focus structure of the sentence, much as the "cleft" glosses in (7) suggest. These sentences are suitable replies to different questions:

(9) a. *háí-sh*   *yisínídlągd*
         who-Q   3ACC-2sNOM-believed
         'Who did you believe?'   (Suitable reply: 7a)

     b. *háí-sh*   *shooshádlągd*
         who-Q   1sACC-3NOM-believed
         'Who believed me?'   (Suitable reply: 7b)

Navajo lacks obligatory Wh-movement. Both Wh-words and strong pronouns have inherent focus. When both are added to a verb-sentence, the strong pronoun is preferably leftmost, in a Topic position, regardless of the grammatical relation of the coindexed weak pronoun.

(10) a. *háí-sh   yínízhí*
          who-Q   3ACC-2sNOM-called
          'Who are you calling?'

      b. *ni   háí-sh   yínízhí*
          you   who-Q   3ACC-2sNOM-called
          'Who are *you* calling?'

(11) a. *háí-sh   shózhí*
          who-Q   1sACC-3NOM-called
          'Who is calling me?'

      b. *shí   háí-sh   shózhí*
          I   who-Q   1sACC-3NOM-called
          'Who is calling *me*?'

"Strong" pronouns may be coreferent with possessive pronouns and postpositional objects as well as with subjects and direct objects—in short, with incorporated pronouns in any grammatical relation. In (12b), the strong pronoun coindexed with the possessive pronoun is reduplicated for greater emphasis.

(12) a. *shi-má*   b. *shí shí shi-má*
          'my mother'   'It's *my* mother!!'

(13) a. *shá   'ánílééh*   b. *shí shá   'ánílééh*
          1s-for 3ACC-2sNOM-make   I   1s-for 3ACC-2sNOM-make
          'Make it for me.'   'Make it for *me*!'

To summarize: while incorporation "subtracts" focus, making contrastive focus on the incorporated pronoun impossible, adding an independent lexical item makes contrast possible. In Yaqui (or English) the freestanding strong pronouns alternate in A-positions with the incorporated weak pronouns, according to the focus articulation of the clause. In these languages, "strong" pronouns are case marked in A-positions, whether or not there is subject agreement. In contrast, in a pronominal argument language like Navajo, "strong" pronouns are caseless adjuncts, not ordered according to grammatical relation, and co-occur with weak pronouns in any grammatical relation to mark focus. This co-occurrence of pronouns is additive and is analogous to the marking of contrastive focus by adding stress or augmenting an intonation peak.

   If there are languages where only weak pronouns can occur in argument positions and freestanding pronouns serve only to mark contrastive focus, then a language with some other means of marking focus should be able to do without freestanding pronouns. This possibility is realized: there are pronominal argument languages that have no freestanding pronouns at all. Lummi (Straits Salish) has weak pronominal clitics and affixes, as shown in (14). The ACC object is a pronominal suffix, and the NOM subject is a second position clitic.

(14) k^wə *niŋ-t-oŋəł-lə* '=sx^w
       help-TRAN-1pACC=PAST=2sNOM
       'You helped us.'

While Straits Salish has no freestanding pronouns, it has a paradigm of deictic lexical roots that mark the phi features of person and number. These roots never serve as subjects or direct objects; only pronominal arguments, as in (14), appear in these positions. The person-deictic roots differ from the pronominal arguments as follows: (a) they appear in sentence initial position, as the lexical head of a main clause; (b) they appear with a determiner, as head of a subordinate nominalized structure; (c) they are exclusively third person in syntax; and (d) they have inherent focus. Their distribution is shown in (15):

(15)   a.   nə k^w=yə x^w=ø   cə k^wə niŋ-t-oŋə ł
            YOU=MODAL=3ABS   DET help-TRAN-1pACC
            'It must be *you*, the [one who] helped us.'

       b. k^wə niŋ -t-ŋ =ł   'ə cə nə k^w
            help-TRAN-PASS=1pNOM   OBL DET YOU
            'We were helped by the [one who is] *you*.'

Example (15a) shows a person-deictic root as lexical head of a main clause; Lummi has no copula. Example (15b) shows this root with a determiner, as lexical head of an oblique agent adjunct to a passive clause. Oblique agents have focus in Salish (and perhaps universally).

In the following excerpt from a text, the first sentence has a weak second person singular pronoun. This referent is put in focus by the use of a deictic root in the second sentence.

(16)   stomə š=sə =sx^w
       warrior =FUTURE=2sNOM
       'You will be a warrior.'

       nə k^w=ø   cə   stomə š   ti 'ə   'ən-sx^w 'ełə
       YOU=3ABS   DET warrior this   2sPOSS-place
       'It's *you* who will be your village's warrior (the warrior for your village).'
       (Charles, Demers, and Bowman, 1978)

Winnebago also lacks freestanding pronouns, but employs a somewhat different strategy to mark focus. There are incorporated (morphophonologically complex) pronominal arguments.

(17) a. *haŋe*   'I bury him'
      b. *raŋe*   'you bury him'
      c. *ŋe*   'he buries him'

A deictic or demonstrative particle is added to the verb to create a construction with contrastive focus on the subject.

(18) *ne:-c'ə -ha-na*
      DEICTIC-instead-1sgSubj-sleep
      '*I* slept, instead.' (Lipkind, 1945)

11.2   Transitivity as a Functional Head in Pronominal Argument Languages

In the Navajo, Salish, and Winnebago examples, we have seen the verb inflected for both subject and object arguments. A feature commonly seen in pronominal argument (PA) languages is the overt marking of transitivity, and the presence of weak pronouns at functional projections in INFL that mark both the subject and object arguments. In Navajo, valence or transitivity is overtly marked in a functional head, the so-called classifier prefix to the verb root. In (19b), the *-ł* classifier marks the verb-sentence as transitive.

(19) a. *ch'iyáán   yíchxǫ'*
          food   3NOM-ruined
          'The food is ruined.' (Unaccusative)

      b. *ch'iyáán   yiyíí-ł-chxǫ'*
          food   3ACC-3NOM-TRAN-ruined
          'He ruined the food.' (Transitive)

We do not assume that the weak pronouns undergo movement into their A-positions, but that they are base generated at argument positions introduced by the functional projections where their case is checked. These functional heads correspond to auxiliary or "light" elements that determine argument structure (Jelinek and Willie 1996). McDonough (1990) argues for an incorporated auxiliary in Navajo immediately preceding the verb stem where aspect and the subject are marked together in "portmanteau" elements. The verb stem is composed of the root and the so-called classifier, which marks valence. Objects, McDonough argues, are clitics that are attached more loosely to the Subject/Aux/Verb complex. Aspect is exceptionally rich and complex in Navajo, and there are a number of entailments among values of voice, transitivity, and aspect.

11.3 Subject Agreement and Object Clitics

We need to distinguish pronominal argument languages from languages with two other widely distributed features of argument structure: a) subject agreement, and b) object clitics. These latter two features frequently co-occur, producing a kind of subject/object asymmetry that is exemplified in languages such as Spanish, Chichewa (Bresnan and Mchombo 1987), and Egyptian Arabic (Jelinek, in press). In these languages, the verb agrees with both definite and indefinite subjects. However, direct object clitics differ significantly from AGR phenomena in that they never cooccur with *indefinite* NPs. The following examples are from Egyptian Arabic:

(20) a. *kalt (it)-tiffaaHa*
      ate:1sNOM (DET)-apple
      'I ate (the)/an apple.'

    b. *kalt-aha*
      ate:1sNOM-3fsACC
      'I ate it.'

    c. *kalt-aha,*   *it-tiffaaHa*
      ate:1sNOM-3fsACC the-apple
      'I ate it, the apple, (that is).'

    d. **kalt-aha,*   *tiffaaHa*
      ate:1sNOM-3fsACC apple
      'I ate it, an apple'

In (20c), an intonation break identifies the definite NP as an "afterthought" adjunct. Example (20d) is excluded, as is (21b), In Spanish.

(21) a. *La comí, la manzana.*   b. **La comí, una manzana.*
      'The apple, I ate it.'   [*an apple, I ate it]

This contrasts with the situation in Navajo and other PA languages, where we do not see this subject/object asymmetry. Third person pronouns, both subject and object, may cooccur with either definite or indefinite NPs:

(22) a. *bilasáana yíyą́ą́'*   b. *bilasáana ła' yíyą́ą́'*
          apple   3ACC-1sNOM-ate   apple   one 3ACC-1sNOM-ate
          'The apple, I ate it.'   'One/an apple, I ate it.'

The default reading of NPs in Navajo is definite, but they may be given an indefinite reading in certain contexts, i.e. in existential constructions. Complex
NPs may be marked indefinite by the inclusion of a cardinality expression, as in
(22b). Nominals on either definite or indefinite readings may be linked to third-
person subject or object pronouns in Navajo, subject to certain constraints imposed by the Inverse voice, to be specified in section 11.4.3. In pronominal argument languages, arguments (the weak pronouns) may not be dropped, but
adjuncts (strong pronouns and nominals) need not be added.

11.4   Nominal Adjunction and Direct/Inverse Voice in Navajo

Like strong pronouns and Wh-words, nominals are adjuncts to the Navajo verb-
sentence. Nominals may identify a familiar referent that is "new" in the context.
Compare:

(23) a. *yisisdlą́ą́d*
          3ACC-1sNOM-believed
          'I believed him/her.'

      b. *bí*   *yisisdlą́ą́d*
          he/she   3ACC-1sNOM-believed
          'I believed *him/her*.'

      c. *'ashkii*   *yisisdlą́ą́d*
          boy   3ACC-1sNOM-believed
          'I believed him, the boy.'

Nominal adjuncts are licensed by a coindexed pronominal argument in the verb-
sentence; they must match this pronoun in phi-features. Jelinek (1984) and Willie (1991) argue that NP adjuncts, like relative clauses, are predicated of pronominal heads, and that the pronoun + adjunct form a complex discontinuous
argumental expression at the level of the interpretation of the sentence.

   When a non-third-person strong pronoun and an NP are both added to a transitive sentence in Navajo, either order of the adjuncts is acceptable. The phi-
features of the non-third-person pronoun determine coreference. Again, the word
order where the strong pronoun is leftmost is preferred, regardless of the grammatical relation of the coreferent weak pronoun.

(24) a. *shí 'ashkii sétał*
      I   boy   3ACC-1sNOM-kicked
      'It was *I*, I kicked the boy.'

   b. *shí 'ashkii siztał*
      I   boy   1sACC-3NOM-kicked
      'It was *me*, the boy kicked me.'

Both strong pronouns and nominals may have strong contrastive focus, marked with a focus particle.

(25) *'ashkii=ga'*   *yisisdlą́ą́d,*   *ni*   *'éí'*   *at'ééd*
      boy=FOCUS   3ACC-1sNOM-believed   you   DEM   girl

   yisínídlą́ą́d
   3ACC-2sNOM- believed
   'It was the *boy* I believed; as for you, you believed the girl.'

The focus particle *=ga'* typically follows the leftmost word. Strong pronouns and nominals may receive additional focus under the scope of an adverbial quantifier.

(26) a. *t'áá shí   t'éiyá 'ashkii   yisisdlą́ą́d*
      just   I   only   boy   3ACC-1sNOM-believed
      'Only *I* believed the boy.'

   b. *t'áá 'ashkii t'éiyá yisisdlą́ą́d*
      just   boy   only   3ACC-1sNOM-believed
      'I believed only the *boy*.'

However, a strong pronoun is incompatible with a nominal under the scope of *only*; conflicting focus markers would be present.

(27) a. **shí t'áá 'ashkii t'éiyá shédléézh*
   b. **t'áá 'ashkii t'éiyá shí shédléézh*

Perkins (1978) gives an analysis of a particle marking contrastive constituent negation in Navajo, and Willie and Jelinek (1996) discuss other focus particles.

   We have seen that strong pronouns in Navajo are employed to mark focus, do not show case marking, and do not have a fixed position in the clause marking a grammatical relation. However, there is a construction type in Navajo where the order of NP adjuncts is fixed: transitive sentences with two third-person arguments. Note that it is only with these *exclusively third-person* transitive sentences that contrasts in phi-features will not suffice to fix coreference between the weak pronouns and any NP adjuncts. When two NP adjuncts are present, the sentences are interpreted as follows:

(28) a.   *'ashkii   'at'ééd   yiyiiłtsą́*
           boy   girl   3ACC-3NOM-saw
           'The boy saw the girl.'

      b.   *'at'ééd   'ashkii   yiyiiłtsą́*
           girl   boy   3ACC-3NOM-saw
           'The girl saw the boy.'

This fixed order of the NPs suggests that word order is marking grammatical relations. And the fact that the sentence is grammatical without the nominals has been attributed to "multiple agreement" and pro-drop.

(28) c.   *yiyiiłtsą́*
           3ACC-3NOM-saw
           'She/he saw her/him.'

Evidence against multiple agreement and pro-drop, and in support of the claim that nominals are adjuncts, is provided by the analysis of complex sentences in Navajo. Let us begin with relative clauses.

11.4.1   Relative Clauses in Navajo.

Hale and Perkins (1976), and Platero (1974) pointed out problems raised by the following construction type.

(29) *'adą́ą́dą́ą́'   'ashkii   'at'ééd   yiyiiłtsą́-nę́ę̨   yidoots'ǫs.*
      yesterday   boy   girl   3A-3N-saw-REL   3A-3N-will kiss
      'The boy who saw the girl yesterday will kiss her.'

In this complex sentence, the arguments of the relative clause and the following main clause are obligatorily coreferential. We could account at least for coreference of the subject arguments, if we assumed that the NP *'ashkii* is the main clause subject, and that the relativized and main clause verbs show agreement with this subject. The problem is that both the lexical NPs are internal to the relative clause, which is under the scope of the temporal adverb *'adą́ą́dą́ą́'* 'yesterday'; the main clause has Future time reference. On a "pro-drop" and agreement analysis, we would have to assume an initial *pro* (the head of the relative) that would be coreferential with the NP *'ashkii* within the relative clause.

(30) *[pro ['adą́ą́dą́ą́' 'ashkii 'at'ééd yiyiiłtsą́nę́ę]] pro yidoots'ǫs.
                    S   O   V

This violates Condition C of the binding theory and ought to exclude the reading given. Suppose, however, that the relative clause, a derived nominal, is an adjunct.

(31) The boy$_i$ who saw the girl$_j$ yesterday, he$_i$ will kiss her$_j$.

Now Condition C is irrelevant, and we need to account for coreference of both arguments across the two clauses in some other way. In each clause, the verb is inflected for both arguments. Our claim is that this inflection corresponds to incorporated weak pronouns, discourse anaphors. Within the relative clause, the NPs are adjuncts to the verb-sentence and are coindexed with the pronominal arguments that license them. The entire relative clause, including any NPs present, is in turn an adjunct that provides discourse antecedents for the main clause incorporated pronouns. Hale (1973a, 1983) identified adjoined relative clauses in Australia, and they are common in Native America.

The constraint does not apply if a nominal appears in the second clause, introducing a new referent.

(32) 'adą́ą́dą́ą́'   'at'ééd   yiyiiłtsą́-nę́ę   Baa'   yidoots'ǫs'
      [yesterday   girl   3A-3N-saw-REL] Baa'   3A-3N-will kiss
      'The one$_i$ who saw the girl$_j$ yesterday, he$_i$ will kiss Baa'$_k$.'

The "relativizing" enclitic -nę́ę (-yę́ę) can in fact occur with simple nominals and be glossed 'aforementioned'. The following example is from Young and Morgan (1987):

(33) mą'ii   gałbáhí   yę́ę   yich'į' dah diilghad   jiní
      coyote   rabbit   afore. 3-to off 3NOM-started to run 4NOM-say
      'Coyote started to run towards (this) aforementioned gray rabbit, it is said/they say.'
      [Coyote, this aforementioned gray rabbit, he started to run towards it, they say.]

Or, it can be used to refer to someone who is deceased:

(34) shicheii-yę́ę
      my grandfather-former
      'my late grandfather'

The obligatory coreference between the adjoined and main clause arguments that we see in (29) is found in *all* complex sentences in Navajo in transitive clauses with exclusively third-person arguments[1]. An example with an adjoined temporal clause:

(35) a. *Jáan Kii   yiztał=go*   *néidíílts'in*
          John Kii   3NOM-3ACC-kicked=COMP 3ACC-3NOM-hit
          'When John$_i$ kicked Kee$_j$, he$_i$ hit him$_j$.'

      b. *yiztał=go*   *néidíílts'in*
          3ACC-3NOM-kicked=COMP, 3ACC-3NOM-hit
          'When he$_i$ kicked him$_j$, he$_i$ hit him$_j$.'

This constraint does not apply when an intransitive clause is included. Here, coreference between some argument of the adjoined temporal clause and the pronominal subject of the following main clause is possible but not obligatory.

(36) *Jáan Kii   yiztał=go,*   *yóó'eelwod*
      John Kii   3ACC-3NOM-kicked=COMP, 3NOM-ran away
      'When John$_i$ kicked Kee$_j$,he$_{i,j,k}$ ran away.'

This looks just like discourse anaphora in languages with subject agreement and object clitics.

(37) *Cuando Juan le pegó a Pablo, se fué corriendo.*
      'When John$_i$ hit Paul$_j$, he$_{i,j,k}$ ran away.'

The Navajo constraint on coreference exemplified in (29) and (35), which does not apply in Spanish, is stated in (38):

(38) In sequences of transitive clauses with all third person arguments, there is obligatory coreference between the two pronominal arguments of the first clause and the two pronominal arguments of the second.

In the next section, we argue that this unusual constraint on coreference across clauses in Navajo follows from the "voice split," the well-known *yi-/bi-* alternation in the language. Either one or the other value of the voice alternation must be present whenever the conditions for it are met: in transitive sentences with exclusively *third*-person arguments. The voice alternation is excluded where there is a first-, second-, or "fourth"-person argument, and in intransitive sentences; that is, it occurs only where the phi-features of the weak pronouns will not suffice to fix coreference unambiguously.[2] The voice alternation determines the topic/focus articulation of the clause, and thus determines the interpretation of a nominal or strong pronoun appearing in the focus position to the left of the verb complex. This makes word order relevant to the interpretation of the sentence, despite the non-argumental status of the nominals.

11.4.2   The Navajo Inverse Voice

The well-known *yi-/bi-* alternation in Navajo, described in a pioneering paper by Hale (1973b), may be identified as a voice alternation. (Gender is an artifice employed here to mark coindexing.)

(39) a. Q. *haa-sh   yít'iid*
             what-Q   3ACC-3NOM-did
             'What did she$_i$ do?'

      b. A. *yiztał*
             3ACC-3NOM-kicked (Direct)
             Focus$_j$-Topic$_i$-V
             'She$_i$ kicked him$_j$.'

(40) a. Q. *haa-sh   yidzaa*
             what-Q   3ACC-3NOM-happened
             What happened to him?

      b. A. *biztał*
             3ACC-3NOM-kicked (Inverse)
             Topic$_j$-Focus$_i$-V
             ['He$_j$ was kicked by her$_i$.']

In (39b), the agent is topic, and the patient is part of the focus. In (40b), the *bi*-pronoun appears in the Inverse construction, and marks a *topicalized patient*. These sentences do not mean the same, even when no nominals are present. There is a change in the mapping between grammatical relations and topic/focus structure. The inverse is not a passive; it is a transitive with two direct arguments. However, the passive (in brackets in the examples here) is often the "best available" gloss, since the passive and inverse both make the patient topical.

Krifka (1991) identifies a "particularly vexing problem" of analysis in connection with the following construction type:

(41) *SUE KISSED John.*   (TOPIC-COMMENT; Krifka 1991)

Krifka observes: "There is a reading where *Sue* and *kissed* seem to form a simple focus, at least semantically; (41) may be an answer to

(42)   *What happened to John?*

where the focus is equivalent to *was kissed by Sue*" (1991:152). Krifka identifies this sentence type as a Topic-Comment construction, as opposed to a Focus-Background construction, since a comment (the string *Sue kissed* in this example) need not be a syntactic constituent. In contrast, a focus must be a constituent, and a background need not be.

The Navajo inverse, like Krifka's example in (41), makes the patient topical. Krifka also notes that the passive is often the best paraphrase for topic-comment sentences like (41). However, the Navajo inverse and direct do not differ in surface syntactic constituency; they differ only in topic/focus structure, as shown in (39b) and (40b). Partee (1991) notes that in a topic-comment construction, there is a requirement that the topic be established in the discourse. This requirement applies to the referent of the *bi*-object pronoun in Navajo. The inverse construction, like ergative constructions, has a special marked status in universal grammar, since it violates a thematic hierarchy whereby agents are topical in transitive sentences. The Navajo inverse may be regarded as a grammaticalization of a topic-comment construction like (41).

Nominals in Navajo third-person transitive sentences are interpreted as follows. A nominal immediately preceding the inflected verb is in the focus position. Whether this nominal is coindexed with the agent or patient pronominal argument depends upon the *yi-/bi*-alternation.

In both (43) and (44), the nominal *łį́į́'* is in the focus position. In (43) the following patient pronoun has focus in the verb-sentence, and serves as an anaphor to the nominal. In (44), equivalent to Krifka's example, the focus nominal immediately precedes the *topicalized patient* pronoun, and coreference is excluded. By virtue of its position, the nominal has focus; it cannot be coindexed with the explicitly topicalized pronoun *bi-*, the patient, and by default is coindexed with the focused agent pronoun.

(43)   The Direct (*yi-*) Construction

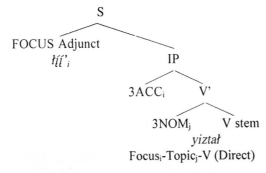

łį́į́' *yiztał*
horse   3ACC-3NOM-kicked (Direct)
FOCUS Focus-Topic-V
'He kicked it, [the horse]ꜰ.'

(44)   The Inverse (*bi-*) Construction

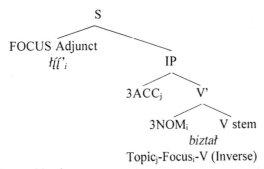

łį́į́' *biztał*
horse   3ACC-3NOM-kicked (Inverse)
FOCUS Topic-Focus-V
'He was kicked by it [the horse]ꜰ / [The horse]ꜰ kicked him.'

We noted that there is no direct/inverse alternation in constructions that include a non-third-person argument. As shown in examples (7) and (45), the phi-features of non-third-person incorporated pronouns determine unambiguously their coreference with strong pronouns.

(45) a.   *shí   sétał*
          I   3ACC-1sNOM-kicked
          '(It was) *I*, I kicked him.'

b. *shí   siztał*
   I   1sACC-3NOM-kicked
   '(It was) *me*, he kicked me.'

Nominals in Navajo are never coindexed with first- or second-person pronouns. In (45), the strong pronoun has contrastive focus, whether it is an adjunct to the subject or object pronoun. The pre-verbal position is a focus position, not an object position, for both nominals and strong pronouns.

Now consider sentences with two adjoined nominals, not common in discourse. The position immediately preceding the verb is the focus position. A nominal must be coindexed with a pronominal head. By default, an "outer" nominal must be coindexed with the pronoun that is not coindexed with the inner nominal; it is a "topic-adjunct", or reintroduced topic.

(46)

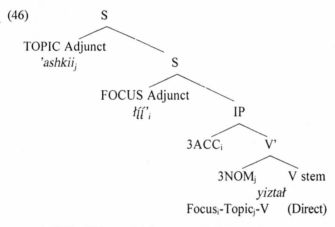

'ashkii   łį́į́'   yiztał
boy   horse   3ACC-3NOM-kicked (Direct)
TOP-ADJ FOCUS   Focus-Topic V
'The boy, he kicked [the horse]꜀.'

(47)

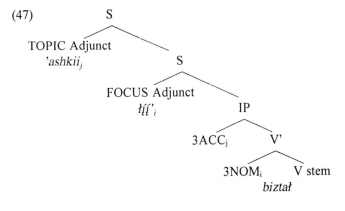

Topic_j-Focus_i-V   (Inverse)

'ashkii	łį́į'	biztał
boy	horse	3ACC-3NOM-kicked (Inverse)
TOP-ADJ	FOCUS	Topic-Focus V

'The boy, he was kicked by [the horse]_F.'

"Outer" nominals are coindexed with the topic pronoun, whether agent or patient. In sum: in each voice alternate, the NP in the focus position is coindexed with the focus pronoun of the verb-sentence.

Finally, coindexing across the arguments of a sequence of two third person transitive clauses is as follows. The two pronominal arguments of the first clause (and their adjuncts, if any) must be coindexed with the two pronominal arguments of the main clause, as we saw with Platero's relative clause example (29) above. The voice alternation obligatorily operates over the topic/focus structure of *both* clauses in the sequence. Compare (48), the structure for the complex sentence shown in (35b), where the agent is topic in both clauses, with example (49) where the second clause is inverse.

(48)

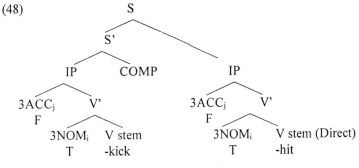

yiztał=go   *néidííłts'in*
3ACC-3NOM-kicked=COMP,   3ACC-3NOM-hit (Direct)
'When he_i kicked him_j, he_i hit him_j.'

(49)

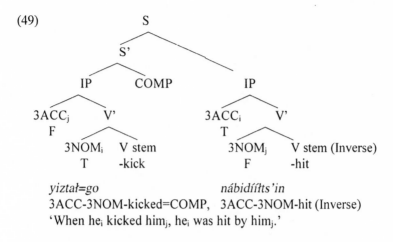

yiztał=go   nábidíiłts'in
3ACC-3NOM-kicked=COMP,   3ACC-3NOM-hit (Inverse)
'When he$_i$ kicked him$_j$, he$_i$ was hit by him$_j$.'

In sum: in each voice alternate, the focus pronoun of the first clause is coindexed with the focus pronoun of the second.

It is important to note that there can be no more than one occurrence of inverse *bi-* in a clause, since there can be no more than one voice alternation in a
clause. Also, complex sentences in Navajo cannot contain more than one relative
clause. Relatives cannot be "stacked" in Navajo, nor can each argument in a
transitive clause be coindexed with a separate relative; these are long-standing
puzzles in the analysis of Navajo. These constraints on multiple relatives preclude multiple topic switches.

Additional evidence on the adjunct status of nominals is provided by the fact
that the direct/inverse voice alternation *must* apply with oblique objects as well,
as long as all arguments are third person.

(50) a.   *dibé   łįį'   yitah   yígháah*
           sheep   horse   3-PP   3-join (Direct)
           'The sheep went among the horses.'

      b.   *dibé   łįį'   bitah   yígháah*
           sheep   horse 3-PP   3-join (Inverse)
           'The horse went among the sheep.'
           (As for the sheep, the horse, among them it joined).

The topical oblique object pronoun *bi-* in the postpositional phrase in (50b)
marks the phrase as disjoint in reference with the preceding focus nominal. The
leftmost nominal *dibé* does not form a syntactic constituent with the postpositional phrase, although it is coindexed with the *bi-*postpositional object. Some
postpositions and their objects in Navajo are procliticized to the inflected verb;
others remain detached. The verb and any preceding post-positional phrases form
a noninterruptable constituent, the Maximal Verb Complex (Willie 1991), that
is the domain of the voice alternation. This complex determines the interpreta-

tion of the adjoined nominals, even with respect to number, as in (50). (Nouns in Navajo are not marked for number, aside from a half-dozen words referring to humans.)

11.4.3 Definiteness and the Inverse

An important property of inverse constructions in Navajo is identified by Willie (1991), who argues that the preferred reading of a Navajo noun is definite (outside of existential contexts, etc.) unless it is overtly marked indefinite. The examples in (51—53) show that in a direct transitive, either argument can be definite or indefinite.

(51) *'ashkii   'at'ééd   yizts'ǫs*
      boy   girl   3ACC-3NOM-kissed
      'The boy kissed the girl.'

(52) *'ashkii   léi'   'at'ééd   yizts'ǫs*
      boy   a   girl   3ACC-3NOM-kissed
      'A boy kissed the girl.'

(53) *'ashkii   'at'ééd   léi'   yizts'ǫs*
      boy   girl   a   3ACC-3NOM-kissed
      'The boy kissed a girl.'

(The particle *léi'* can also have a specific reading in some contexts, as with English *a, an* (see Diesing 1992), but this is not the reading we are concerned with here.) Compare the inverse forms in (54—56):

(54) *'ashkii   'at'ééd   bizts'ǫs*
      boy   girl   3ACC-3NOM-kissed (Inverse)
      'The boy, the girl kissed him.'

(55) *'ashkii   'at'ééd   léi'   bizts'ǫs*
      boy   girl   a   3ACC-3NOM-kissed (Inverse)
      'The boy, a girl kissed him.'

(56) * *'ashkii   léi'   'at'ééd   bizts'ǫs*
      boy   a   girl   3ACC-3NOM-kissed (Inverse)
      ['A boy, the girl kissed him.']

For the inverse, an indefinite reading of the antecedent for the agent pronoun is permitted, but an indefinite reading of the antecedent for the highly pre-suppositional topicalized patient *bi-* is excluded.

Willie also shows an interesting contrast in the interpretation of Wh-words in the direct/inverse voice alternation. There is no obligatory Wh-movement in Navajo, but there may be focus (leftward) movement of the Wh-word. The particle *-sh* encliticized to Wh-words has inherent focus, and usually occurs after the first word in the sentence.

(57) a. *háí-sh   yizts'ǫs*
          who-Q   3ACC-3NOM-kissed (Direct)
          'Who did he kiss?'

      b. *háí-sh   bizts'ǫs*
          who-Q   3ACC-3NOM-kissed (Inverse)
          'Who kissed him?'

When a Wh-word and a second nominal are adjoined, both adjuncts have focus, and the following ambiguity arises with the direct construction:

(58) a. *Jáan háí-sh yizts'ǫs*
          John who-Q 3ACC-3NOM-kissed (Direct)
          'As for John, he kissed who?'

      b. *háí-sh   Jáan   yizts'ǫs*
          who-Q   John   3ACC-3NOM-kissed (Direct)
          1) 'Who was it, that kissed John?' Or:
          2) 'Who was it, that John kissed?'

In (58a), the first adjunct is a topic, and no focus movement and ambiguity are present. The second reading of (58b) shows optional focus movement of the Wh-word + Q to the leftmost position in the sentence. Now compare (59), the inverse construction with a topicalized patient pronoun.

(59) *háí-sh   Jáan   bizts'ǫs*
      who-Q   John   3ACC-3NOM-kissed (Inverse)
      'Which one (of you) was it, that was kissed by John?'

A Wh-word coindexed with a *bi*-pronoun is given a presuppositional "which one" reading; the questioned patient in (59) must belong to a presupposed set, which includes the addressee. It is "D-linked", in the sense of Pesetsky (1987). When a presuppositional reading is not intended, the direct form, as in example (58), is employed. The inverse does not permit optional focus movement of the Wh-word:

(60) a. *Jáan háí-sh   bizts'ǫs*
          John who-Q   3ACC-3NOM-kissed (Inverse)
          'As for John, he was kissed by whom?'

     b. *háí-sh   Jáan   bizts'ǫs*
          who   John   3ACC-3NOM-kissed (Inverse)
          1) 'Which one (of you) was kissed by John?'
          2) *'John was kissed by whom/which one?'

The *bi*-pronoun marks a topic/focus inversion that is incompatible with focus movement of the Wh-word.

11.4.4 The Animacy Hierarchy

In most of the examples of the voice alternation that we have seen so far, either the direct or inverse form can be used, depending on which argument is topical. However, if the two third-person referents differ along an animacy scale, it is conventional to make the more animate or human referent the topic. Compare (61, 62):

(61) a. *ł̨į́į́'   tsé   yiztał*
          horse rock   3ACC-3NOM-kicked (Direct)
          'The horse kicked the/a rock.'

     b. *?* tsé   ł̨į́į́'   biztał*
          rock horse   3ACC-3NOM-kicked (Inverse)
          ['the rock was kicked by the/a horse']

(62) a. *?* ł̨į́į́'   'ashkii   yiztał*
          horse boy   3ACC-3NOM-kicked (Direct)
          ['the horse kicked the/a boy']

     b. *'ashkii   ł̨į́į́'   biztał*
          boy   horse   3ACC-3NOM-kicked (Inverse)
          'The boy was kicked by the/a horse.'

The less animate referents here are typically not topical, are more apt to be new information. Speakers vary in respecting the hierarchy, and its use is declining now under language loss. Making a less animate or volitional patient topical is clearly ruled out when this patient is indefinite or new information, not established in the discourse, since the inverse requires a specific patient. The use of the inverse form here can be understood as a way of ensuring that agents low on the animacy scale are focused as new information, while the high-ranking, definite patient is made the topic.

Additional evidence on the adjunct status of nominals is provided by lexical/semantic constraints on the plausible interpretation of sentences that include nominals. When the lexical features of the transitive verb entail an animate agent and an inanimate patient, a focus nominal need not be coindexed with the patient/focus of a *yi-* verb.

(63) *'ashkii   yiyííłta'*
      boy   3ACC-3NOM-count plural objects
      'It was *the boy* who counted them.' (*The boy* counted them).

Since inanimate objects do not count boys, this sentence poses no problems of interpretation. An example with a postpositional phrase, where the preceding animate nominal is plausibly interpreted as coindexed with the agent pronoun:

(64) *'asdzą́ą́   yii'   yiyííłbéézh*
      woman   3-in   3ACC-3NOM-cooked
      'It was the *woman* who cooked it in it.' (e.g., food in a pot)

In these examples, the animacy hierarchy makes it impossible to include a nominal corresponding to the inanimate topic in the position preceding the animate focus nominal, and the use of the direct form is permitted, although it is not preferred. If the preverbal position marked a grammatical relation, an object position, then we might expect (64) and (65) to be ruled out entirely.

There are a few special contexts where the animacy hierarchy and the voice alternation may be set aside. If the sentence makes reference to natural forces endowed with supernatural powers in Navajo culture, such as the lightning or the rainbow, the animacy scale may be irrelevant (Willie 1991; Thompson 1996). And, if a first-, second- or fourth-person possessor argument is present, it can disqualify the sentence as an environment for the voice alternation.

(65) *shilį́į́'*   *'ashkii   yiztał*
      1sPOSS-horse   boy   3ACC-3NOM-kicked
      'My horse kicked the boy.'

Thompson (1996) cites the example shown in (66). In this example also the first person possessor pronoun excludes the voice alternation:

(66) *díí   sis   shizhé'é   'áyilaa*
      this   belt   1sPOSS-father   3ACC-3NOM-made
      'My dad made this belt.'

A comparison of (65 and 66) shows that word order does not mark grammatical relations in these sentences lacking the voice alternation.

11.4.5 The Inverse and Generics

We have seen that in complex sentences with adjoined temporal or relative clauses in Navajo, the constraint stated in (38) applies. In these constructions, the voice alternation can mark a switch across clauses in the topicalized argument. Complex sentences with direct verb forms can be used in generic statements in Navajo:

(67) *łééchąą'i mą'ii yił didił=go*   yiyiiłhash
     dog   coyote 3-PP 3NOM-catch=COMP 3ACC-3NOM-bites (Direct)
     'When a dog$_i$ catches a coyote$_j$, it$_i$ bites it$_j$.'

However, inverse forms cannot be used in generic statements. Since the topicalized patient is definite/specific, it excludes a generic reading. Example (68) is about a specific coyote and a particular event.

(68) *łééchąą'i mą'ii yił deezdééł=go*   bishxash
     dog   coyote 3-PP 3-caught=COMP 3A-3N-bit (Inverse)
     'When the dog$_i$ caught the coyote$_j$, it$_i$ was bitten by it$_j$.'

Constructions with relative clauses cannot be generics in Navajo, whether direct or inverse. Relatives are presuppositional:

(69) a. *łééchąą'i mą'ii yił deezdééł=yéę*
         dog   coyote 3-PP 3-caught=REL (Direct)
         yiyiiłhash
         3A-3N-bite DIRECT
         'The dog$_i$ that caught the coyote$_j$, it$_i$ is biting it$_j$.'

     b. *łééchąą'i mą'ii yił deezdééł=yéę*
         dog   coyote 3-PP 3-caught=REL (Direct)
         biiłhash
         3A-3N-bite INVERSE
         'The dog$_i$ that caught the coyote$_j$, it$_i$ is being bitten by it$_j$.'

The adjoined relative clause in Navajo refers to a backgrounded proposition, to information and referents established in the discourse: "aforementioned." The relative need not be past time, but it is presupposed, familiar information.

11.4.6   Coreference and Possessive Noun Phrases

A second constraint on anaphora in complex sentences in Navajo is exemplified
in (70).[3]

(70)

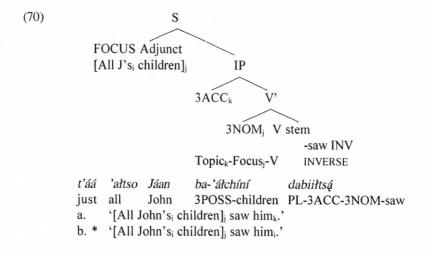

t'áá   'ałtso   Jáan   ba-'áłchíní   dabiiłtsá
just   all   John   3POSS-children   PL-3ACC-3NOM-saw
a.   '[All John's$_i$ children]$_j$ saw him$_k$.'
b. *   '[All John's$_i$ children]$_j$ saw him$_i$.'

This constraint is stated in (71):

(71)   Coreference between possessive arguments internal to a complex NP and
       the pronominal arguments of a following verb-sentence is excluded.

For most speakers, coreference of this kind is impossible; for others, it is
strongly dispreferred. What prevents the noun internal to the complex NP in
(70) from serving as the discourse antecedent for an incorporated pronoun in the
verb-sentence? This would be a perfectly natural reading for an apparently parallel construction in a language like Spanish, with subject agreement and object
clitics:

(72)   *Todos los hijos de Juan lo vieron.*
       '[All John's$_i$ children]$_j$ saw him$_{i,k}$.'

Compare a passive gloss for the inverse construction in (70):

(73)   [all John's$_i$ children]$_j$,   he$_k$ was seen by   them$_j$.
       FOCUS Adjunct   Topic   Focus

The passive gloss points up the fact that the patient argument of the inverse verb is the topic. Although the complex possessive NP is higher on the tree than the weak pronouns, it cannot provide discourse antecedents for both of them. It is necessarily an adjunct to one of the verbal arguments, and use of the inverse marks the complex POSS NP as disjoint in reference with the topicalized patient of the following verb sentence. The inverse cannot treat the two arguments of the POSS NP as it would the two pronominal arguments introduced at functional projections in an adjoined clause. POSS NPs have internal arguments, but unlike clauses, they do not have topics—and the inverse marks a switch in the mapping between grammatical relations and topic/focus structure.

It follows from the generalization in (71) that anaphora involving third-person arguments in "picture nouns" in Navajo is excluded. In "psych" verb constructions in Navajo, the Experiencer is typically a postpositional object (Jelinek and Willie, 1996). A sentence corresponding to:

(74)   a. [*Pictures of John$_i$*]$_j$ *please him$_i$.*
       b. [*Pictures of himself$_i$*]$_j$ *please John$_i$.*

would be expressed as a complex event.

(75)   *Jáan*   *'abi'diilkeed=go*   *bił*   *nizhóní*
       John   3-PASS-pictured=COMP   3-with   3-good
       'When John$_i$ is photographed, it pleases him$_{i,j}$.'

There are no simple nouns corresponding to 'picture' or 'photograph'. Since the first clause in (75) is an intransitive, the direct/inverse alternation cannot apply, and reference of the Experiencer postpositional object *bi-* is not fixed (this is an intransitive clause, and *bi-* does not mark the inverse here). The deictic "fourth" person can be used to force coreference.

(76)   *'aho'diilkeed=go*   *hwił*   *nizhóní*
       4-PASS-pictured=COMP   4-with   3-good
       'When that person$_i$ is photographed, it pleases that person$_i$.'

The fourth person in Navajo, like first and second, cannot enter into the direct/inverse alternation, and is employed in a variety of discourse contexts. It is often used as an impersonal, and does not ordinarily cooccur with an NP, but may do so in certain construction types that resolve ambiguities or force coreference. The fourth can be used in this way with complex possessive NPs:

(77) Jáan t'áá 'ałtsoní ha-'áłchíní   dahoołtsą́
      John just all   4POSS-children   PL-4ACC-3NOM-saw
      'John$_i$, just all that person's$_i$ children$_j$ saw that person$_i$].'
      (All John's$_i$ children]$_j$ saw him$_i$.)

The fourth-person pronouns, both subject and object, are exclusively definite and refer primarily to humans, as with the *bi*-pronoun.[4]

11.5   Reflexives and Reciprocals

Anaphors that are bound within the verb-sentence in Navajo appear in the verb prefix array. They are invariant as to person or number, and the resulting inflected verb is overtly marked intransitive by the use of the *d-* or *l*-classifier. There are no independent pronouns or nominals that are coreferent with a reflexive or reciprocal that may be adjoined to the sentence—that is, there are no freestanding 'self' or 'each other' forms. Any constituents of this kind would be blocked by the case filter, since the verb is morphologically intransitive.

11.5.1   Reflexives

The reflexive prefix *'adi-* can occur with both singular and plural subjects. The following examples show the contrast between forms with a third person object and a reflexive.

(78) a. *yoolóós*
          3ACC-3NOM-guide
          'He is guiding it.' (Transitive)

      b. *na'ádidlóós*
          around-REFL-3NOM-guide
          'He is guiding himself around.' (Intransitive)
          (as with a blind person feeling his way)

The *d-* classifier is overt in (78b), the intransitive form.

11.5.2 Reciprocals

When the reciprocal anaphor *'ahi-* is used, the subject is necessarily two or more in number.

(79)   *'ahiidleesh*
       RECIP-1dlNOM-painting
       'We two are painting each other.'

Since the reflexive and reciprocal prefixes derive intransitive constructions, Navajo has no way to place contrastive focus on the incorporated "self" argument. Adding a freestanding pronoun simply places focus on the agent, which is of course coreferent.

(80)   *t'áá   shí   'ádéshgish*
       just   I   REFL-1sNOM-cut
       '*I'm* the one who cut myself/me.' (Intransitive)
       [*I cut *myself/me*]

11.5.3 Logophoric Anaphors

Reflexive or reciprocal possessors may appear as arguments of nominals in the preverbal focus position. Examples from Young and Morgan (1987):

(81)   *'ádáyi'*   *ni'sétsi*
       REFL POSS-throat-in   around-1sNOM-poked
       'I swabbed my [self's] throat.'
       [I poked around in my throat]

A reciprocal with a first-person dual subject:

(82)   *'ałkék'eh*   *yiiltsą́*
       RECIP POSS-foot way   3ACC-1dlNOM-saw
       'We saw each other's footprints [path].'

In (83), with all third-person arguments, the higher, leftmost nominal is the antecedent for a reciprocal possessive pronoun in the focus nominal.

(83)   *tsídii   'ahiłtsiits'iin*   *néiniłtash*
       bird   RECIP POSS-head   3ACC-3NOM-peck
       'The birds are pecking each other on the head.'
       [The birds, each other's heads, they are pecking them.]

These "logophoric" anaphors differ from the true reflexive anaphors given in (78) to (80). Example (81) contains an oblique adjunct. The verbs in (82) and (83) are transitive, with a third person object; thus, they permit a complex nominal adjunct containing a possessor argument in the focus position. Young and Morgan note that this construction type is confined primarily to body parts and related items such as clothing and footprints.

Logophoric possessor anaphors pose a number of problems for the binding theory. Partee and Bach (1981) argue that the correct generalization is that pronouns are disallowed, and anaphors required, only when the anaphor and its antecedent are coarguments of the same lexical head. Reinhart and Reuland (1993) and Pollard and Sag (1992) come to the same conclusions concerning the problems raised by anaphors that appear to be exempt from Principle A—that is, do not require a local binder. These problem cases, including anaphors in "picture" NPs, and possessor reciprocals, they classify as logophoric anaphors, which need only to have a discourse antecedent, and do not require to be A-bound, as in the following:

(84) *John was furious.*
      The picture of himself in the museum had been mutilated.

Consider the following example from Japanese, where the suffix *-wa* marks a constituent as a topic. In double topic constructions, it is possible to have a logophoric anaphor in the "lower" topic.

(85) *Sakenomi-tachi-wa   otagaino   kuruma-wa   dameni shita.*
      drunkards-TOP   each other's cars-TOP   wrecked
      (Speaking of) the drunkards, (as for) each other's cars, they wrecked them.

The possessor pronouns in the Navajo examples in (81) to (83) are not arguments of the verb, but of the nominal. Their syntax is consistent with that of the class of anaphors across languages that require only discourse antecedents. The Navajo reflexives that are A-bound are incorporated into the verb-sentence, like the other pronominal arguments.

11.6   Summary on Nominal Adjuncts and Focus in Navajo

We have considered the following lines of evidence bearing on the claim that nominals in Navajo are not in A-positions but are adjuncts ordered according to the focus structure of the complex sentence:

(86) a.   Adjoined clauses provide discourse antecedents for weak pronouns
            in the following main clause.

b. Independent "strong" pronouns can appear in the focus position immediately preceding the verb-sentence, whatever the grammatical relation of the coindexed Pronominal Argument.

c. Coindexing in the direct/inverse is focus-to-focus, both with simple nominals and adjoined clauses.

d. Optional focus movement of Wh-words produces a word order that does not correspond to putative grammatical relations.

e. True reflexive/reciprocals are A-bound within the verb-sentence.

f. Lexical semantic features of verbs and nominals place constraints on plausible construals.

These features provide evidence that Navajo is a Pronominal Argument language, where nominals are ordered according to topic/focus structure.

11.7 Adverbial Quantification in Navajo

Some recent work on quantification in natural language (Bach et al. 1995, Jelinek 1995a) demonstrates an association between quantifier type (determiner versus adverbial) and argument type across languages. In Navajo, weak quantifiers appear as predicates.

(87) *táá' niilt'é*
three 1pNOM-be
'We are three (in number).'

Strong quantifiers are unselective adverbials (Lewis 1975).

(88) *'ałtso 'iishį́į́'*
all ['a-]-1s-dyed black
'I finished dyeing (black).' (Activity complete)

The verb in example (88) includes underlyingly the prefix '*a*-, said to mark an indefinite object. This prefix derives an intransitive construction which describes an activity, an "anti-passive" form that excludes a referential object. In contrast, example (89) contains a third-person object pronoun.

(89) *'ałtso yiishį́į́'*
all 3-1s-dyed black
'I finished dyeing it/them black.'
Or: 'I dyed all of it/them black.'

These examples illustrate the variable scope of the adverbial quantifier.

In (88), the activity construction, there is no object pronoun that the quantifier may have scope over; it takes scope over the action (scalar interpretation). In (89), the quantifier may have scope over either the action or over the object argument. Faltz (1995) argues that Navajo quantifiers are "floating"—that is, not in construction with nouns, and constituting adjuncts in their own right.

For example (70), the preverbal string containing the quantifier can be construed as one or two complex nominals. Example (90) shows the one nominal construal that we have been looking at above. Example (91) shows the reading with two nominals.

(90) [*t'áá*   *'altso*   *Jáan*   *ba-'álchíní*   ]   *dabiiłtsá*
      [just   all   John   3POSS-children]   PL-3ACC-3NOM-saw
      Focus Adjunct   Topic-Focus-V
      'He$_k$ was seen by [all John's$_i$ children]$_j$.'

(91) [*t'áá*   *'altso*]   [*Jáan*   *ba-'álchíní*   ]   *dabiiłtsá*
      [just   all   ]   [John   3POSS-children]   PL-3ACC-3NOM-saw
      Topic Adjunct   Focus Adjunct   Topic-Focus-V
      'They all$_k$ were seen by [John's$_i$ children]$_j$.'

When the string is interpreted as two nominals, the first is an adjunct to the topicalized patient, as in (91). If the quantifier is immediately before the verb-sentence, a different reading is possible.

(92) [*Jáan*   *ba-'álchíní*   ] [*t'áá 'altso*   ]   *dabiiłtsá*
      [John   3POSS-children] [just   all]   PL-3ACC-3NOM INV
      Topic Adjunct   Focus Adjunct T-F-V
      '[John's$_i$ children]$_j$ were seen by all of them$_k$.'
      (They all$_k$ saw John's$_i$ children$_j$.)

Related ambiguities arise with the direct forms.

Determiner quantification is absent in Navajo. Determiner quantification in lexical argument languages such as English precludes the ambiguity in quantifier scope seen in Navajo, but requires the presence of syntactic constituents (NPs) that do not correspond to the constituent structure of the associated tripartite semantic structure; NPs with a determiner quantifier contain both the quantifier and the restriction on that quantifier. This association between quantifier type and argument type has been claimed to be present in Straits Salish, Navajo, Mohawk, and Asurini do Trocara (Bach et al. 1995). Whether this association holds generally across languages is an empirical question yet to be answered.

11.8   Concluding Remarks

Baker (1996) argues that the "macro-parameter" underlying polysynthesis is the requirement that every theta role of a head be related to a morpheme in the word containing that head. The goal here has been to go beyond stating that the presence of weak pronouns in INFL in Navajo is obligatory. We identify these pronominal arguments as discourse anaphors and show how they fit into the topic/focus articulation of the Navajo clause. We have argued that "polysynthetic" or more generally Pronominal Argument languages—a class that includes languages with AUX or INFL clitic strings, such as Warlpiri and Straits Salish—are discourse configurational languages.[5] We do not assume that the weak pronouns undergo movement to their argument positions in INFL, but that they are base generated at the functional projections where their case is checked. In contrast, nominals have no grammatical or direct case and are excluded from the subject and object argument positions introduced at the functional projections.

For many polysynthetic languages, word order is said to be "free"; what is meant by "free" is that nominals are not ordered according to grammatical relations. A summary of the evidence on Navajo as a discourse configurational language was given in (86). If two disjoint nominals appear in a transitive sentence in Navajo, the first is in the topic position and the second is in the focus position. The direct/inverse voice alternation always coindexes focus-to-focus, but in the inverse clause, there is a switch in the mapping between grammatical relation and focus structure. In early transformational treatments of Navajo syntax, the inverse was called "subject/object inversion."

(93) a.   *'ashkii   'at'ééd   yizts'os*
           boy   girl   3ACC-3NOM-kissed (Direct)
           'The boy kissed the girl.'

      b.   *'ashkii   at'ééd   bizts'os*
           boy   girl   3ACC-3NOM-kissed (Inverse)
           'The girl kissed the boy.'

The problem here is that the glosses given are inadequate. We know the truth conditions, we know who got kissed, but we don't know how to use (93b) appropriately in context. More accurate glosses would be:

(94) a.   *'ashkii   'at'ééd   yizts'os*
           boy   girl   3ACC-3NOM-kissed (Direct)
           'The boy kissed the girl.'

      b.   *'ashkii   at'ééd   bizts'os*
           boy   girl   3ACC-3NOM-kissed (Inverse)
           'The girl kissed the boy.' (Krifka's example)

There is a change in the topic/focus structure of the verb-sentence from (94a) to (94b). The patient (*bi-*) is the backgrounded topic in (94b). This produces a switch in the coindexing of nominals, which always appear in topic, focus order.

Navajo differs from some Northern Athabaskan languages, where NPs are in argument positions. Dogrib (Saxon 1984) and Slave (Rice 1989) have incorporated object pronouns which are mutually exclusive with all object NPs, definite or indefinite. There are cognates of the *yi-/bi-* object pronouns in these languages; however, their function and distribution varies along with argument structure (Saxon and Rice 1992, Thompson 1996). In Babine-Witsuwit'en, object clitics are excluded only with *indefinite* object NPs (Gunlogson 1995). This is reminiscent of the situation in Spanish or Arabic. These Canadian Athabaskan languages have determiner quantification, while Southern Athabaskan does not.

There are language universal links between grammatical relations and topic/focus structure that underlie correspondences and parametric variation of this kind across languages. In the default topic/focus articulation of the clause in universal grammar, subjects are typically old information that is presuppositional and backgrounded. In contrast, objects are part of the focus, the new information, either as indefinites or as definites that are "new" in the context (Diesing 1992). In languages with subject agreement, familiar subjects can be adequately identified by their phi-features, and we see "pro-drop." There is less discourse motivation for dropping objects, part of the new information, than in "subject drop." Some languages permit the dropping of object NPs in lexical contexts where they are largely predictable, as in cognate object constructions. Diesing and Jelinek (1995) argue that pronouns are presuppositional elements that must be raised out of the VP before logical form, in order to avoid a type mismatch. Pronominal Arguments are a syntactic option that a language may select in order to place pronouns at functional projections in INFL, so that the distribution of pronouns in the overt syntax corresponds to positions that they must assume by LF.

If word order differences are employed exclusively to show the topic/focus articulation of the clause, then grammatical relations must be marked in a different component of the grammar—via the case-marked pronominal arguments. A system with weak pronouns in A-positions co-occurring with nominal adjuncts which are ordered according to the topic/focus structure of the clause produces a certain amount of redundancy. Compare the situation in Czech and Hungarian. In these languages, nominals are in A-positions, as shown by their overt case marking, but they "scramble" or are reordered to reflect topic/focus relations. There is subject agreement and object clitics. In such a grammar, there is no need for incorporated weak pronouns, since case marking on the arguments suffices to identify grammatical relations.

The redundancy seen in pronominal argument languages is the price paid for using word order exclusively to mark focus and backgrounding. This "dual representation," the presence of coindexed pronouns and nominals, has been claimed to be simply an areal feature. However, pronominal argument systems appear in many language areas and show features that can be accounted for in terms of a particular grammaticalization of topic/focus structure.

Notes

We are greatly indebted to Emmon Bach, Andrew Barss, Fernando Escalante, Aryeh Faltz, Ted Fernald, Hisako Ikawa, Eva Hajičova, Hen Hale, Joyce McDonough, Barbara Partee, and Petr Sgall for comments and helpful discussion of these topics. None is responsible for our errors.

1. Speas (1990) analyzes this coreference in complex sentences in Navajo as parallel processing and attributes it to universal principles of discourse anaphora.
2. In contexts where the voice alternation is excluded, bi- is the ordinary object and possessor pronoun.
3. We thank Ken Hale (personal communication) for drawing our attention to the problem posed by sentences like example (71).
4. Willie (1991) gives an extended treatment of the syntax and discourse functions of the fourth person in Navajo.
5. The term "head-marking," as we understand it, also does not include second-position clitic strings.

References

Bach, Emmon, Eloise Jelinek, Angelika Kratzer, and Barbara Partee (eds.). 1995. *Quantification in Natural Languages*. Dordrecht: Kluwer.

Baker, Mark. 1996. *The Polysynthesis Parameter*. New York: Oxford University Press.

Bresnan, Joan and Sam Mchombo. 1987. Topic, Pronoun and Agreement in Chichewa. *Language* 63:741–82.

Charles, Al, Richard Demers, and Elizabeth Bowman. 1978. Introduction to the Lummi Language. Unpublished manuscript. University of Arizona.

Diesing, Molly. 1992. *Indefinites*. Cambridge, Mass.: MIT Press.

Diesing, Molly, and Eloise Jelinek. 1995. Distributing Arguments. *Natural Language Semantics* 3:123–176.

Escalante, F. 1990. Voice and Argument Structure in Yaqui. Ph.D. dissertation, University of Arizona, Tucson.

Faltz, Leonard 1995. Towards a Typology of Natural Logic. In Bach et al. (eds.).

Gunlogson, Christine. 1995. Pronominal Prefixes in Babine-Witsuwit'en. Master's thesis, University of Washington.

Hajičova, Eva, Barbara Partee, and Petr Sgall. 1995. Topic-Focus Articulation, Tripartite Structures, and Semantic Content. Unpublished manuscript. Charles University, Prague.

Hale, Kenneth. 1973a. The Adjoined Relative Clause in Australia. In R. M. W. Dixon (ed.), *Grammatical Categories in Australian Languages*, N.J.: Humanities Press.

Hale, Kenneth. 1973b. A Note on Subject-Object Inversion in Navajo. In B. Kachru et al. (eds.), *Issues in Linguistics: Papers in Honor of Henry and Renee Kahane*, 300-309. Chicago: University of Chicago Press.

Hale, Kenneth. 1983. Warlpiri and the Grammar of Non-Configurational Languages. *Natural Language and Linguistic Theory* 1:5–47.

Hale, Kenneth, and Ellavina Perkins. 1976. *The Structure of Navajo: Course Notes.* Tucson: University of Arizona.

Jelinek, Eloise. 1984. Empty Categories, Case, and Configurationality. *Natural Language and Linguistic Theory* 2:39–76.

Jelinek, Eloise. 1989. Argument Type in Athapaskan: Evidence from Noun Incorporation. Paper presented at the AAA-CAIL, Washington, DC.

Jelinek, Eloise. 1995a. Quantification in Straits Salish. In Bach et al. (eds.).

Jelinek, Eloise. 1995b. Pronoun Classes and Focus. Paper presented at the Workshop on Focus, University of Massachusetts, Amherst.

Jelinek, Eloise. In press. Agreement, Clitics and Focus in Egyptian Arabic. In Ur Shlonsky and Jamal Ouhalla (eds.), *Studies in Semitic Syntax.*

Jelinek, Eloise, and Fernando Escalante. 1991. Focus and clitics in Yaqui. Paper presented at the Uto-Aztecan Conference, University of California, Santa Cruz.

Jelinek, Eloise, and MaryAnn Willie. 1996. Psych Verbs in Navajo. In Jelinek, Eloise, Sally Midgette, Keren Rice, and Leslie Saxon (eds.), *Athabaskan Language Studies: Essays in Honor of Robert Young,* Albuquerque: University of New Mexico Press, 15–34.

Kiss, Katalin E. Identificational vs. Information Focus. *Language* 74:245-273.

Krifka, Manfred. 1991. A Compositional Semantics for Multiple Focus Constructions. In S. Moore and A. Wyner (eds.), *Proceedings from Semantics and Linguistic Theory I,* (Cornell Working Papers in Linguistics, No. 10), 127–158.

Lewis, David. 1975. Adverbs of Quantification. In E. L. Keenan (ed.), *Formal Semantics of Natural Language,* Cambridge: Cambridge University Press.

Lipkind, W. 1945. *Winnebago Grammar.* New York: King's Crown Press.

McDonough, Joyce. 1990. Topics in the Phonology and Morphology of Navajo. Ph. D. dissertation, University of Massachusetts, Amherst.

Partee, Barbara. 1987. Noun Phrase Interpretation and Type-Shifting Principles. In J. Groenendijk, D. de Jongh, and M. Stokhof, eds., Studies in Discourse Representation and the Theory of Generalized Quantifiers, GRASS 8, Foris Dordrecht.

Partee, Barbara. 1991. Topic, Focus and Quantification. In S. Moore and A. Wyner, eds, *Proceedings from Semantics and Linguistic Theory I,* (Cornell Working Papers in Linguistics, No. 10), 159–188.

Partee, Barbara, and Emmon Bach. 1981. Quantification, Pronouns, and VP-Anaphora. In J. Groenendijk, T. Janssen, and M. Stokhof (eds.), *Formal Methods in the Study of Language.* Mathematisch Centrum. Amsterdam University.

Perkins, Ellavina. 1978. The Role of Word Order and Scope in the Interpretation of Navajo Sentences. Ph.D. dissertation, University of Arizona, Tucson.

Pesetsky, David. 1987. Binding Problems with Experiencer Verbs. *Linguistic Inquiry* 18:126–140.

Platero, Paul. 1974. The Navajo Relative Clause. *International Journal of American Linguistics* 40: 202-246.

Pollard, Carl, and Ivan Sag. 1992. Anaphors in English and the Scope of the Binding Theory. *Linguistic Inquiry* 23(2):261–304.

Reinhart, Tanya, and Eric Reuland. 1993. "Reflexivity" *Linguistic Inquiry* 24:657-720.

Rice, Keren. 1989. *A Grammar of Slave.* Berlin: Mouton de Gruyter.

Saxon, Leslie. 1984. Dogrib Pronouns. Ph.D. dissertation, University of California, San Diego.

Speas, Margaret. 1990. *Phrase Structure in Natural Language. Studies in Natural Language and Linguistic Theory.* Dordrecht: Kluwer.

Thompson, Chad. 1996. The History and Function of the *yi-/bi-* Alternation in Athabaskan. In Jelinek, Eloise, Sally Midgette, Keren Rice, and Leslie Saxon (eds.), *Athabaskan Language Studies: Essays in Honor of Robert Young,* Albuquerque: University of New Mexico Press, 81-100.

Willie, MaryAnn. 1991. Navajo Pronouns and Obviation. Ph.D. dissertation, University of Arizona, Tucson.

Young, Robert, and William Morgan. 1987. *The Navajo Language: A Grammar And Colloquial Dictionary,* Revised edition, Albuquerque, N.M.: University of New Mexico Press.

12

THE FUNCTION AND SIGNIFICATION OF CERTAIN NAVAHO PARTICLES

Robert W. Young and William Morgan

Published in 1948 by the Education Division of the United States Indian
ice, the brochure entitled *The Function and Signification of Certain Nc
Particles* was designed as an aid to frustrated teachers of English to N
students of that period.[1]

Although Article 6 of the Navajo Treaty of 1868 committed the federal
ernment to provide educational facilities for "every thirty children betweer
ages of six and sixteen) who could be induced or compelled to attend sch
interest on the part of tribal members was understandably low at the time
funds were lacking. As a result, nearly a century passed before school oppo
ties became universally available to the tribe.

Wartime experiences during the 1940s acted as catalysts to stimulate in
in learning English on the part of tribal members, with the result that, afte
war, the nation suddenly faced the gargantuan task of carrying out treaty ol
tions for a backlog of Navajo children and young people, illiterate in En
and monolingual in Navajo, that had reached thousands. To cope with the
lem a crash program was launched, beginning in 1946, designed to pr
basic language and work skills to a segment of the population that othe
would face life disadvantaged.

Few teachers involved in the crash program had personal experience witl

288

language other than English—much less with Navajo—nor did they have special training in second-language teaching techniques.

All languages possess means of one kind or another with which to shade meaning—including the complex intonational system employed by English. The simple statement "this is my car" contrasts sharply with "*this* is my car," "this *is* my car," or "this is *my* car." Voice pitch and stress subtly modify the meaning of the utterance, although its component words remain. Mastery of this system came slowly and painfully for many Navajo students—especially those teenagers and young adults who were beyond the age when language is readily acquired.

Even after students mastered the rudiments of English phonology they often spoke in monotones. The intonational patterns of English were elusive, and the teachers, lacking knowledge of the Navajo language, searched in vain for explanations. Rising inflection to mark yes/no questions, for example, seemed quite "natural" to the teachers, but the students failed to respond as expected.

The explanation, of course, lay in the first-language experience of the students: the Navajo language does not employ the same intonational patterns as English for the purpose of shading meaning. Many nuances, rendered by voice inflection and stress in English, are rendered by particles in Navajo. Navajo is a "tone language"—one in which low/high (falling/rising) voice pitch is fixed as an inherent feature of all noun, verb, pronominal, and postpositional stems, as well as many of the adverbial morphemes that function prominently in the derivational system.

Low tone is unmarked graphically, but high tone is written by placing an acute accent over the vowel: *ni* 'you' contrasts with *ní* 'he/she says'. Contrasting vowel length (duration) is also a distinctive feature of Navajo phonology—long vowels are written as doublets. *Bitǫ'* 'his/her water' contrasts with *bitoo* 'its juice'. Falling and rising tone patterns .are restricted to long vowels and diphthongs, as in *níígo* 'he/she saying' and *hágoónee'* 'that's all, good-bye'.

The speaker cannot convert *ni* 'you' to question status by rising inflection—*ní* means he/she says. Nor can *bitoo'* be uttered as *bitóo'!*, an exclamation, because the low tone of its component syllables is fixed. English "you" can be converted to question status by raised inflection, to produce *you*?

In the Navajo sentence *'ashkii 'ólta'góó dah diiyá* 'The boy left for school', the final word ends in a high tone, but the sentence cannot be construed as a question—it is a simple statement. To convert the sentence to question status Navajo employs a yes/no question particle *da'* or an enclitic *-ísh* or both together, as *'ashkiísh 'ólta'góó dah diiyá* 'Did the boy leave for school?' or *da' 'ashkiísh 'ólta'góó dah diiyá* 'Did the boy leave for school?'

In the sentence *dlǫǫ' 'a'ą́ą́lwod* 'The prairie dog ran into the hole', the final syllable is low in tone, and it cannot be converted to question status by rising inflection to produce *'a'ą́ą́lwód*. *Dlǫ'ísh* (or *da' dlǫ'ísh*) *'a'ą́ą́lwod* is required for 'Did the prairie dog run into the hole?'

Contrariness to fact is usually conveyed by a peculiar intonational pattern in English, but in Navajo this feature is expressed by the particle *hanii*, Thus, the simple statement *nát'oh naháłnii'* 'I bought cigarettes' is reversed by the addition of *hanii* to produce *nát'oh hanii naháłnii'*. A literal translation might be 'it wasn't cigarettes that I bought,' but spoken English would more likely use intonational stress to mark contrariness to fact. The English speaker might say "I didn't buy ciga*rettes!*" with rising intonation on *-ettes* (*tó dilchxoshí naháłnii'*

'I bought soda pop'). Similarly, *Yootóógóó hanii niséyá* 'I didn't go to *San*ta Fe'—*Na'nízhoozhígóó niséyá* 'I went to Gallup'. And *jįįdą́ą́' hanii nahodoołtį́į́ł hwiinidzin ńt'éé'* 'People *expect*ed it to rain today (but it didn't).'

The particles *ga'* and *ląą* and, in some contexts *yee'* connote emphasis. Thus, in reply to *háílá yik'íníyá* 'who found it', someone might raise his hand, to be contested by the true finder who exclaims *shíga'*, '*I* found it, *I'm* the one who found it!' Similarly, *shíyee'*, '*I'm* the one'. And in reply to the query *háíyee' bééhonohsin* 'which one of you two knows it', a knowledgeable person might respond with an emphatic *shíłą́ą́!* 'I do!'

The particle *yee'* functions as an intensifier in contexts of the type *'awéé' 'áłts'íísí yee' bik'íníyá* 'I came upon a *little tiny* baby'—in contradistinction to *'awéé' 'áłts'íisí léí bik'íníyá* 'I came upon a little baby'. *Yee'* corresponds to high inflection in English "*little tiny*."

To a limited extent Navajo shares with English the emphasizing technique of vowel lengthening, but the pitch is already high, in Navajo. Thus, *'ahbíní* 'morning' takes the shape *'ahbíííní* 'very early in the morning' in *t'ah'ahbíííínígo ńdiish'na'* 'I got up very early in the morning'. *'Áłts'ísí* 'it is little' takes the shape *'áłts'íííísí yee'* with the meaning 'teeny-tiny,' as in *mósí yázhí 'áłts'íííísí yee' bik'íníyá* 'I found a little teeny kitten'.

Kóne' hółchxon can be translated as 'it stinks in here', but it cannot be modified to emphatic status by lengthening *hół-* to produce *hóoołchxon*. Emphasis must be supplied by the particle frame *doondó —— da*, as in *doondó' kóne' hółchxon da!* 'It really *stinnnks* in here!'

Some noun, verb, and other stems can be semantically intensified in Navajo by inserting heavily aspirated *x* or its voiced correspondent *gh* between the initial consonant and the vowel. Such intensification usually includes pejorative overtones. *chííl* 'snowstorm' contrasts with intensive *chxííl* 'awful snowstorm, blizzard'; *sǫ'* 'such-and-such star' contrasts with *sǫ'* 'star'; *'ałtso* 'all' contrasts with intensive *'atsxo* 'every bit, completely'; intensive *dzghąądi* 'right here' contrasts with *dząądi* 'here'; and intensive *jooshłxá* 'I hate him, detest him' contrasts with *jooshłá* 'I dislike him'.

Although *The Function and Signification of Certain Navaho Particles* was designed, nearly a half century ago, as an aid to teachers of English, it may still serve students of the Navajo language as an introduction to the system employed by that language to modify meaning—a system that is often subtle and as difficult for English speakers to master as the intonational patterns of English were for Navajo young people in the past.

[The original pamphlet follows.–Eds.]

The Function and Significance of Certain Navaho Particles

All languages possess intricate mechanisms for the purpose of shading and varying meaning, as well as for giving linguistic expression to attitudes on the part of the speaker. Specific words or groups of words may be used for this purpose; or voice intonation and emphatic stressing of certain words may subtly impart variations of meaning to the basic idea conveyed by the group of words themselves. The simple statement "this is my car" may acquire many shaded meanings not inherent in the component words, depending on the manner in which they are uttered. Tone of voice and general demeanor of the speaker may connote any of a number of emotional aspects: disgust, incredulity, surprise, anger and the like. Again, the meaning of the above sentence can be even more subtly altered by stressing one or another of the words. "*This* is my car," "this *is* my car," "this is *my* car," "this is my *car*," etc. do not convey precisely the same idea, even though the component words remain unchanged. So common is this use of relative loudness and intonation in English that when a person speaks in a monotone without using the techniques available for expressing his attitude and emotions we complain that his speech is "colorless" or "without expression."

In Navaho, many attitudes and emotions on the part of the speaker may be expressed or hinted at in manners analogous with or identical to those employed by English. Anger, excitement, fear, incredulity, disgust, etc. may be patent in the manner of speaking, while the relative importance of some ideas in comparison with others may be brought out by stress (relative loudness). However, on the whole, the Navaho language does not lend itself to employment of variable word and sentence intonation to the same degree and in the same manner as English.

In the first place, Navajo is a tone language, in the sense that its vocabulary is composed of elements in which the relatively fixed tonal quality of each constituent syllable figures as an integral part of the pronunciation thereof. As a generalization we can say that each syllable has a relatively fixed high or low tone (which may become a falling or rising tone under certain circumstances). In fact the matter of tone may often be the only distinguishing characteristic between two otherwise homophonous words. Compare, for example, *nílí*, you are: *nilį́*, he is; *yídlo*, you are laughing: *yidlo*, he is laughing; *'azéé'*, mouth: *'azee'*, medicine.[2]

Secondly, Navaho carefully distinguishes vowel length, fundamentally in the two categories of short and long. Relative vowel length often serves to distinguish meaning, as in *hólne'*, you are telling: *hóólne'*, that you might tell, *náhásdlį́į'*, (impersonal) it reverted to a former status: *nááhásdlį́į'*, (impersonal) it again became. In some instances Navaho employs the technique of prolonging a vowel by way of indicating exaggeration or intensification, in a manner similar to *li* of English "a li-i-i-ttle bit," but Navaho is more restricted in the use of this technique than English. Navaho examples are: *'átts'íísí yee'*, it is very small: *'átts'ííííísí yee'*, it is very very small; *t'iįhdígo*, a little bit, to a small degree: *t'įįįįhdígo*, a very very little bit; *t'ah 'ahbínígo*, while still morning: *t'ah 'ahbííííínígo*, while still very very early in the morning.

In Navaho an intensive or depreciative, often voicing an attitude of disgust, exasperation, or lack of esteem, is indicated by insertion of *x* or *gh* in the stem of the word. Thus *shash*, bear: *shxash*, confound bear; *dzạadi*, here: *dzghạadi*, right here, confound it! *jooshłá*, I hate him: *jooshłxá*, I hate him (with an intense hatred). In general, *x* follows a voiceless consonant, and *gh* follows a voiced consonant for this purpose (including *g*, *d*, *b*). In some instances such an intensive pronunciation is clumsy or impossible, and consequently is not used. The following list of words will exemplify this matter more fully:

> *'awéé'*, baby > ——
> *bijááad*, his leg > *bijghááad*
> *bik'ah*, its fat > ——
> *bilíí'*, his horse > *bilghíí'*
> *bimá*, his mother > —— (*bimá ni'*)
> *bitł'aa'*, his rump > *bitłx'aa'* (*bitłx'xaa'*)
> *bizhí*, his voice > *bizhghí*
> *chin*, filth > *chxin*
> *ch'ah*, hat > *chx'ah* (*chx'xah*)
> *dibé*, sheep > *dibghé*
> *diné*, man > —— (*diné ni'*)
> *dlǫ́ǫ́'*, prairie dog > *dlghǫ́ǫ́'*
> *dził*, mountain > *dzghił*
> *dił*, blood > *dghił*
> *gah*, rabbit > *gghah*
> *hosh*, cactus > *xosh* (*x* is exaggeratedly aspirate)
> *hooghan*, home > ——
> *ké*, shoe > *kxé*
> *łíí'*, horse > *łxíí'*
> *sǫ'*, star > *sxǫ'*
> *tsin*, wood > *tsxin*
> *ts'in*, bone > *tsx'in* (*tsx'xin*)
> *tłah*, ointment > *tłxah*
> *yaa'* > ——
> *zas*, snow > *zghas*

At best, translation from one language to another is a matter of *approximating* the meaning expressed by the original. The accuracy, or degree of approximation varies with the degree of cultural and linguistic difference or similarity between the two peoples. If the concept being translated is entirely foreign to the group into whose language it is being translated, then the rendition may turn out to be only a very rough approximation. Where the same concept is held in common by both groups, the translation may be very accurate. If two groups are closely related culturally and linguistically, the difficulties attendant upon translation are minimized.

The same factors are involved in the matter of learning a new language. We learn French with relative ease because we hold so much in common, culturally and linguistically, with the French people. On the other hand we learn Chinese or Navaho with difficulty because we have so little in common with these peoples. By the same token it is hard for them to learn our language.

Even after we learn enough to get along well in a foreign language, we often have great difficulty in mastering the mechanisms employed by that language to express the more subtle shadings and gradations of meaning. We commonly have a feeling of frustration at being unable to express ourselves satisfactorily in the new language, and we may not clearly understand many things which are said to us, because we employ different techniques in our native tongue for varying meaning, and are hard put to discover corresponding mechanisms as they exist in the new language. This is especially true if we are acquainted only with a standard literary form, and are without experience in the colloquial form of the foreign tongue. Where a literary form of the language exists, it is always at variance with the everyday speech of the people, and even a considerable knowledge of one does not completely open the door to the other. The literary form often employs terms and syntax not used in colloquial speech, and the language of everyday life is often characterized by use of words and expressions which purists attempt to disown. Our dictionaries list many everyday terms and expressions as "colloquialisms" or "slang." Many more are not even listed, and in fact some of them are fads which go from our language as suddenly as they entered it. Into this latter category fits the terminology we refer to as "jive talk." However, for the purely practical purpose of learning a new language in order to make more effective one's associations with the people who speak it, our experience must be broad enough to include the colloquial forms.

The colloquial forms of all languages are rich in expressions which either replace a less common term, or which more or less subtly vary its meaning. Often the group of words which compose an "idiomatic expression" lose to all intents and purposes their customary individual meanings; the complex as a whole renders a certain meaning, but the component parts thereof do not signify exactly what they would appear to mean. Thus we say "Take off!" or "Beat it!" to mean "Go away," without reference to the literal meaning of "taking off" or "beating" something. Similarly, we say "He had a close shave," with a meaning entirely different from the literal one. The Navaho say "*Nihá ha'íídiz*, he accomplished something for us;" but the literal meaning is, "He twisted something (rabbits) out for us." (Reference is to a mode of hunting rabbits by twisting a rough-pointed stick into their fur and hide, and then pulling them from their holes.)

Again, a particle or a group of particles may be used to render a meaning or a shade of meaning so subtle that it escapes the novice entirely. Or peculiar voice pitch, word and sentence intonation, and other such variations in utterance may characterize a given language. It is relatively easy to master those elements of a foreign language which are analogous or similar to familiar corresponding features of one's native tongue, and it is comparatively easy to gain understanding of the usual name and action words; but a full understanding of such elusive aspects of the foreign language as sentence tone, seemingly nonsense particles, extended word meanings (idiomatic expressions) and the like comes only with much study and experience in the new language. Yet, a functional knowledge of all these elements is requisite for a satisfactory practical knowledge of a language. Without such knowledge one is unable to convey his thoughts, attitudes and emotions in the manner and with the degree of completeness to which he is accustomed when speaking his native tongue. And there is no frustration more acute than the desire to express oneself attended by an inability to discover the words or mechanisms wherewith to satisfy that desire.

Many of our Indian children come to school from homes where English is not spoken. They are faced with the necessity of learning to use a new form of speech which is linked with a set of foreign cultural institutions and a different way of thinking, doing and behaving. To a great extent these children find themselves studying the foreign language and culture subjectively, for they are still within their native environment. They are urged, and in former times were forced, to use English as a medium for conveying their thoughts. Yet, their knowledge of English gained in the classroom is not adequate to meet their everyday needs on the playground and in other associations with their class-mates. The result is that they use the native language for satisfying conversation with fellow-tribesmen, and often remain taciturn or confine themselves to brief exchanges in English with whites.

Only colloquial English can meet their needs with regard to expression in that language. The language of the textbooks and of the classroom is necessary, but it is not per se complete. Anyone who attempts to carry on an informal conversation in Spanish after a few years of formal study in a classroom will understand the reasons for which the Navaho school child is reticent about using or attempting to use English for other than formal needs. English simply does not satisfy his needs for expression. It cannot hope to satisfy them until he has a reasonably full mastery of the colloquial forms of the language. This includes not only the colloquial terminology, but all the peculiar uses to which we put stress, voice pitch, word and sentence intonation and the like. In many instances Navahos who have spoken English for years belie their ignorance of many of these features that characterize spoken colloquial English by their inability to supply corresponding forms for the English in terms of their own language, or adequately translate certain expressions from their own language into English. Their inability is often due to limited knowledge of English, rather than to any actual lack in one or the other language of a means for expression.

The school teacher can accomplish much by way of helping children to gain a useful, satisfactory knowledge of English by herself analyzing the differences that distinguish the two languages, and thus discovering the problems the child faces in gaining an adequate knowledge of our language. The child's willingness to use English will depend upon the degree to which it satisfies his needs for expression; this factor is dependent largely upon practice and experience in spoken English, in association with native speakers, but by understanding something of the linguistic problems involved, the teacher can evolve many time saving devices which will make her teaching more rapid and more effec-tive.

The present pamphlet, dealing with certain Navaho particles, will be of use to the teacher in discovering some of the linguistic problems involved in teaching English to Navahos. Other publications, such as THE NAVAHO LANGUAGE, can provide the basic knowledge of structure, morphology and syntax of Navaho needed as a foundation for the formulation of efficient teaching techniques.

It is our plan to publish also a vocabulary and phrase-book of colloquial Na-vajo expressions with their corresponding English meanings, as well as a hand book to acquaint teachers with the problems involved in teaching the sounds of English to Navajo beginners. Even a small knowledge of "how it is said or done by Navajos" can be a valuable tool to the white teacher in evolving a more rapid and effective way of teaching English words and their usages.

In the present pamphlet we make free use of colloquial English wherever necessary to render the best possible equivalent for the Navajo form.

Robert W. Young
Specialist in Indian Languages

'áłt'ąą, after all; in spite of; unfortunately; "darned if"; how come? (The latter in conjunction with *ha'át'éegoshą',* why?)

'Áłt'ąą yoodláá', he drank it **after all** (As when a person had previously decided not to drink it, but for one reason or another drank it anyway.)

Ha'át'éegoshą' 'áłt'ąą dah diniyá, How come you're going **after all**? (As when a person had previously decided against going, but subsequently changed his plans.)

Gah t'áadoo ła' yiissiihí t'óó 'ahayóí niséłtseed, dóó mą'ii yííníiłdongo 'áłt'ąą sésiih, I killed a lot of rabbits without missing a one, and **in spite of that** when I shot at a coyote I missed it (or colloquially, "---- and when I shot at a coyote **darned if** I didn't miss it.").

Shiwoo' diniihgo biniinaa 'azee'ííł'íní' bich'į' déyáá ńt'éé' 'áłt'ąą shiwoo' neezk'e', I was going to go to the doctor for my toothache, but "**darned if**" my tooth didn't stop aching.

Shíká 'adoolwoł nisin ńt'éé' 'áłt'ąą t'áadoo níyáa da, I wanted him to help me, but **unfortunately** he did not come.

Ha'át'éegoshą' 'áłt'ąą doo yáníłti' da, **How come** you stopped talking? (As when a braggart suddenly stops talking upon the appearance of someone who knows him.)

-'as, an enclitic attached to a noun or verb to connote a feeling of scornful disbelief. English usually achieves the some shade of meaning by pronouncing the word loudly with a peculiar intonation, and often with lengthening of one or more of the vowels.

Gah'as, A ra-a-a-bbit!! (As when one tells a long tale concerning his hunting exploits, leading his listeners to assume that he killed big game; but they exclaim in scorn when it develops that he bagged only a paltry rabbit.)

Deesk'aaz'as, Co-o-o-ld!! (What do you mean "cold?")

'áyąą; 'áyaańda, no wonder.

'Ayóígo deesk'aaz, 'áyąą (or 'áyaańda) dinistsiz, It's cold, **no wonder** I'm shivering.

Hoozdo hoolyéedi deesdoi sha'shin. 'Áyaańda (or 'áyąą) diné bi'éétsoh t'áá gééd ndaakai, I guess it's warm in Phoenix. **No wonder** people go around without their coats.

Shitł'aajį'éé' 'íídláád lá, 'áyaańda ('áyąą) shaa yídloh, I see that (V. *lá*) my trousers are torn, **no wonder** you're laughing at me.

In conjunction with interrogative enclitic *-shą' ('áyaańdashą')* the meaning is **why? what makes you think so?**

Tséhootsooídi yas t'óó 'ahayóí nahalin, There seems to be lots of snow at Fort Defiance. *'Áyaańdashą',* What makes you think so?

Díí nástáán 'ayóo ndaaz nahalin, This log looks awfully heavy. *'Ayańdashą',* Why? What makes you think so?

'azhą̖ —— ndi, This combination of particles renders the meanings **even though; no matter how.**

'Azhą́ shibéeso hólǫ́ǫ ndi t'áadoo ła' baa nínil da, **Even though** I had money, I didn't give him any.

'Azhą́ nízaajį' ndi 'ałchin, He can smell, **no matter how** far (away he may be).

'azháánee' —— *ndi,* (V. *-nee'*).

---

ch'į́įgóó; ch'ínígóó, everything possible (but in vain). (Roughly a combination of the concepts expressed individually by *łą́ą́góó,* in many ways, many things, plus *ch'ééh,* in vain.)

Ch'į́įgóó baa ntséskees, It's **no use** for me to think about it (I am considering it from every angle but without result).

Ch'į́įgóó ch'ééh tádííyá, I went everywhere (looking for something) **but no luck**.

Diné 'ániid daaztsánígíí t'áá 'íiyisíí t'áá ch'į́įgóó ch'ééh bá 'áhóót'įįd, **Everything possible** was done (to save) the man that just died; they did **everything they could** to save the man that just died (but everything they did was to no avail).

Chidí sits'ą́ą' hashtł'ish yiih yilwodgo t'áá ch'į́įgóó ch'ééh 'íít'įįd, I did **everything possible** to get my car out of the mud (but in vain).

---

da, an enclitic particle with several connotations, as illustrated below:

a) as a conjunction with the meaning **as, such as**, often joining a series of nouns which exemplify a preceding statement. (In this instance compare the usage of *da* as a distributive prefix on verbs.)

Nihisiláago t'áadoo le'é t'óó 'ahayóígo deinízin, jó 'éí bee'eldǫǫh da, bee'eldǫǫh bikǫ' da, 'ée' da, dóó bee na'anishí (da), Our soldiers need many things, **such** as guns, ammunition, clothing and implements.

Dini' t'áá bíhólníhígíí' 'ádá ndiiltsił, tsídii da, We will kill some game for ourselves, **such as** birds.

b) expresses uncertainty and indefiniteness, as English **some** in sometime, someplace.

Hahgoda 'índa nich'į' niná'deeshdléél, I'll pay you back **some**time.

Háájída shį́į́ shił dooldlosh, I'll go **some**where (on horseback at a trot).

Háadida shį́į́ náá'ahiidiiltséél, We'll see each other again **some**place.

'Azee'ííł'íní yáadida jéí 'ádįįh bits'ą́ą́dóó hólónígíí nii' hóló shiłní, The doctor told me I have **some**thing awful in me that causes tuberculosis.

Bighandi yáadida yíyą́ą', I had **some** awful (nasty) things to eat at his house. *Jó 'éí ch'osh ditł'ooí dóó t'áadoo le'é díigi 'át'éego,* Caterpillars and things like that.

c) used in conjunction with the interrogative enclitic *-shą',* the meaning is similar to English (**I**) **wonder**.

Háadidashą' 'ásht'į́, **I wonder** where I am?

Yáadidashą' 'át'į́, **I wonder** who he is?

Háájídashą' shich'ah silį́į', **I wonder** what became of my hat? (i.e. I wonder which direction my hat (became) went?)

Hastiin sání yę́ędashą' háájí silį́į', **I wonder** what became of the old man?

d) used in conjunction with proclitic *doo* to negativize.

Doo yá'áshǫǫ da, It is **no** good.
Doo shił yá'át'éeh da, I do **not** like it.

---

daashą' 'át'é (ibid *haashą' 'át'é*),   an expression translatable as **why sure; of course**.

Nikiníyáá łą́ą, daashą' 'át'é, **Why sure** I'm going home. (As one exclaims when another person refuses to believe that one actually intends to do as he says.)

Daashą' 'át'é 'áłtsé 'íyą́, **Why sure**, (go ahead and) eat first.

Ni'niidlíísh, Are you cold? *Daashą' 'át'é deesk'aaz ndó'*, **Of course**, because it (weather) is cold.

Dooládó' nilį́į́' neesk'ah da, My but you have a nice fat horse. *Daashą' 'át'é*, **Of course** (what did you expect?).

---

daashin,   a particle serving to indicate that one is uncertain in his recollection, and is asking for confirmation or correction in regard to that which he is trying to recall. It corresponds to the English **was it, wasn't it**, in usages such as the following:

Shash Bitoodi daashin niiłtsą́ą ni', **Wasn't it** at Fort Wingate that I saw you?

Dini' daashin daolyé, **Was it** *dini'* that you called them?

Dini' game daashin 'óolyé, **Was it** "game" (animals) that *dini'* means?

-dą́ą́',   an enclitic of variable meaning. (See also *ládą́ą́'*; *yę́ędą́ą́'*.)

   a) translatable as **ago, last**, when attached to nouns, or to verbs used in a nominal sense.

Naaki nááhaiídą́ą́', Two years **ago**.

Shį́įdą́ą́', **last** summer.

   b) attached to perfective or neuter verb forms the meaning is **if, in case**.

Dichin sínílį́į́'dą́ą́' dibé sits'ą́ą́' díílghał, **If** you get hungry, eat one of my sheep (lit. eat a sheep away from me).

Nił łikandą́ą́' baa hólne', **If** you like it, say so.

Béeso nee 'ásdįįdą́ą́' ła' na'deeshnił, **In case** you run out of money I'll lend you some.

---

de',   a proclitic meaning **here, hither**; used only with commands.

De' ninááh, Come **here**!

Ła' de' nohhááh, One of you (two or more) come **here**!

De' ní'aah, Bring it **here**! (a single roundish object)

---

doo,   a proclitic used in conjunction with *da* or *-góó* to negativize. (See *da; -góó*.)

---

dooládó' —— da lá,   a combination of particles translating the English (**it**) **certainly is; my but it is**, etc.

Dooládó' ndaaz da lá, It **certainly is** heavy!

Dooládó' deesk'aaz da lá, **My but it's** cold!

---

doondó' —— *da*; *doo ndi* —— *da*; *doondó' ndi* —— *da*,   these particle combinations translate **not even, won't even.**

Doondó' daatsaah noolin da, He doesn't **even** look sick (let alone act sick). (Note the peculiar intonation of the word "look" in the English version.)

'Awéé' doondó' **(or** *doo ndi*) *yidlóoh da,* The baby isn't **even** cold (much less suffering in any other way).

Doo 'adlą́ą da dóó doo 'asdzání yaa yinít'į́į da dóó doondó' ndi ná'áłt'oh da, He doesn't drink, he doesn't go with girls, and he doesn't **even** smoke.

---

doochǫǫł,   **repulsive; ridiculous.**

Hastiintsoh t'áá 'áłahji' bi'éé' yik'íhidizheeh łeh, 'áko doochǫǫł 'ájít'į́ dooleeł daniidzin, Mr. Tso is always spitting on his clothing, and we think **it's ridiculous!**

Doochǫǫł 'át'éego ha'éé' bik'íhizhdizheeh dooleeł, **It's ridiculous** for one to spit on his clothing.

Doochǫǫł 'át'éego 'ák'íhidíjeeh, **It's ridiculous** the way you spit on yourself.

---

doosha' —— *lá,*   a combination of negativizing proclitic *doo,* interrogative enclitic *-sha',* and enclitic *lá,* connoting an attitude of determination, and translating English **I'll see that; I'll make sure that; I'll take care that,** etc.

Doosha' gah t'áá gééd náshdááh lá, **I'll see to it that** I do not return without a rabbit.

Doosha' niiłhash lá, **I'll see that** it doesn't bite you.

Doosha' 'ákónáánásh'nééh lá, **I'll see that** I do not do that again.

---

doosha' léi' —— *lá,*   similar in meaning to *doosha'* —— *lá.*

Doosha' léi' 'ashkii tó biiłhéé lá, I'll **see to it that** the boy does not drown.

Doosha' léi' t'áadoo 'awáalya yah 'aninááh lá, I'll **see to it that** you do not go to jail.

Doosha' léi' 'awáalya yah 'aninááh lá, **I'll see to it that you** go to jail.

---

doo t'áá k'ad —— *da,*   this combination is used with perfective mode forms of the verb to give the meaning **(I) do not want to.**

Doo t'áá k'ad siláago sélį́į' da, **I do not want to** be a soldier.

Doo t'áá k'ad naa ní'ą́ą da, **I do not want to** give it (a single roundish object) to you.

Doo t'áá k'ad 'ákǫ́ǫ́ niséyáa da, **I do not want to** go there.

---

doo yéé —— *-í,*   this combination of the proclitics *doo* and *yéé* with the relative enclitic *-í,* connotes admonishment or threat. It is much like the English expression, "it is a good thing for (you) that."

Doo yéé niiłtsání, **It's a good thing (for you) that** I didn't see you (you're just lucky that I didn't see you).

Doo yéé shaa yánĩłti'go ndiséts'ą́'í. Niyéłhį́į́ shį́į́ doo ńt'éé', **It's a good thing** I didn't hear you talking about me. I probably would have killed you.

Doo yéé shináát 'ádíníní, You hadn't better let me hear you say that! I wish you had said that in my presence.

Shaa nánít'į́ jiní; doo yéé 'íídą́ą́' 'ákwe'é naasháhí, I heard that you were talking about me (lit. it is said that you were bothering me); **it's a good thing for you that** I wasn't there at the time.

---

doozáagi, how long? how much longer? This particle expresses an attitude of impatience.

Doozáagi 'íłhosh, **How long** are you going to sleep? (Come on, get up!)

Doozáagi 'ahíł hołne', **How much longer** are you two going to talk? You two certainly can talk a long time!

---

doozhǫǫgo, a decent, a half way decent.

Doozhǫǫgo shikin hólǫ́ǫ laanaa, I wish I had **a decent** home.

Doozhǫǫgo yee dahináa dooleeł, They will make **a decent** living on it (by means of it).

Doozhǫǫgo da'íítta'ígíí, Those who have **a decent** education.

---

dó' —— -ísh łí, a combination of the enclitic *dó',* also, interrogative enclitic *-ísh,* and enclitic *łí,* serving to express an attitude of uncertainty, wonder or apparent probability.

Na'nízhoozhígóó dó' díníyáásh łí, **Could it be that** you're going to Gallup? **Do you happen to** be going to Gallup?

Béeso dó' nee 'ádinísh łí, **Could it be that** you are out of money? Say, you're not broke, are you?

Ndaaz dó'ísh łí, **Could it** be heavy? **I wonder if** it is heavy (as one might say before trying to lift it)?

Shik'éí dó' ńlį́įsh łí, You **might (could)** be one of my relatives.

-ee, (possibly related to the postposition *-ee,* by means of), adverbializes certain nouns, verbs and particles.

Ńlóhee hashniih, I know the Hail-**way** (ceremony).

Díí hastiin béshee haniih, This man knows the Flint-**way**.

* Tąądee yigááł,* He is walking slow**ly** along.

T'áá na'ńle'ee naalnish, He works slopp**ily**; he does sloppy work (throwing things about in disorder).

T'óó na'ńle'ee yigááł, He is walking careless**ly** along; he is bungling along (knocking things aside without caring).

Dibé t'áá ła' bizhi'ee kingóó dadíníilkał, Let's throw all the sheep together in one group and drive them to market (*bizhi',* their body; *t'áá ła' bizhi'ee,* in a single body).

Naabeehó dine'é t'áá ła' bizhi'ee daazlį́į́', The Navaho tribe united (became single-bodied**ly**).

T'áá 'ádíláahee nahałtin, It's raining torrents (it's raining in a rough manner. Cp. *she'ádíláah,* I'm full of mischief.).

T'áá 'ádíláahee shich'į' haadzíí', He spoke gruff**ly** to me.

Hashkéhee k'ehgo nihich'į' yáálti', He really bawled us out; he really told us off (he spoke to us in a mean, angry manner).

---

ga', an enclitic particle serving to emphasize and particularize a noun or pronoun to which it is attached. In spoken English we express this by word stress and voice pitch, and in written English it is commonly represented by italic type.

'Éí ga' shí 'ásht'į́, **I'm** the one who did it (not he or someone else).

Díí ga' łį́į' nizhóní, **This one** is the pretty horse; **this** is the prettiest horse (not one of the others).

Shí ga', No, it is **I**; no, **I'm** the one (as when one person states that he is going to do a certain thing and another person disagrees, saying emphatically that **he** is the one who will do it).

Nda ga', **No-o-o! Emphatically no.** (Often heard as *ndagha'*, or *dagha'* in rapid speech.)

-gi, this enclitic is essentially a locative, meaning **at** in the sense of a general, less closely defined area than *-di*, also translating **at** (but in the sense of a specific, closely defined place). When *-gi* is attached to a 3rd person indefinite verb form (usually a continuative or durative imperfective) the meaning is **the art of, how to**. Both usages are exemplified below.

Tsintahgi 'ałhosh, He is sleeping in (**at**) the forest.

Europe hoolyéegi, In Europe; **at** the place called Europe.

Kwe'é sézínígi, Here **where** I am standing; here **at** the place where I am standing.

'Atł'óogi yínashiniłtin, She is teaching me **how to** weave.

Naabeehó bizaad bee yáti'gi yínashineeztą́ą́', He taught me **how to** speak Navaho.

Na'ałkǫǫ'gi bínandínéeshtįįł, I will teach you **how to** swim.

-gi 'át'éego, this combination of enclitic *-gi* and the participialized verb *'át'é*, it is, is translatable as **like** with reference, not to appearance (in which case *nahalin, noolin*, etc. are used), but to likeness or sameness in quality, action, character, etc. The following examples will illustrate.

Shígi 'át'éego doo bił łikan da, **Like** me, he doesn't like it.

T'áá shí yáshti'ígi 'át'éego yáłti', He talks just **like I** do.

Nigi 'át'éego shił hóyéé', I'm lazy **like** you are.

-gile' 'át'é, a combination used with forms of the optative to give the meaning **easily, without effort**.

Kwii dázh'dółtł'ingo tó dah siyį́įgo 'ájóléhégile' 'át'é, one could **easily** make a lake here by damming it up.

Díí bee'eldǫǫh bee bįįh jiyółhéłígile' 'át'é, one could **easily** kill a deer with this gun.

-góó, attached to nouns translates **to, toward** (with reference to motion to a place). Thus:

'Ólta'góó déyá, I am on my way **to** school.

Na'nízhoozhígóó diit'ash, Let's go **to** Gallup (we dual).

When the place to which *-góó* refers is a general instead of a specific place, the translation is usually **along, in**, and in some instances *-góó* is not translated in English. Below several examples are given, each contrasted with a similar example in which *-góó* is replaced by *-gi* in order to provide a fuller understanding of the former.

Tábąąhgi sézį́, I am standing on (**at**) the shore (water's edge).

Tábąąhgóó yisháál̥, I am walking **along** the shore.

Yikáa'gi dah sitį́, He is lying on (**at upon**) it.

Yikáá'góó naat'a', He is flying about (**in the general area**) above it.

Dził̥gi shighan, My home is **at** the mountain.

Dził̥góó naashá, I am walking about **in** the mountains.

Naadą́ą́' bitahgi sézį́, I am standing (**at**) amongst the corn.

Naadą́ą́' bitahgóó naashá, I am walking about (**along**) among the corn.

When *-góó* is attached to a verb nominalized by relatival enclitic *-í*, the resultant form is translatable as **to where**. The other locative enclitics, *-gi* and *-di*, can be similarly used, translating **at the place where**.

Deeyáhágóó doo shił bééhózin da, I do not know (**to**) where he is going.

Kéyah Bolivia wolyéhégi, **At the place** called Bolivia; in the country called Bolivia.

The particle *góó* can replace negativizing enclitic *da* and adverbializing enclitic *-go* in such usages as:

Doo'ákót'éégóó 'áłyaa or *doo'ákót'éego 'áłyaa da*, It was not made correctly.

'Éí kéyah doo bikáá' 'anit'ą́ą́góó (or *'anit'ą́ą dago*) *biniinaa Naabeehó t'áá bíni'ídi 'át'éego 'ádayiilaa lá*, Because things will not grow (mature) on that land I found that the Navahos just let it lie (without using it).

Ha'asídí nihééhósin léi' doo nihaa ná'áhodíłt'į́įgóó t'óó nihił ch'í'ní'éél, Inasmuch as the watchman knew us, we sailed out without his paying any attention to us.

(See also *t'áadoo ——— -góó*)

-go,   this enclitic is widely used to participialize and adverbialize. Its uses are sketched below.

1. *-go* adverbializes other particles:

'Éí beego nááś diikah, With that ('that withly') we (pl.) will go ahead (progress).

Diné t'óó 'ahayóígo nabi'diztseed, Many people were killed.

2. *-go* participializes verbs, rendering such meanings as **when, as, while**.

'Atiingóó yisháałgo shiiłtsą́, He saw me (**while** I was) walking along the road.

Mą'ii hastiin yiyiiłtsą́ągo dah diilwod, **When** the coyote saw the man it started to run.

-go 'át'é,   a combination used with future tense forms of the verb to denote indubitable capacity of the subject to perform the act denoted by the verb.

Díí tsé dah dideesh'áałgo 'át'é, I **can** lift this rock.

Nik'ehdideeshdleełgo 'át'é, I **can** whip you (in a fight).

Nahodooltį́įłgo 'át'é, It is going to rain (for certain).

In the above combination *haz'ą́* can replace *'át'é* without altering the meaning.

Nik'ehdideeshdleełgo haz'ą́, I **can** whip you (in a fight).

Nahodooltį́įłgo haz'ą́, It is going to rain (for sure).

-go da, a combination roughly equivalent in meaning to English **about, around**, but with the added connotation that the decision is up to the person addressed.

Łį́į́' táa'go da shaa nínííł, Give me **about** three horses (the exact number is up to you).

'I'íí'ą́ago da shaa díínááł, Come to see me **around** sundown.

-go da 'át'é, this combination is similar to that described above, except that the enclitic *da* modifies the meaning to express a potential **might**, instead of positive **can**.

Na'nízhoozhígóó deesháałgo da 'át'é, I **might** (possibly) go to Gallup.

T'áadoo déyáa da nahodooltį́įłgo da 'át'é nisingo biniinaa, I did not go because I thought it **might** rain.

Shizhé'é 'át'įigo da 'át'é nisin, I thought it **might** be my father.

(*Sha'shin nisin* is practically synonymous with *-go da 'át'é*.)

---

haalá t'áá 'éiyá —— ni', a combination usually translatable as **now let's see**. It indicates that one is trying to recall something momentarily forgotten. The examples will serve to illustrate.

Haalá t'áá 'éiyá yinílyée ni', **Now let's see**, what was your name? (As when one is confronted by a person whose name he should be able to recall, but which has slipped his mind.)

Haalá t'áá 'éiyá jiił'įih ni', **Now let's see**, what does one do? (As when a person 'gets stuck' on a machine which he has momentarily forgotten how to operate.)

Haalá t'áá 'éiyá yit'ée ni', **Now let's see**, how did it look? (One cannot remember its appearance offhand, although he recalls having seen it previously.)

---

haahláyéé, a combination the force of which is similar to that described for *doo yéé —— -í*. It connotes an attitude of admonishment or threat. It will be noted that the 3a. form of the verb (i.e., that form with 3a. personal pronominal *ji-* as subject) is required, even though the admonition may be addressed to a 2nd person. *Yéé* may be repeated at the end of the sentence or omitted, as we have indicated by (*yéé*).

Haahláyéé ch'įíghááh (*yéé*), **Don't dare** come out.

Haahláyéé 'ajiiłhosh (*yéé*), **Don't dare** go to sleep.

Haahláyéé 'iijiłhash (*yéé*), **Don't dare** bite.

---

haashą' 'át'é, (ibid *daashą' 'át'é*). *Daa* and *haa* are synonymous.

---

hágoónee',   a combination of *hágo* and *-nee'* (V. *-nee'*) translatable as **well, well all right then** in most usages.

Hágoónee' t'áá 'ákódí shahane', **Well**, that's all I have to say (as in closing a letter).

Hágoónee', k'ad nikiníyá, **Well**, I'm going home now.

Hágoónee', béeso shaa ní'aah, **Well all right then**, give me a dollar (a person says as he finally gives in to another).

Hágoónee' shichei, **Well good-bye** grandfather (one says in taking leave).

---

hanii,   a particle that denotes contrariness to fact.

Doo hanii kingóó díníyáa da nisin, I thought that you weren't going to town (but I see that you are).

Doo hanii kót'éego'ánfléeh da, Why don't you do it this way? (Instead of the way you are actually doing it.)

Shí hanii 'ásht'{, I didn't do it (in denial to a direct accusation).

Shí hanii t'éiyá Bilagáana bizaad shił bééhózin, I'm not the only one who knows English (despite appearances to the contrary).

Bá naashnishígíí bighangóó shił nát'áazhgo háájí da bił 'ałnáá'á'ołgo hanii 'ákǫ́ǫ́ shił 'ałnánát'ash dooleeł niizį́į́', When the man I work for brought me home with him, I (mistakenly) thought that he would take me with him in his boat wherever he went (but he did not). (in this example *niizį́į́'* translates I thought, and *hanii* indicates that what I thought was contrary to fact.)

Nihił ha'az'éelgo tó haashį́į́ yit'éego nihik'i dziiłhaalgo t'áá hanii 'ádíji' 'íłį́į́ ńt'éé', When our boat reached shore a great wave struck us, and I thought that was the end (but I survived). (*'íłį́į́ ńt'éé'*, it was thought; it appeared that.)

Ni hanii, Not you. (As when a number of individuals are getting into a car at my invitation, but one individual whom I had not included tries to enter also.)

Shighandi nánísdzáago doo naagháhí da lá, 'áádóó sha'áłchíní yę́ę hanii 'ałtso daneezná niizį́į́', When I returned home I found no one there, and I thought my family must all have died (but discovered that they had not at a later date).

Díí jí hanii nahodoołtį́įł 'íłį́į́ (or *hwiinidzin*) *ńt'éé'*, It looked like (i.e. it was thought that it would) rain today (but it did not).

Shibéeso hanii hólǫ́ǫ nisin ńt'éé', I thought I had some money (but discovered that I had none).

-ii',   an enclitic that functions as a conjunction between two verbs that express closely related or consecutive actions. (*-ii'* is also attached to *dooda*, no, to give *doodaii'*, or, or else.)

Yah 'ííyáii'neezdá, He came in **and** sat down.

Tsin ła' néidiitą́ii' náshidííłhaal, He picked up a stick **and** hit me.

-ísh,   (the vowel of *-ísh* commonly assimilates to the final vowel of the word to which it is attached.) An interrogative enclitic, usually attached to the first word in an interrogative phrase, clause or sentence. It may be used in conjunction with proclitic interrogative *da'*, which serves to introduce a question, though *da'* is not necessary in most instances. The function of *-ísh* is to indicate a question. Cp. *-shą'*, *-sh*.

(*Da'*) *dichiní sh nílį́*, Are you hungry?

(*Da'*) *Dinétsohí sh yiní lyé*, Is your name *Dinétsoh*?

'Adą́ą́dą́ą́'ash doo Na'nízhoozhígóó nisíníyáa da, Didn't you go to Gallup yesterday?

Doósh nił yá'át'éeh da, Don't you like it? (*doo + í sh > doósh*)

-jį',   with nouns and pronouns this enclitic is used with the force of English **up to, as far as**. With verbs it translates **until**.

Kinjį' niníyá, I went **as far as** the house.

Nánísdzáajį' shidibé shá baa 'áhólyą́, Take care of my sheep for me **until** I return (i.e. up to I have returned).

Néíní dzáajį' ná yíní shtą' dooleeł, I will hold it for you **until** you return.

---

jó,   a proclitic particle translatable as **as I now know, I see that, well, because you see**, etc.

Kingóó shił díí'ash, Take me to town. *Doo bihónéedzą́ą́ da*, It is impossible. *Ha'át'éegoshą'*, Why? *Jó shichidí bikee' deesdǫǫh*, **Well, because** my tire is flat.

Béeso sha'díínił, Lend me some money. *Hahgoshą'*, When? *Jó k'ad*, **Well,** right now.

Jó nił bééhózingo Bilagáana bizaad doo diists'a' da, **Well, as you know,** I cannot understand English.

---

lá,   this enclitic denotes primarily that the idea which it modifies has just occurred to one, just been discovered, or just been brought to one's attention. It is often translatable by English phrases such as **I find, I found, I discovered**. In other instances English uses voice pitch and word stress of a particular type to express *lá*.

Díí tsé 'át'éé lá, This (I find) is a **rock**. (One just discovers the fact and exclaims after having thought it to be something else.)

Shíká nahadláá lá, **I found out** that there was a ceremony going on for me (i.e. after me, in the sense that the ceremony was designed to bring me back. Cp. *Shik'i nahadlá*, there is a ceremony going on over me.)

'Atiingi chidí léi' yiiłtsą́ą́ lá, **It just occurs to me** that I saw some car (i.e. one I cannot identify) on the road. (V. *léi'*.)

T'áá 'aaníí shibéeso t'óó 'ahayóí ndí t'áadoo biniiyéhé da lá, Actually I had a lot of money, but I **found it to be** useless (because I had no place to spend it).

Dichin shi'niiłhį́, I'm hungry. *Shí dó' lá*, (I find that) I am too. (It just occurs to one that he also is hungry, but he had not thought of the fact until the other person mentioned it.)

Jó t'áá bééhózíní léi' 'ádíníí lá, There was nothing to (solving) that—what do you mean **ha-a-rd**?

Jó t'áá bééhózíní lá, (I found) that was easily solved; I found that to be easy; there was nothing to that.

Lá often replaces interrogative enclitic *-shą'* to ask questions relating to who, what, why, where, when, which way, etc. In this usage *lá* often makes the question less direct, and indicates a desire for the other person's opinion in the matter.

'Áádóó 'aláaji' sizínígíí háajigo lá da'diil'oł níigo shaa níyá, And the (ship's) captain came up to me saying 'which direction shall we sail?' (i.e. which direction do you think we should sail?)

Háajigo lá yá'áhoot'ééh lá níigo tsinaa'eeł yíchxǫ'go tó biih yílį́į́ léi', He said 'I wonder which direction is best' inasmuch as the boat was wrecked and water was leaking in.

Háí lá 'ánít'į́, Who are you? (One asks thus in a milder, less blunt manner than would be the case with interrogative -shą'.)

Ha'át'íí lá hádíní'į́į́', What are you looking for? What the heck are you looking for?

Háadi lá 'ádeiit'į́, Where are we (dist. pl.)?

Díkwíí lá ninááhai, How old are you?

Háágóó lá, Where to? (i.e. where are you going?)

---

ládą́ą́',   a combination of the enclitics lá and dą́ą́', translatable as **if, in case, in the event that**. (V. dą́ą́').

T'áadoo le'é biniinaa nétł'ah ládą́ą́' doo 'áadi deesháał da, **In case** I am held back by something I will not get there.

Nahałtin ládą́ą́' doo deesháał da, **In the event that** it rains, I will not go.

Doo nahałtin ládą́ą́' deeshááł, **If** (provided that) it doesn't rain I will go. (Note that negative enclitic da is omitted).

---

lágo,   there are two distinct particles, one composed of lá plus adverbializing -go, the other an optative (negative) particle.

1. lá + go:

Dibé t'áá daaztsą́ą́ lágo bik'íníyá, I found that the sheep was already dead when I came upon it.

Lágo with future tense or imperfective mode forms of the verb translates **before**.

Poland neeznáá yiską́ągo bik'ehodidoodleeł lágo Russia bisiláago łahdę́ę'go Poland yiih yiizą́, Ten days **before** Poland was conquered Russian soldiers invaded Poland from the other side. (Lit. when in ten days Poland will be conquered Russia's soldiers moved into Poland from the other side.)

Neeznáá yiską́ągo na'akai dooleeł lágo hataałii bi'niitsą́, Ten days **before** the ceremony (yé'ii bichei) the medicine man got sick. (Lit. when in ten days there will be a ceremony the . . . .)

Łį́į́' táá' yiską́ągo dadootsaał lágo bí'diiłid, I branded the horse three days **before** it died. (Lit. when in three days the horse will die I branded it.)

Chidí k'adę́ę yichxǫǫh lágo nahátnii', I bought a car just about the time (just before) it fell to pieces. (Lit. when the car is about to go to pieces I bought it.)

2. Lágo with forms of the optative mode expresses a negative wish or desire, which may also function as a negative imperative (remote rather than immediative in force).

Haóódziih lágo, Would that you do not speak; would that you say nothing; say nothing.

Nahółtą́ą́' lágo, Would that it doesn't rain; I hope it will not rain (at some in the future).

lá jiní, an expression used largely by children, and roughly equivalent to **let's play like, let's pretend that.**

Shash niidlį́į́ lá jiní, **Let's play like** we're bears, (Lit. we find that we are bears it is said.)

Kin góne' siikéé lá jiní, **Let's pretend that** we're in the house; we'll **play like** we (dual) are (sitting) in the house. (Lit. we find that we are sitting in the house it is said.)

---

lą́ą, an emphatic enclitic, usually expressed by stress or peculiar intonation in English.

Hastiin Nééz lą́ą hádadíníit'į́į́', We (dist. pl.) are looking for Mr. Nez (not for someone else).

Bįįh lą́ą haashzheeh, I am **deer**-hunting (not hunting something else).

Daashą' 'át'é yah 'adiikah lą́ą, Why sure, we (pl.) will go in.

Nikiníyáá lą́ą, daashą' 'át'é, Certainly I'm going home. (As when another person refuses to believe that you are serious.)

---

laanaa, an optative particle expressing a wish or desire. It is usually translatable as **would that,** and used in conjunction with optative, imperfective or neuter forms of the verb.

Díí Bilagáana bibéeso t'óó 'ahayóí lá. Bibéesooígíí shíí' laanaa, I found that this white man has a lot of money. I wish I had his money. (Lit. I wish his money would become mine.)

Mexico hoolyéhígíí hoostse' laanaa, Would that I might see Mexico; I wish I might see the place called Mexico.

Díí dził bąąhgóó shash ndaakai laanaa, I wish there were bears on this mountain; would that bears lived on this mountain.

'Ákóyinishyée laanaa, I wish that were my name; would that I were named thus. (*Laanaa* is never used in a negative sense. If the last example were made a negative *laanaa* must be replaced by *dooleełę́ę́ < dooleeł+yę́ę́. Doo 'ákóyinishyée da dooleełę́ę́,* I wish that weren't my name.)

Often, in expressing a wish, the (optative mode) form of the verb is in 3a. person (pronominal *ji-* subject) although one may not be referring to a third person actually. This construction is similar to English **I wish that one could; would that one might.**

Ńléi tsé bikáa'gi 'ajółhosh laanaa nisin, I wish that one could go up on top of that rock and go to sleep.

---

la', an enclitic particle that expresses a feeling of consternation, puzzlement or surprise. (See also *t'óó la'; t'ah doo la'* —— *da.*) *La'* often represents such English phrases as **I don't see why it is; I can't understand why.**

Ch'ééh la' baa ntséskees, **I don't know why it is, but** I simply get no place thinking about it; **I don't know why, but** I simply can not make up my mind about it.

Ch'ééh la' ńdiish'aah, **I don't know why, but** I can't lift it.

Shi'éé' la' t'óó baa yánísin, **I don't know why, but** I'm ashamed of my clothes.

'Asdzą́ą́ la' silį́į́' lá, **Why,** she's a grown lady. (As one exclaims upon seeing a young lady, now grown, whom he had not seen since (her) childhood.)

---

le', an optative particle used with optative, imperfective, neuter and progressive forms of the verb. It is usually translatable as **let** (it be thus); **I wish that.**

'Adinídíin le', **Let there be** light.

Tó shigodta'go neel'ą́ago yishdlosh le', **Let** me be trotting along with the water up to (between) my knees; I **want to be** (or **wish** I were) trotting along with water up to my knees.

K'ad Na'nízhoozhídi naasháa le', **I wish** I were in Gallup now (Lit. now at Gallup I am walking about would that).

K'ad ta'neesk'ání ła' yishą́ą́ le', **I wish** I were eating a melon now (Lit. now a melon I am eating it would that).

Tó diłhił ła' séł'ą́ą́ le', **I wish** I had some whisky on hand.

---

le' 'át'éégóó, a combination of enclitic *le',* the verb *'át'é,* it is, and enclitic *-góó,* This combination is used with optative mode forms of the verb to express what is roughly equivalent to **proof against** in English. It indicates that conditions are such that the act denoted by the verb cannot possibly be carried out.

Shiníbaal doo tó biníkáoogeeh le' 'át'éégóó 'ííshłaa, I made my tent **so no** water **could** leak through it; I made my tent water**proof.**

Doo ha'át'íi da yiníkáooya' le' 'át'éégóó bidziilgo tsin neelkáalgo 'áyiilaa jiní, It is said that he made a stockade **so** strong **that nothing could** get through it.

---

léi', an enclitic attached to or used with nouns, verbs and other particles with variable meaning.

1. Attached to or used in conjunction with nouns, *léi'* indicates that the noun in reference is strange to, or outside the experience of the speaker. It corresponds, in this usage to English **a certain, some, some —— or another.**

'Atiingi chidí léi'yiiłtsą́, I saw **some** car on the road; I saw a **strange** car on the road.

'Adą́ą́dą́ą́' hastiin léi' bitsii' 'ádingo shaa níyá, Yesterday. **some** bald-headed man (of unknown identity) came up to me.

Tooh ńlį́į́ léi'gi níyá, He came to a **certain** (unidentified) river.

Hastiintsoh 'asdzání léi' yá'ázyeh, Mr. Tso married a **certain** young lady (with whom the speaker is not acquainted). (Note that *'asdzání* denotes a young lady, while *'asdzą́ą́* would indicate an elderly woman.)

Naghái 'asdzą́ą́ léi' Hastiintsoh be'esdzáán 'át'é, That lady is Mr. Tso's wife. (Here *léi'* is not translated. The woman is being pointed out and neither the speaker nor the person spoken to may be acquainted with her; or the speaker, but not the person spoken to, may be acquainted with her.)

Naghái łééchąą'í léi' 'ayóo hashké, That dog is really mean. (The speaker has had previous experience with the dog in reference, but the person spoken to has not.)

2. *Léi'* is sometimes used in place of *ła',* a, an.

Tsin léi' néidiitą́ or tsin ła' néidiitą́, He picked up a stick.

3. *Léi'* is used as a conjunction, sometimes replacing *-dago biniinaa* (I couldn't) **because, inasmuch as, in view of the fact that.**

Doo shitah hwiináa da léi' (or *dago biniinaa) shibee'eldǫǫh ch'ééh dah diishtįįh,* **In view of the fact that** I was weak I couldn't lift my gun.

'Ahbínígo tó 'ásdįįd léi' biniinaa ni' bikáa'ji' hajizh'áázh, tó bíká, They (dual) went ashore in the morning to get water **because** the supply had become exhausted. (Here *léi'* replaces *-go.)*

'Azhą́ 'ayóigo níyol ndi shił yá'áhoot'ééh tónteel bííghahgi léi', Even though it is windy, I like the place **because** it is beside the sea.

Shichidí bikee'yá'ádaat'ééh léi' Mexicogóó bee deesháał niizį́į́', **Inasmuch as** my tires were good I thought I'd go to Mexico.

Łóó' hahadleehígíí 'ayóo yiishchįįh léi' bá naashnishígíí doo t'áá shídin łóó' ha'al'eełgóó naagháa da, **In view of the fact that** I know a lot about fishing, my boss never goes on a fishing trip without me (the trip being by boat).

$500. yoosbą́ą́ lágo bibéeso t'óó 'ahayói léi' háájí da shił nináá'doo'oł niizį́į́' jiní, **Inasmuch as** he had made $500, and had a lot of money, he thought he would make another (round trip) voyage somewhere. (If *léi'* is replaced by *-go biniinaa* the meaning becomes obligatory: he **has** to make another voyage because of his earnings and financial condition.)

łá'í ndi, a combination of *ła',* a, one; *-í,* relatival enclitic; and *ndi,* but, even. It translates English **not even one; not a single one.**

Bilagáana bizaad łá'í ndi doo nei'áa da, He doesn't know a **single** word of English. (Lit. he doesn't carry even one word of English about with him,)

Béeso łá'í ndi doo naash'áa da, I haven't **even one** dollar.

łeh, a particle employed commonly with imperfective, repetitive, usitative (wherein it is redundant), and progressive forms of the verb to indicate that the act denoted by the verb is performed customarily or habitually. In English we commonly employ the word **always** for this purpose, or omit expression of habituality by a specific word.

Chidí 'áłchíní bee naagéhígíí doo ba'jóolíí' 'át'ée da daanii łeh, People are **always** saying (i.e. customarily say) that the buses used for carrying the children are not dependable.

'Ahbínígo t'áá 'áłch'į́įdígo nináháłtį́įh łeh, It (usually) rains a little bit in the morning.

Bee'eldǫǫh naashtin łeh, I (always) carry a gun.

---

na'ńle'dii, a particle which, in certain usages, indicates that an event turned out in an unexpected manner to one's disappointment or misfortune. (See also *na'ńle'ee* under *-ee.)*

Na'ńle'dii tó hániyá, tóhą́ą 'ásdįįd lá, I went for water, **but to my dismay** I found the water all gone.

Naalyéhé báhooghandi t'ah doo dá'deelkaałdą́ą́' nisingo na'ńle'dii tsį́į́ł shiisxį, Thinking the trading post would not be closed I rushed (to get there), **but to my dismay** (or **but I was out of luck).**

-nee', an enclitic used with certain pronouns and other particles. It sometimes connotes a 'wait and see' attitude. The examples given below will illustrate its usage. It will be noted that when -*nee'* is attached to certain other particles, the final vowel of which is low in tone, the tone of that vowel becomes a rising tone (thus *haa* + *nee'* > *haánee'*; *hágo* + *nee'* > *hágoónee'*).

Hágoshı́ı́ 'ákónı́lééh; haánee' yit'ée dooleeł, All right, do it that way; **we'll see** what happens. (*Haa yit'é*, how it is; *haánee' yit'é*, (we'll) wait and see how it is.)

Haánee' nóolin dooleeł, **We'll just wait and see how** it looks. (As when several persons are describing an object, and there is difference of opinion regarding its appearance. One person says it is pretty, while another says it is ugly. A person who did not see it personally, decides to wait and see for himself.)

Haánee' hoot'ée dooleeł, **We'll wait and see how** it (the place) is (I am ready to accept what people say about the place, but I decide to wait and see before making up my mind).

Díkwíínee'bą́ą́h'ílı́ı́ dooleeł, **We'll wait and see how much** it is worth.

Háínee' hodínóołnééł, **We'll wait and see who** wins.

Ha'át'íínee' 'át'ée dooleeł, **We'll wait and see what** it is (as when one finds a box and shakes it. One person conjectures that it contains shoes, while another says it sounds like a bottle. So one says 'we'll wait and see').

'Akonee', There, see. (You maintain that it is one way, and another person disagrees. You turn out to be correct, and triumphantly exclaim "akonee").

-*nee'* is attached to *'azhá*, even though, to connote one's unwillingness to perform an act which he cannot escape, and elicit the sympathy of his listeners. Compare:

'Azhá hadoh bik'ee ti'hwiisénii' ndi Hoozdogóó náádésdzá, Even though I suffered on account of the heat, I am going back to Phoenix.

'Azháánee' hadoh bik'ee ti'hwiisénii' ndi Hoozdogóó náádeeshdáál, Even though I suffered from the heat, I'll go back to Phoenix. (The same attitude is expressed in English by pronouncing "I'll go back to Phoenix" in a tone of resignation.)

-*nee'* attached to *-zhá* (Cp. *t'áá bízhání*, he alone) expresses a feeling of envy. It is roughly equivalent to colloquial English **you're lucky**.

'Áadi da'ółta'ígíí' dabízhánee' dóó shı́ı́ yee dah danéét'aah dooleeł, Those who go to school there **are lucky**, and they will probably be proud of it.

Nízhánee' béeso naa yílwod, **You're lucky** receiving money (I wish I had received some too).

---

ni, an emphatic enclitic, usually attached to a verb, and used in conjunction with enclitic *lá* which is attached to a preceding noun or pronoun. It is noteworthy that **ni** does not produce the characteristic lengthening and (or) change of high to falling tone of the preceding stem vowel occasioned by other enclitics.

Díí lá tsé 'át'é ni (**not** *'át'ée ni*), This, I find (V. *lá*), **is a rock**. (One picks up a rock and someone asks what you are doing with that orange. You then state emphatically that what you have is a rock.)

Kingóó lá déyá ni, I'm **going to the house**. (As in reply to the query, *Háágóóshą' déyá nínízin*, Where do you think you're going?)

Shí lá yiiłtsą́ ni, **I** discovered it (**not you**).

Shí lá k'ad Na'nízhoozhígóó déyá ni, Now **I'm** going to Gallup. (You have gone so now **I'm** going to go.)

Shí lá t'éiyá mạ'ii yiiłtsạ́ ni, I saw a coyote (regardless of the fact that **you** maintain that it was something else).

---

ni', an enclitic attached to nouns and perfective mode forms of the verb. With nouns the meaning of *ni'* is similar to that of *ńt'éé'*, and usually indicates that the object named is deceased or no longer in existence. With verbs *ni'* indicates a past event or act which is recalled to mind. In some instances it is translatable as a pluperfect in English.

Shizhé'é ni'yee shił hoolne' ni', **I remember that** my **late** father told me about it. My **late** father **had** told me about it.

Kóhoot'éédą́ą́' kohgo deesdoi ni', **I recall that** last year at this time it was hot. Last year by this time it **had** become hot like this.

Shibee'eldǫǫh dahidiitą́ą ni' ——, **I recall that I** hung up my gun ——. I **had** hung up my gun (As when one is telling a story and tells something like: "And that night there was an earthquake. My gun fell down and nearly struck me on the head—I (recall that I) had hung my gun up—so I etc.")

Sitsilí t'ah 'ahbínígo kintahgóó dah diiyáa ni', My younger brother **had** (I recall) started off to town in the morning.

-shạ'; *-sh*, an interrogative particle attached to nouns, pronouns, participialized or nominalized verbs, and to other particles. It does not serve, like *-ísh*, to merely interrogativize an otherwise declarative sentence, and is never used with, or as an equivalent of, the proclitic *da'* (V. *-ísh*; *da'*). *-shạ'* is used with the interrogative pronouns to ask who, where, whence, whither, how, why, how about, what about, etc.

Háíshạ' (*háísh*) *'át'į́*, Who is he?

Dííshạ' (*díísh*) *ha'át'íí 'át'é*, What is this?

Háágóóshạ' (*háágóósh*) *díníyá*, Where are you going?

Ha'át'ííshạ' (*ha'át'íísh*) *nínízin*, What do you want?

Ha'át'éegoshạ' (*ha'át'éegosh*) *t'áadoo díníyáa da*, How come you didn't go?

Shíshạ', How about me?

Haashạ' (*haash*) *yínidzaa*, What happened to you? (How did you do it?—an injury.)

Tł'éédą́ą́'shạ' *haa yínít'įįd*, What happened to you last night? What did you bring upon yourself last night?

Hashideel'į́'goshạ' *haa hodoonííł*, What if he finds out about me? If he finds out about me what will happen?

'Azee' daji'aałígíí jiyį́įhgoshạ' *haa jit'ée łeh*, What usually happens to one when he eats peyote?

---

shį́į́, a dubitative enclitic, usually translatable as perhaps, probably, possibly. In Navaho, when referring to such variables as future weather conditions or other events which it is to be presumed will take place, *shį́į́* indicates that **possibility**, rather than certainty attaches to one's statement (since appearances or intentions with relation to futurity are often misleading). *Shį́į́* attached to certain pronouns makes them indefinite, as *háíshį́í*, someone, (lit. who-probably), *ha'át'ííshį́í*, something (lit. what-probably).

Yiską́ągo nahodoołtį́į́ł shį́í, It will **probably** rain tomorrow.

Haashį́í néelą́ą́' nááhaiídą́ą́', A great number of years ago (lit. how-probably many years ago).

Haashį́í nízahgóó 'eelwod, It ran a considerable distance (lit. how-probably much farther it ran).

Haashį́í yidéetą́ą́' silį́í', It became very deep (lit. how-probably deep it became).

Łeezh háájíshį́í tó bił 'adahaaz'ééł, Time after time the water washed the soil away (somewhere) (háájíshį́í, what-direction-probably; an indefinite direction).

---

shoh, (not to be confused with *shoo*, look!) This particle indicates that an incident has been suddenly recalled to mind, after having been momentarily forgotten. It is usually translatable as **oh, by the way**.

Shoh, 'atiingi chidí léi' yiiłtsą́ą ni', **Oh, by the way**, I just remember that I saw a strange (V. *léi'*) car on the road.

Shoh, díí jį́ t'áá 'éiyá nda'iilyée ni', **Oh, by the way**, (I remember) this is pay-day. (Cp. *ni'*)

---

t'áá 'áłdįį; t'áá 'íítdįį; t'áá 'íítdįįł yit'éego (t'áá 'íítdįįłit'éego), in some locutions these particle combinations render the idea **in reserve; in readiness, at one's disposal**, and in others the meaning is similar to that of English **likely**.

Bee'eldǫǫh t'áátá'í t'áá 'áłdįį (or t'áá 'íítdįįłit'éego) ninítá, I left one gun where I could get at it (in case I needed it).

Chidí bikee', t'áá 'íítdįįłit'éego 'ii' séł'á, I have a tire in (my car) **just in case** (I should need it).

Ch'iyáán t'áá 'íítdįįłit'éego bá 'ííshłaa dóó dah diiyá, I left some food for him and departed. (*T'áá 'íítdįįłit'éego bá 'ííshłaa*, I left it for him; I left it at his disposal or for his use.)

T'áá 'áłdįį (or 'íítdįį) doo 'ákwii hadááyáa da, I am not **likely** to get off (as from a train) at the wrong place. (Note the verb *hadááyá*, I got off, in the perfective mode.)

T'áá 'áłdįį (or 'íítdįį) yee 'ádił 'adeesdǫǫh, He is not **likely** to shoot himself with it. (*Yee 'ádił 'adeesdǫǫh*, he shot himself with it.)

---

t'áadoo —— -i, *t'áadoo*, in conjunction with an imperfective mode form of the verb relativized by enclitic *-í*, translates **before**, in the sense of **immediately before**.

T'áadoo 'áadi nisháhí shee nikihonííłtą́, **Before** I got there it started to rain on me.

T'áadoo yiistséhí náshidííłts'in, **Before** I saw him he hit me.

T'áadoo'ákǫ́ǫ́ disháhí nádzá, **Before** I went there he came back.

Used in conjunction with a durative or continuative imperfective, progressive or repetitive verb form, *t'áadoo —— -í* renders an immediate (negative) imperative. It demands that the person addressed discontinue an action already started.

> *T'áadoo yídlohí,* Don't laugh! Quit laughing!
>
> *T'áadoo yáníłti'í,* Don't talk! Quit talking!
>
> *T'áadoo tł'óodi naninéhí,* Quit playing outdoors!

---

t'áadoo ―― *-ígo t'éiyá,* a combination of *t'áadoo* (without); relatival enclitic *-í* (the one); participializing and adverbializing *-go,* and *t'éiyá* (only). It is most commonly used in conjunction with a durative imperfective verb form, to render the meaning **only if (you) do not; only on condition that (you) will not** (do that which is denoted by the verb).

> *T'áadoo nchaaígo t'éiyá 'ákǫ́ǫ́ nił deesh'ash,* I'll take you **only if** you do not cry.
>
> *T'áadoo háiida bił hólne'ígo't'éiyá díí łį́į́' naa deeshtééł,* I'll give you this horse **only on condition that** you won't tell anyone.

---

t'áadoo ―― *-góó; t'áadoo* ―― *-góógo,* a combination of particles used with perfective mode forms of the verb to give the meaning **unless.**

> *T'áadoo nahóółtą́ą́góógo shinaadą́ą́' 'ałtso dadoogą́ą́ł,* My corn will all dry up **unless** it rains.
>
> *T'áadoo lą'í yidzaazgóógo dą̨ągo ch'il doo ńdahodoodleeł da,* **Unless** it snows a lot the plants will not come back up in the spring.
>
> *T'áadoo 'azee'ál'į́įgóó díníyáágóógo jéi'ádįįh yéigo ndí'nóołhééł,* **Unless** you go to the hospital your tuberculosis is going to start to become really serious (lit. start killing you hard).

---

t'ahádą́ą́', possibly composed of *t'ah* (still; yet), *-á- < -í* (relatival enclitic), and *-dą́ą́'* (ago; past). The meaning is **right now before it is too late; now's the time to.**

> *T'ahádą́ą́' tó yígeed łá' 'ádadiilníił,* Let's make a ditch right now **before it's too late.**
>
> *T'ahádą́ą́' tsinaabąąs chizh ła' bee nijóyéłígi le' 'át'é,* **Now's the time** to get some wood with that wagon (before it's too late and the wagon is no longer available).

---

t'ah doo ―― *da,* *t'ah,* (still, yet) used in conjunction with negativizing *doo* ―― *da,* and an imperfective mode form of the verb, translates **never,** in the sense that one has never performed the act denoted by the verb. It could also be more literally rendered as **not yet.**

> *T'ah doo 'ákǫ́ǫ́ disháah da,* I have **never** gone there (lit. I am still not in the act of starting to go there).
>
> *T'ah doo shash ła'yiistséeh da,* I have **never** seen a bear (lit. I am still not in the act of seeing a bear).
>
> *T'ah doo bįįh ła' sisxée da,* I have **never** killed a deer.
>
> *Bįįh t'ah doo sisxée da ńt'éé',* I had **never** killed a deer (lit. it used to be that I am (was) still not in the act of killing a deer).

***t'ah doo la'*——— *da*,** a combination of particles used with a semeliterative verb form, and similar in meaning to English (**I**) **wonder why** (**I**) **never** ——— **anymore.** (V. *la'*.)

T'ah doo la' náá'áshdlą́ą da, **Golly, I never** take a drink any more (and I wonder why, or wonder at the fact). (lit. I wonder why I am still not drinking again.)

T'ah doo la' náánéístséeh da, I **wonder why I never** see him **anymore.**

T'ah doo la' shaa náánídáah da, **Why is it that** you **never** come to see me **any more?**

***t'áá ká*,** a combination of particles used with optative mode forms of the verb to express a negative command, in the sense of **see that** (**you**) **do not** (perform the act denoted by the verb).

T'áá ká haóódziih, **See that you do not** say anything!

Sodizin báhooghan góne' t'áá ká ná'óólt'oh, **See that you do not** smoke in church!

(Cp. *t'áá káágóó,* in the open air; outdoors, as in *t'áá káágóó 'iiłhaazh,* I slept outdoors.)

***t'áá shǫǫ*,** a combination of particles translatable as **it's a good thing; boy, it's a good thing that;** (**I'm**) **glad that.**

La' t'áá shǫǫ díį' béédááhai, **It's a good thing that** some of them are four years old.

T'áá shǫǫ shá niiltła, **I'm sure glad that** he stopped for me.

Nihe'ena'í t'áá shǫǫ t'áadoo danihiiłtsą́ą da, **Boy, it's sure a good thing that** our enemies didn't see us.

***t'áá shǫǫ da*,** a combination of particles used to express an idea similar to that expressed by English **at least; the least** (**you**) **could do; the least** (**you**) **can do.**

T'áá sáhí 'ííníyą́ą'. T'áá shǫǫ da 'íyą́ shididííniił, You ate by yourself. **The least you can do is** ask (tell) me to eat.

T'áá shǫǫ da t'óó nits'ą́ą' 'ashą́. Jó doo shich'į' ndííléeł da lá, **The least you can do** is give me a meal. Look, I know you're not going to pay me.

(Cp. *t'áá shǫǫdí,* please; at least.)

***t'áá shǫǫ*——— *lá*,** a combination of particles that expresses a feeling of relief when one discovers that his fears were groundless. It is comparable to English **whew; boy,** accompanied by an appropriate sentence tone and manner of speaking.

T'áá shǫǫ t'ah naashjaah lá, **Whew,** I still have them. (As when one puts coins into a holey pocket, and suddenly remembering the condition of the pocket he frantically searches therein to see if the money has fallen out. *T'áá shǫǫ lá* expresses the feeling of relief that he experiences upon finding the money still there.)

---

t'óó la', a combination of particles that serves to express the fact that appearances would lead one to believe something that is not necessarily true. It corresponds to English **looks**, enunciated with a peculiar emphasis, or written in italics.

Díí ké t'óó la' 'álts'íísí nahalin, This shoe **looks** too small (but it may not prove to actually be too small).

Díí béeso t'óó la' be'elyaa nahalin, This dollar **looks** like a counterfeit (but it may not be).

T'óó la' bíyó deesk'aaz, It **seems** to be a bit cold (weather).

---

t'óó tsé'édin (<t'óó tsé 'ádin, merely no rocks??), a term meaning **become continually worse; get more intensive.**

Bee nihich'į' 'ańdahazt'i'ii t'óó tsé'édin danéeséél nahalin, Our problems seem to grow **continually worse.**

'Ólta' nihitah hólónígíí t'óó tsé'édiní da nihits'ą́ą́' 'ałch'į' 'ańdaalne'go 'át'é, Our schools continue (to make matters worse for us by closing) to close on us.

'Ałní'ní'ą́ago t'óó tsé'édin nikihoníłtą́, At noon it began to rain **harder** (worse than ever).

'Adą́ą́dą́ą́' 'atiin doo hózhǫ́ yá'áhoot'éeh da ńt'éé'. Jį́įdą́ą́' t'éiyá t'óó tsé'édiní da hashtł'ish hazlį́į' lá, Yesterday the road wasn't very good. Today it **got worse** with mud (got muddier).

---

tsididįįį', **a profusion of (duties); too many things.**

Tsididįįį' yizhnít'į́igo t'óó hoł 'áhádįįh, When a person has **too many things** to do he gets confused.

'Át'ah 'índa 'ahił hodiilnih, k'ad tsididįįį' yinísht'į́, 'éí bąą, I can't talk to you now because **I'm swamped** (with work).

---

yee', an enclitic used often as an intensive, and sometimes translatable by English **really; in truth; very; extremely.**

'Álts'íísí yee', He is **really** little (very very little),

Shí yee' 'ádíshní, I'm **really** the one who said it. (One admits that he was actually the one who said it after another person was falsely accused.)

Shí naat'áanii nishłį́, I'm the boss. Shí yee', I am. (Like colloquial English, "That's what **you** think, **I'm** the boss.")

'Eii yee' shí, **Hey**, that's **mine**; that is really mine. (As when someone pockets one's property and starts away with it.)

Dooda yee' 'azlį́į', Things became hopeless; things became terrible. (lit. emphatically **no** came to pass; (what was) by all means no happened. Cp. dooda yee', absolutely no (not)!)

Yee' is also used in expressions such as the following:

1. *haashíyee'*, let's (do a thing) and see what the result will be; let's just try it and see what happens.

Haashíyee' 'ahíłká 'ańdaajah, Let's help one another (and just see what the result of our cooperation will be).

Haashíyee' 'aadę́ę́ chidí shił bídíyííł, Give my car a push and let's see what happens (maybe it will start).

2. *haa'íyee'*, let's see (do it so I can see; let me *see or find out for* myself).

Haa'íye't'áátáhádi ch'ínáádiníldóóh, Let's see you smile (once) again.
Haa'íyee' haalá níníłdáás, Let's see how heavy you are.
3. *k'adee'*, now's the time; now's a good time (to).

K'adee' ńléi mą'ii bił 'azhdoołdǫǫh, Now's a good time to shoot that coyote (because he is standing still, or other conditions are just right).

K'adee' yidzaazdą́ą́' gah hajólzheehígi le' 'át'é, Now since it snowed is a good time to hunt rabbits. (V. *-gi le' 'át'é*.)

---

yę́ę; yéeni', an enclitic used with several meanings, as listed and exemplified below. Initial *y-* is often elided, and the vowel of *yę́ę* assimilates to the final vowel of the preceding word. Thus *shimá yę́ę > shimáhą́ą; tó yę́ę > tóhą́ą* (not *tóhǫǫ*), etc. Words that do not normally end in a final *-h* (i.e. words ending in an open syllable) often take a final *-h* before *-ę́ę*.

1. Used with nouns, the force of this enclitic is similar to that of *ni'; ńt'éé'*. I.e. it signifies that the object expressed by the noun has ceased to exist, is dead or gone.

Shizhé'é yę́ę yee shił hoolne', My **late** father told me of it.
Shimáhą́ą yee shił hoolne', My **late** mother told me of it.
2. In narrative *yę́ę* attached to a noun or verb indicates that the object or action expressed thereby has already figured in the foregoing part of the account. In this sense *yę́ę* may be translated as **the one that, that which** (in a past sense); **the aforementioned; this, these** (as in colloquial English).

'Áko gah neistseedę́ę biwos dah sinilgo nikinádzá, So then he started back home with the rabbits he had killed slung over his shoulder. (*-ę́ę* indicates that the rabbits and his act of killing them had already been mentioned.)
3. Attached to a future tense form (including *dooleeł* when it is used to futurize another verb), *yę́ę* expresses a wish, hope or desire on the part of the speaker that the act or state denoted by the verb be realized. (V. *laanaa; lágo*.)

Nahodoołtį́łę́ę (< *nahodoołtį́ł*, it will rain + *yę́ę*), I wish it would rain; I hope it rains.

Bįįh diyeeshhéłę́ę, I wish I could kill a deer; I hope I will kill a deer,

Doo Bogus Check yinishyée dooleełę́ę, I wish that my name were not Bogus Check. (Note that the optative particle *laanaa* cannot be used to express a negative desire or wish. However, in a positive sense either *laanaa* or *dooleełę́ę* can be used, with a distinction in the shade of meaning: *James yinishyée laanaa*, I wish (would that) my name were James; *James yinishyée dooleełę́ę*, I hope my name will be James; I wish I could be called James.)

---

yę́ędą́ą́' (-ę́ędą́ą́'; -'ą́ądą́ą́'), a combination of the particles *yę́ę* and *-dą́ą'* (V. *dą́ą'*) used with perfectives, neuters, continuative, or durative imperfective verb forms in the sense of when (in a past sense).

Shizhé'é hináhą́ądą́ą́' t'áá kwe'é nihighan ńt'éé', When my father was living our home was right here.

Dichin síníłį́'ę́ędą́ą́' dibé ła' sits'ą́ą yíníłghal, When you got hungry you ate one of my sheep (lit. . . . ate a sheep away from me).

With imperfective mode forms of the verb, (preceded by *t'ah doo ——— da*, still not) *yę́ędą́ą́'* is equivalent to before; prior to.

T'ah doo yiistséhę́ędą́ą́ doo wooshdlą́ą da ńt'éé', Before I saw it I didn't believe it (lit. when I was still not in the act of seeing it I did not believe it).

Notes

1. This is a new introduction written by Robert Young for this book. The original pamphlet is reproduced here with only minor changes for presentation and a few substantive corrections that were made by Robert Young. The original document spells *Navajo* at times with *h* and at times with *j*, a variation that was common before the Navajo government adopted *Navajo* as the official spelling. We have retained the original spelling alternations for their historical interest. It may be significant to someone sometime to know that Young and Morgan at one time spelled it both ways.

2. In chants, prayers and songs, not only tone quality but vowel lengths are often altered in a peculiar way. Likewise, in ordinary speech, words or groups of words may be uttered at a lower or higher voice level than those which precede or follow, for purposes of emphasis, to indicate direct quotation, etc. *Jiní* means he (one) says, it is told, it is said, and in narrative the sequence *jiní jiní*, he says, it is said, often occurs. In this instance the first *jiní* (he says) is always uttered at a higher tone level or "octave" than the second *jiní* (it is said; it is told; according to the story, etc.)

13

SACRED AND SECULAR ISSUES IN
NAVAJO EDUCATION

Theodore B. Fernald and Paul R. Platero

This chapter is a report on the language and culture discussion that took place at the Athabaskan Conference on Syntax and Semantics at Swarthmore College on April 26, 1996. We will attempt to express the nature of the dialogue and represent the main ideas that emerged in a neutral, unbiased manner. The goal here is to lay out some of the main issues so that the dialogue can continue and involve additional people. By agreement with the participants, the views represented here will not be attributed to any individual, but to the discussion as a whole. Certainly there is no one who will agree with everything that is in here, since conflicting views are expressed. The group did not seek to achieve a consensus but to initiate discussion of these considerations.

13.1 The Issues

Since the 1970s there has been a serious decline in the transmission of Navajo to the youngest generation. It is estimated that 80% of Navajo preschool children could speak Navajo in the early 1970s. Platero (to appear) reports a 1992 study he conducted which found that only 45.7% of Navajo preschoolers could speak Navajo. Only 17.7% were monolingual in Navajo. Thus, despite the fact that the Navajos constitute the largest population of indigenous North Americans, the Navajo language is undergoing a drastic decline in use. Although adults constitute a significant population of Navajo speakers, the median age in the Navajo Nation is 19 years, and when there is a serious decline in the use of a language among young children it is clear that the language is threatened.

The reasons for this decline are many, ranging from official opposition in the past by the U.S. government to economic pressures to speak English to an inability of the Navajo government to launch and sustain programs that would strengthen the status of the language. To address all these issues would require more time and imagination than we were able to muster, so we chose to examine a particular problem in detail and to discuss a particular sort of strategy for addressing it.

One factor that makes it difficult to teach Navajo language and culture in schools has to do with the fact that various religions are represented in the Navajo Nation. Some Navajo parents follow traditional Navajo religion; other parents subscribe to or hold beliefs that are influenced by other traditions: for example, Catholicism, a variety of Protestant denominations, Mormonism, and the Native American Church. It is believed by many that traditional Navajo culture makes no distinction between what is sacred and what is secular. This might mean that any effort to teach any aspect of Navajo culture in the classroom will necessarily involve teaching religion. But teaching religion in schools is problematic since not everyone has the same religious beliefs, and, in addition, it would violate the doctrine of the separation of church and state which could affect public funding for the schools. Occasionally, efforts to teach some aspect of Navajo culture in public schools have led parents to remove their children from the class. Some parents oppose any effort to teach anything about Navajo language or culture in classrooms out of fear that their children might be taught religious principles inconsistent with the family's beliefs. Nevertheless, many Navajos who have adopted other religions still wish to hold on to some aspects of their heritage.

If there were some way to separate the secular from the religious aspects of culture, it would be possible to teach the secular subjects in schools and leave religion as a matter of personal choice. People would continue to respect their religious beliefs, but they would not practice religion in schools. Many questions arise at this point. From the point of view of a traditional Navajo, it may not seem possible to make the distinction between sacred and secular matters. Part of the traditional view is that everything is sacred. For other Navajos, certain traditional practices conflict with the precepts of other religions and others do not. From their point of view, avoiding the conflicting areas in schools might be sufficient to allow the other subjects to be taught. Still others would like the living tradition of Navajo culture to survive through the next century and beyond, but they fear that if it is not possible to teach any aspects of culture in schools, the tradition will not be passed along to the youngest generation.

13.2   The Discussion

These were the issues we chose to discuss. We did not reach a consensus, nor
did we expect to, but we did clarify some of the issues and set the stage for the
discussion to continue.

The discussion began with a panel of four speakers. The panel was followed
by an open discussion. Many of the participants spoke of their own experiences
in schools growing up. Many had experienced the policies of the U.S. government, which was trying to do away with Navajo language and culture. They re-
counted stories of their experiences in government schools where they were not
permitted to speak Navajo. Several had soap put in their mouths when they were
caught speaking Navajo. One classroom had a policy that you would have to
keep your nose inside a circle drawn on the chalkboard if you spoke Navajo. If
you moved your nose for any reason, the teacher would whack you on the legs
with a yardstick.

In the early part of this century, the U.S. government mounted tremendous
opposition to any effort to preserve American Indian languages and cultural traditions. Along with other Indians, Navajo children were shipped as far away as
Chemawa, Oregon and Carlisle, Pennsylvania, to boarding schools run by the
Bureau of Indian Affairs (BIA). The policy was to remove Indian children as far
from home, language, and culture as possible and to try to keep them separate
from others who spoke the same language. This had a devastating effect on other
Indian groups. The effect was less damaging to the Navajo culture, since there
was a large population of Navajo students in all the boarding schools. This at
least made it possible for them to speak with each other in Navajo, but they
were subject to punishment if they were caught.

There is no official opposition anymore (although this may change if efforts
to make English the official language of the United States are successful), but
the Navajo culture is more severely threatened than ever. The government's policies in the past have already done substantial damage that may even (already) be
fatal. Many graduates of schools have become teachers and have continued to
carry out the old BIA plan to rid children of their native language and culture.

13.3   Separating the Secular from the Sacred

Efforts to exclude discussion of all traditional knowledge from the classroom
have the effect of excluding the Navajo language from the classroom as well.
For most people, this is an unintended consequence. If we could draw a line between sacred and secular aspects of culture, language and the study of it would
be included in the secular area. Certainly there are words that are rich in sacred
meaning and cannot be fully understood without a grasp of the sacred tradition.
Discussing such words might not be appropriate for public schools. However,
the study of the Navajo language and grammar is clearly a secular enterprise.
Distinguishing the sacred from the secular would allow Navajo language instruc-

tion in public schools and constitute a major contribution in efforts to preserve the Navajo language.

One of the participants in the conference pointed out that there is a continuum between secular and religious aspects of culture. If we were to try to use this strategy, we would need to identify areas that are clearly secular and those that are clearly religious. There would be many areas left in between. We would have to recommend that those areas also be left out of the classroom and instead be dealt with in private. Any proposal would be controversial, but perhaps there would be some areas of culture that nearly any Navajo parent would agree could be taught in school. For example, pollen offerings, prayers, and chants are clearly sacred matters, and at least certain aspects of the visual arts, music, and philosophy are secular.

Another participant holds the belief that the Navajo culture is a single, unified entity and that one cannot isolate what is sacred from anything else. This person said the Universe has one song and we all sing that one song. It is not possible to divide the culture into parts. However, there is another approach that may allow the culture to be studied in schools. Anglo colleges are able to teach courses in comparative religion without teaching that any one of the religions is actually true. Students do not participate in religious practices, but they are shown how the practices are done and what they are taken to mean. Then students decide for themselves what to think. The difference between learning about religion and being taught to follow its tenets is mainly a matter of pedagogical technique. What the elders teach is meant to be shared. There are schools where the teachers are trusted to pass along cultural knowledge. They have experience with implementing these ideas.

Another participant reasoned as follows: Navajos follow various religions, but the people still have a common identity. What do they all hold in common? The ability to retain *k'e* and language are a common bond among all Navajo people, regardless of religion. *K'e* is a concept of relationships beyond the family that includes the clanship system. When you meet someone, the relationship in the extended family of clans is established. An additional meaning for *k'e* is about harmony and service with other people, animals, nature, the land. It is an all-encompassing concept. If you do not live in accordance with *k'e,* your life falls out of balance and needs to be restored. Even people who went through the BIA boarding schools retained some concept of *k'e*; the most core aspect of Navajo identity survived. But sometimes things change when people have children. What the BIA tried to do to them, they unintentionally do to their children. How can this happen? It may be that parents associate the English language with education due to their own experiences with school, and because Navajo was stigmatized in the BIA schools, some of this attitude remains. This speaker proposed adding to curricula instruction in secular things that every Navajo ought to know: how to bottle-feed a lamb, dig for wild carrots in the spring, make herbs into soup, build a fire. Additional areas of knowledge that should be included are how to build a house, care for livestock, provide for the family, and speak the language.

Another participant pointed out that missionaries drew a line between religion and secular culture based on their own assumptions about the universe, but they drew the line in the wrong place. Missionaries dictated which parts of Navajo culture could be retained by Christians. Navajo people need to do this for themselves. This speaker also said we must have respect for the followers of all religions. Preachers, politicians, language teachers, and medicine men are the orators who have gotten people together in one place and who touch many people all at once. They are the people who preserve the language. We shouldn't alienate any of them because they all serve a purpose.

13.4 Maintaining the Language

Participants in the conference agreed that parents need to be impressed with the fact that Navajo is very hard to learn as an adult. Children have a special ability to acquire language, but this ability is lost as one becomes an adult. One participant argued that some drastic steps must be taken if we are to preserve Navajo. It is not enough to teach people a few phrases. We need to create situations in which people must use Navajo.

There was also a call for efforts to change the attitude some people have towards Navajo and to make it more attractive to use for young people. It was suggested that the language needed to be glamorized. Another participant replied that the language doesn't need to be glamorized; it is perfectly fine as it is. Another said that 'glamorize' may not be the right word to use but that the idea of improving its appeal to young people makes sense. Some felt that improved teaching techniques were called for. However, others thought that the language should be used as a language for popular culture: there need to be books, movies, and television shows in Navajo.

It was also pointed out that Navajo language and culture teachers are in a difficult spot. They are sometimes criticized by Christians for promoting traditional religion, but they are also criticized by traditionalists and neotraditionalists who feel the teachers are setting themselves up unreasonably as experts on the language and the culture. The participants in the conference felt this was an unfortunate situation. Teachers for the most part do the best they can. Unless people with more expertise than the teachers are willing to come forward to do the job, there is no point in criticizing the ones who are willing to try. This kind of criticism is very damaging to efforts to preserve the language and the cultural traditions.

13.5 Conclusion

The participants were for the most part in agreement that it would be a good thing to use Navajo as a language of instruction in public schools, but how to do that was a matter of contention. Is it possible to deal only with secular aspects of culture in public, leaving people free to hold their own religious beliefs in private? If such a separation is not acceptable, can teachers at least expose students to Navajo culture as a subject of classroom study so they can learn about it without actually participating in religious practices that would be objectionable to Navajos of other faiths? These two strategies are not so very far apart. Each involves walking carefully along a fine line, either between the sacred and the secular, or between study and practice. Each strategy has been implemented in an educational setting, and this discussion would benefit from further input from those teachers who walk these fine lines.

On two key points, all the participants in the conference seemed to agree. Navajo people must come to better understand the gravity of the situation. The Navajo language is severely threatened. It will cease to exist except in books unless the people want to preserve it badly enough to continue this discussion and act upon the outcome. The situation will be hopeless unless people are willing to overcome their differences and work very hard to save the language. Even if everyone agrees to the basic objective of preserving the language, it will not be attained if no compromise on a course of action can be reached.

The other crucial point is related to the first. People must understand that Navajo is a modern language and as capable of expressing complex, even scientific, thought as any language is. It is true that much of the access Navajo speakers have to their heritage will be lost if the language is lost. But Navajo is not only a language of the past. It can be a language of the future as well, if the people are willing to work together to preserve it.

As a final note, we would like to point out that everyone concerned about the future of the Navajo culture has a lot more in common with each other than not. We all have the goal of trying to help the Navajo language and culture survive. It would be a shame if our differences were to prevent us from accomplishing what we all want.

Reference

Platero, Paul (to appear). Navajo Head Start Language Study. In Ken Hale and Leanne Hinton (eds.), *A Manual for Language Revitalization*.

SUBJECT INDEX

LANGUAGE INDEX